Luminos is the Open Access monograph publishing program from UC Press. Luminos provides a framework for preserving and reinvigorating monograph publishing for the future and increases the reach and visibility of important scholarly work. Titles published in the UC Press Luminos model are published with the same high standards for selection, peer review, production, and marketing as those in our traditional program. www.luminosoa.org

T0373329

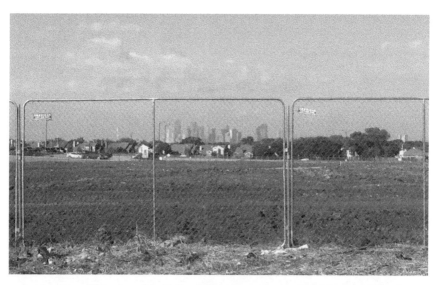

FRONTISPIECE. This view of the Dallas skyline offers a perspective of the potential and promise of the American Dream—a big city, beautiful houses, nice cars, and mature trees—while also remaining just out of reach for the viewer, as it was for many of our interlocutors. *Photo by author.*

Breaking Points

ETHNOGRAPHIC STUDIES IN SUBJECTIVITY

Tanya Luhrmann, Editor

1. *Forget Colonialism?: Sacrifice and the Art of Memory in Madagascar*, by Jennifer Cole

2. *Sensory Biographies: Lives and Deaths among Nepal's Yolmo Buddhists*,
   by Robert Desjarlais

3. *Culture and the Senses: Bodily Ways of Knowing in an African Community*,
   by Kathryn Linn Geurts

4. *Becoming Sinners: Christianity and Moral Torment in a Papua New Guinea Society*,
   by Joel Robbins

5. *Jesus in Our Wombs: Embodying Modernity in a Mexican Convent*, by Rebecca J. Lester

6. *The Too-Good Wife: Alcohol, Codependency, and the Politics of Nurturance in Postwar Japan*,
   by Amy Borovoy

7. *Subjectivity: Ethnographic Investigations*, edited by João Biehl, Byron Good,
   and Arthur Kleinman

8. *Postcolonial Disorders*, edited by Mary-Jo DelVecchio Good, Sandra Teresa Hyde,
   Sarah Pinto, and Byron J. Good

9. *Under a Watchful Eye: Self, Power, and Intimacy in Amazonia*, by Harry Walker

10. *Unsettled: Denial and Belonging among White Kenyans*, by Janet McIntosh

11. *Our Most Troubling Madness: Case Studies in Schizophrenia across Cultures*,
    by T. M. Luhrmann and Jocelyn Marrow

12. *Us, Relatives: Scaling and Plural Life in a Forager World*, by Nurit Bird-David

13. *The Likeness: Semblance and Self in Slovene Society*, by Gretchen Bakke

14. *The Anatomy of Loneliness: Suicide, Social Connection, and the Search for Relational Meaning
    in Contemporary Japan*, by Chikako Ozawa–de Silva

15. *Being Single in India: Stories of Gender, Exclusion, and Possibility*, by Sarah Lamb

16. *The Avatar Faculty: Ecstatic Transformations in Religion and Video Games*,
    by Jeffrey G. Snodgrass

17. *A Life of Worry: Politics, Mental Health, and Vietnam's Age of Anxiety*, by Allen L. Tran

18. *Breaking Points: Youth Mental Health Crises and How We All Can Help*,
    by Neely Laurenzo Myers

Breaking Points

Youth Mental Health Crises and How We All Can Help

‎———‎

Neely Laurenzo Myers

UNIVERSITY OF CALIFORNIA PRESS

University of California Press
Oakland, California

Suggested citation: Myers, N. L. *Breaking Points: Youth Mental Health Crises and How We All Can Help*. Oakland: University of California Press, 2024.
DOI: https://doi.org/10.1525/luminos.205

Library of Congress Cataloging-in-Publication Data

Names: Myers, Neely Laurenzo, author.
Title: Breaking points : youth mental health crises and how we all can help /
    Neely Laurenzo Myers.
Other titles: Ethnographic studies in subjectivity; 18.
Description: Oakland, California : University of California Press, [2024] |
    Series: Ethnographic studies in subjectivity ; 18 |
    Includes bibliographical references and index.
Identifiers: LCCN 2024023388 (print) | LCCN 2024023389 (ebook) |
    ISBN 9780520400610 (paperback) | ISBN 9780520400627 (ebook)
Subjects: LCSH: Young adults—Mental health—United States. |
    Young adults—Mental health services—United States. |
    Psychoses—Treatment—United States. | BISAC: SOCIAL SCIENCE /
    Anthropology / General | MEDICAL / Hospital Administration & Care
Classification: LCC RC451.4.Y67 M94 2024 (print) |
    LCC RC451.4.Y67 (ebook) | DDC 616.8900835—dc23/eng/20240613

LC record available at https://lccn.loc.gov/2024023388
LC ebook record available at https://lccn.loc.gov/2024023389

33   32   31   30   29   28   27   26   25   24
10   9   8   7   6   5   4   3   2   1

For everyone affected by mental health crises:
You are not alone.

CONTENTS

ILLUSTRATIONS

FIGURES

TABLE

Introduction

Under Pressure

So many people are touched by all this stuff, but for some reason or other they don't want to talk about it—in the workplace, in schools, everywhere. I firmly believe that if that comes out, there will be more acceptance, and people will be more prone to open up and say, "Okay, this is really how I feel, and we are in this whole thing together." Because it's a life-changing experience, and it's gonna change your lives obviously, but I would hope that it would be for the better.

—SANDRA (CORRINA'S MOM), AT HOME, WEEK 12

Corrina turned up the volume on her television to drown out the noise of the neighbors carrying on. The apartment walls must be thin, she thought, and her new neighbors always left their television blaring. It was like trying to relax in a hotel room where the person next door was watching the Super Bowl at full volume.

Hours later, longing for sleep, she shut off her TV, but the neighbors' TV droned on. She banged on the walls. No response. She knocked on their door. Nothing.

Corrina curled up on her couch, wishing it would all go away. She buried herself in the pillows. No change. She plugged her ears with her fingers. Still there. She tried her swimming ear plugs. The noises seemed louder.

What the hell?! she thought.

Then, Corinna realized she must have taken some LSD. Her new boyfriend, Colby, had introduced her to the psychedelic in the past few months. She had been stressed trying to take care of her mother, who had been unwell, while also taking a full slate of classes. LSD made her feel better. It made the unusual things happening to her seem more normal—everyone had weird experiences on acid. It felt good to be around other young people who had weird experiences and then get back to life as usual the next day, even if she sometimes did not get back to normal quite as quickly as the others.

She sighed, relieved. Her boyfriend, Colby, could help her with this awful trip, she decided, so she grabbed her car keys to drive to his apartment. However, once she got into her car, she remembered that Colby was out of town. It was summer. She was just there for summer school. So she sat there, in the ninety-plus-degree heat of a Texas summer night, trying to decide what to do. She cracked her driver's side window, but not too far. She did not want someone to grab her.

And then, as she sat there, she began to see all the dots connecting. It was so obvious—how had she not noticed before? Her life was a lie. Her name was not Corrina. She was really an angel named Karina. Her mother, Sandra, was not her mother but rather an evil impostor from "beyond the veil" sent to control her. Her stepfather, Adam, too. Sandra and Adam were fake. They were demons sent to oppress her powers.

Overwhelmed, Corrina banged the steering wheel and hollered. A building resident spotted her while they were trying to park their car. Afraid to approach her, they called the police. It was very dangerous for anyone to sit in a parked car with the engine off in the intense heat.

The police and EMTs responded quickly. Corrina gave them her driver's license when asked and tried to explain that she was an angel. They asked her to please step out of her car. Getting out of the car made sense. She opened the door, and an EMT took her arm and guided her toward the ambulance. They said she needed to be hydrated as soon as possible. She did feel awfully thirsty.

But then, she heard a policewoman spelling her name on the dispatch. C-o-r-r-i-n-a.

The police must be in on it, too! she thought, frantically. *They are saying the wrong name!*

She tried to run away.

The next thing she could remember was waking up and feeling terrified in the Shady Elms emergency room.[1] She had no idea where she was and had never been there before. She thought she might be dead or in between life and death. She knew the demons had put her there.

A few days later, the hospital released Corrina with a new diagnosis: psychosis not otherwise specified. She had not been on LSD; in fact, her substance screen was clear except for cannabis. Her mother, Sandra, picked her up. Sandra was given almost no discharge instructions by the hospital except to give her daughter the prescribed antipsychotic medications.

Between August and November, Corrina stayed with her mother and stepfather in a nice urban neighborhood with mature trees, emerald lawns, and the occasional water feature. Smaller children played in the front yards because pools took up the backyards. Neighbors said hello. But during this time, Corrina mostly stayed inside. She also stopped answering the phone and texting people who knew her as Corrina—they were all part of the evil conspiracy. Sometime in October, Corrina decided to explain everything on her Facebook page. She posted that her real name was Karina, that she was an angel, and that Corrina's life was a lie. For those of her friends not on Facebook, Corrina added posts on Instagram and Twitter.

Then, she abruptly started leaving the house for hours at a time on foot. No one—neither her boyfriend Colby nor her parents (nor Corrina when asked later)—knew where she went. In fits of rage, she sometimes smashed, ripped up, or burned her parents' and her boyfriend's property, including precious, irreplaceable items such as photographs and memorabilia. After wrecking her parents' living room and then her boyfriend's apartment on two separate occasions, Sandra gave her a choice: "We can call the police to get you, or you can let me drop you back off at the hospital, but you need some help."

Corrina did not want to deal with the police again, so she agreed to return to Shady Elms. While she was in the hospital, Sandra went through her car looking for illegal drugs. When she opened the glove box, several unopened bottles of prescription antipsychotic medications fell to the floor. Corrina had not been taking her medication.

At this point, I met and interviewed Corrina for the first time when she enrolled in my study on treatment decision making for young people experiencing early psychosis. I had permission to recruit people from the emergency room for interviews during their inpatient stay, and I followed ethical guidelines to do so, which included a lot of rules.[2] The nurses told Corrina I was coming to meet with her, and so she was waiting to talk in a bright, glassed-in cube, designed so that everyone within a fifteen-foot radius could see but not hear us. She shivered in her thin hospital scrubs. I offered her my blazer, and she draped it over her shoulders. Her stringy, unwashed brown hair fell across her protruding collarbone.

Her hospital unit was loud—open and echoing with the sounds of the television, people talking and shouting, phones ringing—a sensory overload. Corrina startled at every bang and spike in noise. She barely spoke above a whisper. She seemed very worried about "the demons."

A few weeks after she got out of the hospital, I was invited by Corrina's mom to visit their home. My team always did follow-up home visits and interviews in pairs for safety, so a research assistant accompanied me. When we arrived, Corrina sat in a wood-paneled living room darkened with blackout curtains. Her eyes, she said, were sensitive to sunlight. She sat in an oversized, black leather chair. As my eyes adjusted, I noticed a scraggly old terrier snoring at her feet.

Corrina said she was feeling better. A week after she returned home from her last hospitalization, she had awakened from her nap knowing that she was Corrina, not Karina.

"Like Rip Van Winkle!" Sandra joked.

It had taken four months, five different antipsychotic medications, and a nap for her original personality to return. Everything was not magically fine, though. When I asked her how she was doing, Corrina picked at her nail polish.

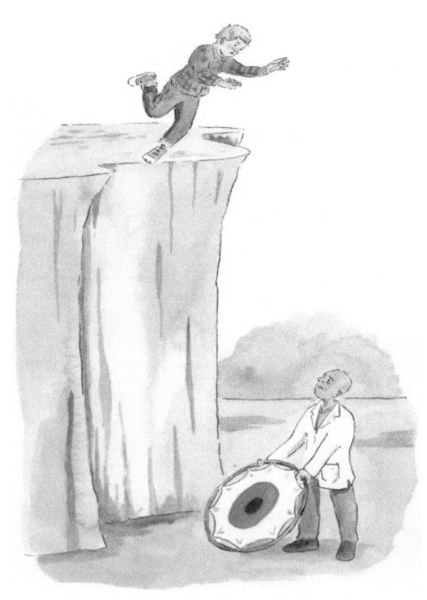

FIGURE 1. Cartoonist Emily Flake's rendering of the situation faced by young persons seeking help for early psychosis. This image shows just how vulnerable young people are, the precarity of the help being offered, and the likelihood that care will "bounce" them into a place that may not be so helpful—and could possibly even be harmful. *From Octavio N. Martinez and Neely Myers, "We Are Failing Young Adults with Psychosis," Hogg Blog, Hogg Foundation for Mental Health, October 19, 2016, https://hogg.utexas.edu/we-are-failing-young-adults-with-psychosis; illustration by Emily Flake.*

"I'm really disappointed. I'm just mad about myself, because I don't understand what to do, and I feel like I've really screwed up a lot of opportunities."

She started to cry.

Corrina had lost months of her life to her mental confusion and had burned many bridges with her school, family, boyfriend, and friends. When Corrina graduated from high school and left home, she was the smart, pretty cheerleader who did lots of volunteer work and was on her way to a good college. Now, rather than being on her way to a happy, independent successful adulthood, she was back at home, with a terrifying diagnosis, little understanding of how she had reached this breaking point, and no clue how to get back on track. Her future, which once looked so bright, now looked disturbingly uncertain.

. . .

The United States—along with much of the Western world—is experiencing what many experts are calling a youth mental health crisis. In 2019, the US surgeon general's general advisory *Protecting Youth Mental Health* warned of a frightening upsurge in adolescent mental health needs—a new threat to America's well-being.[3] Indeed, over the past fifteen years, there has been a forty percent increase in the number of high school students who report feeling so sad and hopeless they could not participate in daily activities, with one in three claiming they felt this way.[4] Nearly half of those high school students who felt hopeless also reported making a suicide plan—a 44 percent increase since 2009. Suicide rates for youths ages 10–24 rose nearly 60 percent between 2007 and 2018, making it the second leading cause of death for this age group.[5] And in 2021, over a third of high school students reported experiencing poor mental health, with a disproportionate impact on Black and Latino youths.[6]

Of course, as we all know, the COVID-19 pandemic did not help. Emergency department usage and psychiatric hospitalizations for young people have risen, as has demand for psychiatric hospital beds.[7] At the same time, over 150 million people—nearly half of the population—live in federally designated mental health professional shortage areas.[8] The costs of this crisis and the lack of access to mental health supports are considerable. Untreated mental health symptoms can lead to poor performance at work and school, interpersonal violence, expensive hospitalizations, and death by suicide—the list goes on.

In addition, young adults are especially vulnerable to experiencing serious mental health concerns—often labeled biomedically as depression, bipolar disorders, and psychotic disorders—that have not yet been identified and so can go unaddressed. These nearly always begin in adolescence, before the age of 25.[9] Psychosis symptoms—such as hearing voices others cannot hear, which can occur across a wide range of diagnoses—often crest at a point known in the clinical literature as a *psychotic break*. For many, psychosis symptoms are episodic and begin as waves, some stronger than others, that eventually become overwhelming—a time I think of as a *breaking point.*

Corrina hit a breaking point and had a psychotic break in her apartment when she heard a television blaring that did not exist and thought that demons posing as loved ones surrounded her. A psychotic break is a complete break with reality, which may include hearing voices, having visions, or fervently upholding ideas that others have trouble accepting as real.[10] These disorienting symptoms of psychosis often begin during a person's early 20s, when they are under tremendous pressure to become a valued, independent American adult. In the United States an estimated 100,000 people experience a first episode of psychosis every year.[11]

Research suggests that there is a "critical period"—a three- or four-month window—after an initial psychotic break when engaging a person in specialty early psychosis care is essential for preventing negative long-term outcomes.[12] This period was the target of this study. Others argue that there is period of up to five years after initial onset when early intervention can help, which is today the target of most early intervention for psychosis programs around the globe. Even so, as of 2022, there were only 381 programs offering specialty early psychosis care in the United States called *coordinated specialty care* (CSC), which was estimated to leave about 75 percent of persons, or more than 75,000 young people, with new cases of early psychosis per year without specialized services in the United States alone.[13] In addition, between 20 and 40 percent of the young adults ages 18 to 35 in the United States who have access to that specialty early psychosis care refuse further treatment.[14]

The study that informs this book used an anthropological approach to understand why young persons who were experiencing a psychotic break were refusing care so frequently during that critical period. Anthropologists have long been interested in the ways people's illness experiences are identified, understood, labeled, and treated in a variety of social contexts, and how people adapt to those experiences. Core anthropological studies of serious emotional distress, for example, include writings on schizophrenia, bipolar disorder, autism, depression, and addiction.[15] Other works focus on adolescents who have been identified as needing mental health care more broadly and the kinds of care offered to them.[16] In addition, the contours, ethics, and variations of Western biomedical approaches to perceived psychopathology as they have been taken up in a variety of social contexts have been well researched.[17] Several notable collections cross over many of these topics in psychological and medical anthropology.[18] These works have collectively taken up questions around psychiatry and mental health in terms of care, ethics, cultural relevance and humility, the social life and power of diagnostic labels and medications, the social and structural determinants of health, and the impacts of both biomedical and local forms of care on the people who use them.

Joining in this scholarly conversation, this book is based on three years of ethnographic research with young persons from culturally diverse backgrounds and their key supporters, research that followed many of them—like Corrina—from their initial hospitalization for a psychotic break back into their homes. My goal was to understand why young people chose to use or to refuse mental health care after a crisis. Effectively helping young people in crisis and, ideally, preventing one before it happens are some of the greatest mental health challenges of our time. This book will address these challenges from a fresh perspective by starting with the everyday experiences of young people and their families during the critical period following their initial hospitalizations. After all, what greater experts are there than those who have been there?

I know firsthand—from experiences in my own family—that psychosis disrupts lives and breaks hearts. Inspired by my family's struggles, for the past twenty years I have been researching how we—as a society, as mental health care workers, and as individuals—can better support people who experience psychosis. What I have learned through my work is that healing from a psychotic break has material, medical, and moral dimensions that require equal attention to promote mental health.

The material dimensions include the spaces and places where people are made to seek mental health support and the resources offered to them, so often shaped by the structural and social determinants of mental health. These determinants include, among other factors, structural racism, lack of employment opportunities with adequate mental health insurance, access to mental health providers, vocational and educational supports, transportation, and housing. All these factors shape a young person's ability to access and use care.

In referring to the medical dimension, I mean the nuts and bolts of care as construed by Western biomedicine and constructed by public health initiatives, which (when done well) can be important resources for people experiencing a mental health crisis and their families. These may include therapeutic supports such as well-informed prescribers, trauma-informed psychotherapists, a place of respite during a crisis, family support specialists, substance abuse counseling, peer specialists, in-home visits, family therapy and education, and alternative health options. At the current moment, many of these basic structures are not available to young persons experiencing early psychosis, a fact that becomes clearer as the book unfolds.

I also highlight the moral dimension, the greatest novel contribution of this book, by pointing to what feminist philosopher Margaret Urban Walker identified as the intimate "moral understandings" developed and shared between people who care about one another, understandings that then reflect their expectations of and responsibilities to one another.[19] Usually such moral understandings are based on shared cultural notions of what is good, beautiful, and true for one's social group at any given moment. These moral understandings, I argue throughout, are seriously compromised by the symptoms of psychosis and then exacerbated by our societal response to them. By using the term *moral*, I am also drawing on an anthropological approach to morality and health that seeks to identify and understand what is life affirming in a specific social context for a specific person, based on the desires and goals they share with the people they care about, and how that process is also key for mental health.[20]

Meeting the expectations of shared moral understandings about what it means to be a "good enough" American adult is crucial for adolescents coming of age in American culture. It is also often the very thing that is compromised between young people and their loved ones during a mental health crisis.[21] Moral understandings need to be repaired when damaged—or, more ideally, protected in the first place. Otherwise, as I demonstrate throughout the book in so many ways, a young person will struggle to have enough moral agency to move forward as an independent adult.

Building on the work of other anthropologists, sociologists, and moral philosophers, I thus define moral agency, the theoretical foundation of my work, as having the wherewithal to aspire, and the intentions and necessary resources to achieve, what one understands to be a good life. Having moral agency means that one person and another have a shared sense that both can uphold their shared moral understandings and so be good enough (if not excellent) to each other, and therefore worthy of an intimate relationship. Being understood as a person capable of being good to another person—in whatever current social context—is essential for the person, their desired relationships, and their vision of a good life to flourish.[22] Having enough moral agency to be seen as a "good enough" person makes possible enriching social connections with desired others, such as romantic partners, friends, family, elders, community groups, and employers.[23] Having relationships with people who see you as a moral agent, allow you to have a relationship with them, and also give you space to try and sometimes fail to be a good person creates opportunities for young people to take meaningful action and move forward in life, at least in the United States.[24]

· · ·

I have been developing my conceptualization of moral agency since 2010.[25] The importance of moral agency for mental health first emerged as a relevant construct after three years of research in a recovery model–based psychosocial rehabilitation agency, Horizons, that failed to help its clients recover in any meaningful way, which was the topic of my first book.[26] The agency's prescribed "journey of recovery" to social belonging and valued citizenship for its "members," as it called individuals with psychiatric disabilities, was based on long-held American moral values about what makes a person good—namely, the ability to independently demonstrate one's rationality, autonomy, and ability to work hard. This set a high bar for the mostly unhoused people with serious psychiatric disabilities whom I engaged. They aspired to lead a good life as others expected but had few resources or relationships with which to get started. Their daily life was fraught in ways that were only exacerbated by a seemingly well intentioned recovery-based mental health policy and practice that ignored the very real structural and relational limitations of their everyday lives.

In 2011, I led another study that asked how primarily African American users of a peer-run public mental health clinic in New York City attempted to "take charge" of their own lives. I found that many of the service users there had long histories of institutional marginalization in "learning disabled" classrooms, foster care, juvenile detention, substance abuse facilities, jails, and mental health service settings.[27] Many had little opportunity to share their life stories in ways that others valued. This work helped me identify what I call *autobiographical power*, or the ability to be at least the editor of your own life story, as essential for a person's sense of moral agency.

Based on this work, I wrote several pieces unpacking further the concept of moral agency, which I could see operating in the stories of people seeking mental health recovery. I elaborated on moral agency as both the intention and means to aspire to a good life that make possible intimate relationships with others. I described how persons who experience a mental health crisis often have a breach in their life narrative, or an Aristotelian *peripeteia*, that erodes their sense of connection to others. After this breach occurs, everyone involved works toward reestablishing that connection by cultivating the person's moral agency, which has three components: autobiographical power, the social bases of self-respect, and peopled opportunities to try and fail.[28] Again, autobiographical power is the ability to at least be the editor of one's own life story in everyday conversations with others.[29] John Rawls's notion of "the social bases of self-respect" highlights the importance of meeting locally valued ideas about what it means to be respected so that you can also respect yourself as a person who belongs.[30] "Peopled opportunities" are social circumstances that enable one to have the opportunity to try (and also sometimes fail) to be recognized as a good, accountable person by others via shared moral understandings that make intimate relationships possible.[31]

Following up on this research, in 2014 a new, National Institute of Mental Health (NIMH)–funded research team that I assembled at Southern Methodist University in Dallas, Texas, began the study that informs this book.[32] This time, my focus was on what guided young persons from primarily ethnoracially minoritized groups' decisions about treatment after an initial emergency hospitalization for a suspected psychotic disorder.[33] The goal was to understand what mattered most to young people ages 18 to 34, and their self-identified key supporters, during the aforementioned critical period—the first few months after an initial hospitalization when engaging in mental health care makes a difference for longer-term outcomes.[34] NIMH researchers work in teams, and I designed this research in partnership with my consultants, who included Michael Compton, a psychiatrist with expertise in African American pathways to care and what contributes to treatment delays for psychosis; psychiatrist and early intervention expert Lisa

Dixon; and the seasoned mental health services researcher and ethnographer Sue Estroff. In addition, as with all NIMH grants, the program officer, Susan Azrin, secured important expertise and feedback from anonymous reviewers on how to best refine my methods and approach. When we received additional funding from the Hogg Foundation for Mental Health Research in 2015, I also added two additional consultants: peer provider and director of the Hope Center, Maggie Caballero, and community psychologist, mental health services researcher, and young person with lived experience Nev Jones.

. . .

Early-intervention research suggests that if young people and their families engage with high-quality, evidence-based mental health supports early enough, they avoid negative long-term outcomes such as homelessness, repeated hospitalizations, and suicide. In this model, psychosis is thought of as similar to cancer: there are "stages" that progress from the earliest phase of social oddities and psychotic-like experiences to a "first break," or complete break with reality.[35] The idea is to catch the illness before it spreads—but, with psychosis, not into the rest of one's body but into the rest of one's life.

Well-designed, compassionate early-intervention programs for young people who have experienced a psychotic break are now typically called coordinated specialty care in the United States and are thought to be cost-effective and prevent longer-term social problems for young people experiencing a mental health crisis.[36] Even so, one recently published (and controversial) paper has suggested the best outcomes may be limited to persons with greater socioeconomic resources,[37] and another has argued that users did not experience long-term, gainful employment as a result of these programs.[38] In addition, research shows that even when these specialty services are on offer, for every ten young adults who experience a psychotic break, up to four or five refuse further mental health care after their initial hospitalization for psychosis, thus putting them at risk for further episodes and worsening outcomes.[39] It may be even more difficult to engage young people with early psychosis from ethnoracially minoritized groups, which have long struggled with systemic and institutional racism, distrust of medical care, and high levels of stigma against people deemed mentally ill.[40]

To explore how to make mental health services for psychosis more appealing to youths experiencing a mental health crisis from a range of cultural backgrounds, my research team engaged with 47 young people—about half of whom self-identified as women and half of whom self-identified as men—ranging in age from 18 to 34. About half also self-identified as Latina/o,[41] one-third as Black,[42] seven white, four South Asian, and one Middle Eastern. In addition, about half were first- or second-generation immigrants—the former meaning they were born outside the United States and the latter meaning one or both of their parents were.[43] We also talked to 19 of the young people's self-identified key supporters—typically a woman and parent, namely their moms. We also interviewed providers of mental health care for Black and Latina/o youths and Black pastors with primarily Black congregants to learn more about the needs and challenges of accessing care for persons from minoritized groups.

This is not to say that the study had a representative sample or that this book offers a definitive account of any of these groups, but I can say with confidence that this book is inclusive and does not focus on white youths. There is a moral imperative to better serve individuals who have been disproportionately impacted by racist policies in the United States (e.g., redlining, overpolicing, the US "war on drugs"), and this book contributes to the literature that responds to this imperative by sharing some of these individuals' experiences when dealing with a mental health crisis. A sample that represents the interests of young persons from a range of cultural backgrounds is important because any broader mental health care reforms must meet the needs of an incredibly diverse nation. It is also important because persons from minoritized groups in the United States experience a higher risk and incidence of symptoms of psychosis and psychotic disorder, and also have more difficulty finding and accessing appropriate services.[44]

The presence of first- and second-generation immigrants in this book is also relevant in that "seeming different" increases one's risk of developing psychosis.[45] A robust literature on immigrants in Europe suggests that immigration increases psychosis risk. In Europe, first-generation migrants face an increased risk of developing mood disorders, and migrants and their children are at an even higher risk for developing psychotic disorders.[46] These phenomena seem associated with social exclusion and minoritized status.[47] Migrating from outside Europe, having Black skin, and being from a socioeconomically "developing" country had the highest impact on psychosis risk.[48] In the United States, the amount of research on immigration and psychosis is limited, but social context clearly shapes the development and experience of psychosis, just as it shapes the development and experience of becoming a valued adult.

Other research finds that Black and Latino individuals are overrepresented in the population of patients diagnosed with psychotic disorders.[49] One study showed that Black children were almost twice as likely to experience schizophrenia, though the higher incidence in this population may have to do with misdiagnosis or socioeconomic disadvantage, and further research is needed.[50] Psychologist Deidre Anglin argues that there may also be a compounding effect of social and environmental stressors related to structural racism and inequality for Black and Hispanic or Latino US populations, such as obstetric complications, police oversurveillance, neighborhood violence, collective trauma, and adverse childhood events, all of which make people more prone to developing psychosis.[51]

Adverse childhood events at the individual, familial, or neighborhood level also increase psychosis risk and can include childhood maltreatment, exposure to violence, the loss or incarceration of a parent, parental unemployment, having a darker skin in a lighter-skinned neighborhood (or vice versa), and perceived discrimination.[52] Many young people in my study talked about these kinds of events. The experience of increased risk of psychosis for sexually minoritized individuals and people with hearing impairments may also be explained by social and environmental stressors related to discrimination and social exclusion.[53]

To the extent possible, we recruited persons from minoritized groups for the study. I and core members of the team—primarily Anubha Sood (a NIMH-funded postdoctoral fellow) and Katherine Fox (an SMU PhD student in cultural anthropology) and eventually, with additional funding from the Hogg Foundation for Mental Health Research, Nia Parson (an associate professor of anthropology at SMU with fluency in Spanish)— recruited nearly all of the young adults enrolled at Shady Elms with the generous support of the hospital leadership, its staff, and its internal review board (IRB). Shady Elms was a psychiatric emergency-only hospital that, according to institutional data from 2014, served 23,000 people in crisis from seven counties in North Texas each year. The hospital reported having about two new first-episode psychosis patients per week. My team recruited and gained consent from those young people, such as Corrina, while they were in the hospital. We then followed up with them after their release in community-based settings to engage them in further interviews and ethnographic home visits over the next several months as they struggled to, as they often put it, "get back to normal."

Anthropologists often use ethnography to understand what everyday life may be like for our interlocutors. What sets ethnography apart from other research methods is its slow accumulation: anthropologists spend a lot of time with the people we are trying to understand, and these engagements occur over a relatively long period. Rather than coming in and administering a survey or questionnaire in a "one and done" approach, an ethnographer may engage someone in an interview or offer a survey, but then will return repeatedly to confirm and refine their observations and interpretations with the help of their interlocutors. Ethnographers are looking not for what someone said once but rather for *iterative* patterns, or repetitions, in what that person and others say over time.

Another hallmark of ethnography is that researchers reflect on the way their own position, or positionality, affects their relationship with the people they are researching. In my case, I asked myself how my role as a white college professor at an expensive local university might affect the ways young persons and their families—with varying levels of education and income and a range of minoritized statuses—interacted with me. How might my presence and the power dynamics between us shape their participation and answers? And how might my own interests and desires—for example, as a family member of someone who experiences psychosis—shape the ways I ask questions or how I understand and interpret what my interlocutors say?

What I love about ethnography is that it allows me to establish a relationship with the people I am trying to understand. I get to know them. They get to know me. In this study, I regularly reminded the people whom I engaged: "Hey, you are the expert on this experience, and it is *your* experience, so *you* tell me. I do not know what it feels like to be a young person with early psychosis or their parent, but you do, and if you are willing to share, then maybe this research can help other people have a better experience by sharing your story." And I meant it. This helped ease the power differential between us.

The members of my research team also brought their own positionalities to the table. I intentionally sought out lab team members who were under 35 (the cut-off age for the study) and who self-identified as persons with lived experience of mental health concerns or as persons from a minoritized group, or both, so that they could bring their lived-experience expertise into the conversations about the data collection and interpretation. Not all the team members met any of these criteria, but I did try.

Early on, the consultants and team members who self-identified as persons from minoritized groups, as well as the staff at the hospital, let me know that the young adults we were trying to recruit were most likely to trust and engage someone who looked like them. Over time, we added several undergraduates to my team, including young persons who identified as being from a minoritized group, both because the young persons seemed to relax around their peers and because the undergraduates could help the rest of us understand youth culture. We also brought on bilingual Spanish-language speakers to translate research documents, conduct interviews with those more comfortable speaking in Spanish, and transcribe the interviews into English. The conversations I had with my team were invaluable in critiquing and shaping the research approach, our follow-up questions and visits, and the way I have thought through the data we collected.

So it is through ethnography, as well as all the various perspectives and experiences that my research team brought to the effort, that we built relationships with the young people and their key supporters over multiple visits, initially at the hospital and then in their home or at a place in the community, such as a Starbuck's Coffee shop, where they felt safe and comfortable, over the course of up to one year. These visits helped my team understand the young persons' experiences over time in their own social context. We were thus able to take our time to explore their hopes, desires, fears, needs, and goals in a place that was comfortable for them, and they had time to trust us enough to share.

This proximity took a toll on the team. It is heartbreaking to see people struggling. Per the ethical research parameters of my project, we were limited to no more than four visits so as not to influence their treatment decisions. We were also supposed to cease following up with them after six months unless they called us first. We thus do not know what happened to those we interviewed over the long run. Therefore, this is not a book of happy endings or finished stories, but of unfolding lives and the ideas they inspired.

One of the most important ideas that emerged from these data, from my perspective, was that paying attention to local forms of moral agency can shed light on what drives young people's decisions about medical treatment, and on how the treatment on offer both helps and hinders American youths in returning to a meaningful life after experiencing a mental health crisis. As I pondered the significance of these data and wrote this book, I came to understand that while many people see psychosis as a breaking point, a rupture from reality and in one's life plan, it could also be a turning point if we offered people the right supports. The good news is that there is a lot we humans can do, and this book points us to a better understanding of how we can help. It is about the United States, but I think it applies to many places—any place where young people are struggling. And, right now, that is everywhere.

. . .

Typically, prior to their initial hospitalizations, the young people in my study were working toward a successful transition to adulthood. In the United States, there is no prescribed, structured, guided rite of passage to adulthood to help an adolescent make that transition. Young people must do it on their own. Thus, the young people I met were socializing and studying and trying to earn a viable income. They needed to establish their moral agency so that they had social credibility as independent adults. Again, moral agency is a person's ability to be seen by intimate others as a "good enough" person in the social context that matters to them, which makes possible the relationships they need to thrive in a culture where everyone is expected to be "self-made."

For young Americans, being healthy enough, attractive enough, and successful enough to secure intimate relationships with others constitutes three common cultural signals of having enough moral agency to thrive. My undergraduate students typically list these three items first when I ask them what it means to be happy. There are other ways to attain moral agency in the United States—participating in community service, belonging to a religious community, caregiving for relatives, becoming an Eagle Scout, serving in the military, rescuing animals, and so forth—but many young people equate an individual's good health, attractive appearance, and success at school or work with being good. American youths must be able to both work hard and play hard and seem healthy, attractive, and successful while doing so. This is the topic of chapter 1.

Some youths achieve these cultural signals of moral agency in high school. They may have been on an athletic team or were part of the band or a cheerleader like Corrina. Perhaps they were popular with peers, engaged in community service, and had good grades. These accomplishments signaled that they were a good-enough person to hire or have as a roommate or a romantic partner—all things most Americans desire as adults. However, when youths leave high school, they are under pressure to prove themselves as moral agents all over again, but this time independently and often in a new place with unfamiliar faces.

A person with enough moral agency to be deemed a responsible, independent adult must have three key capabilities. First, they must have the intention and capacity to exercise autobiographical power, which is the ability to be the writer, or at least the editor, of their own life story. Second, they must be able to seek and secure the social bases of self-respect, and so be recognized by meaningful others as the kind of person they imagine themselves to be. Who we become is relational—it must be mutually agreed upon with the others we want to have in our lives. We must be good enough for the people we want to love us to accept us so we can belong. We first need to affirm that the role we have chosen as the editors of our own lives—be it pop star, stay-at-home mom, or astrophysicist—is the right one for us and that others respect us in that role. I cannot just walk around saying I am an aspiring hip-hop star or news anchor if no one else agrees that it's even a possibility. The third key capability for any person is to successfully negotiate peopled opportunities by practicing one's desired social role with intimate others who are willing to let one try and fail and try again.[54] It is quite likely that someone, especially as they are transitioning to adulthood, won't get it right the first time. So their loved ones have to be patient and give them multiple chances.

It helps to think of this phase in the terms of theater: "All the world's a stage," to borrow from Shakespeare.[55] American youths are expected to fashion their own social role, convince others that they deserve that role, and then seek out opportunities to practice that role with audiences who then decide whether or not they are good at it and so can be respected in that role. Having the ability to do this—to craft oneself into a valued adult in American culture—requires moral agency.

These key components of moral agency—autobiographical power, the social bases of self-respect, and peopled opportunities—are not a given in the United States. They must be earned. It's actually very hard to do, and no one gets a manual or a guidebook. Young people starting the transition to adulthood will have earned some of these components in their home communities as they built up a tentative sense of moral agency before they turned 18 or graduated from high school. But at this point Americans ask their youths to go out and become self-made by finding their own niche—who they want to be—and then making a place for themselves in that niche.[56] We require them to start over in proving themselves to be moral agents, by themselves and to a new audience, by working hard and playing hard.

The American Dream is that anyone can become successful if they try hard enough. But America is not the meritocracy many imagine it to be. Some people get more chances than others. Imagine two young people in their mid-20s—Emily and Andre. Emily is white. Her parents are not rich, but they are comfortably middle-class. Emily is careful to craft a public persona that looks good in the virtual and real worlds. She projects the image of success. She is fit and well dressed. She has a college degree from a reputable university and a nice job at a good company with a solid paycheck. She has her own car, apartment, and a loving girlfriend. Her dog has his own popular Instagram account. Emily "has it all." If she continues to maintain her positive social status in the circles and communities that matter to her, she can tell her own story in her own way. Her loved ones will accept her story as true and respect her for it.

Emily has also been given opportunities to try and fail. And fail she has. When Emily was 18, she was arrested for trying to sell cannabis in a rock concert parking lot to an undercover cop. She was trying to cover the cost of her ticket and hotel room. Emily was convicted but did not go to jail, and her future employers did not hold that against her. People make mistakes, they said. She was young and had no other police record, so why penalize her for it? She spoke her truth, convinced her audience, had chances to try and fail, and became a valued American adult with access to the intimate relationships she needed to thrive. Emily had enough moral agency to live the life she wanted as a socially valued, good-enough adult.

Andre, on the other hand, is Black, and history, research, and common sense indicate that this makes moral agency more difficult for him to access in the majority-white culture of the United States.[57] Due to a long history of social, political, and economic disenfranchisement of Black persons in the United States, his family also has less material wealth to support him than Emily's family. He has struggled since childhood with dyslexia, which went undiagnosed, and so he did not receive the additional educational supports he needed to thrive in school. He wanted to go to college, but his grades were not strong enough for a scholarship, and he could not afford it. With mostly low-income job opportunities available to him, Andre decided to focus on a music career. For a little while, being a musician attracted some women, but no one special to Andre. The band was not making a lot of money, studio time was expensive, and his mom wanted him to get his own apartment, so Andre decided to sell cannabis on the side. Like Emily, Andre was arrested by undercover police, but unlike Emily, he spent three months in jail. Unable to pay rent, he was evicted from his apartment. Upon his release, people were less willing to offer him employment when he reported his record. It was harder to get an apartment after an eviction. His bandmates seemed reluctant to reconnect with him. He became increasingly depressed and anxious.

Andre's chances for making a successful transition to becoming a valued American adult were diminishing. He was losing his ability to become the kind of person he wanted to be. He wasn't telling the story he wanted to tell and was rejected for the roles he tried to take on. He had few opportunities for a second try and was penalized for his failures. Andre did not have enough moral agency to nourish the relationships he needed to live life on his own terms. It was difficult for him to build up moral agency when others were reluctant to give him a chance to try.

All young adults in the United States are trying to become moral agents independently so that they can become people "good enough" to have meaningful lives and relationships. However, the research suggests that many persons from marginalized or minoritized groups of all ages lack moral agency in contexts of transition when they are tasked with proving their moral value all over again with new sets of intimate others.[58] They must work extra hard to reestablish that they are a "good person" in order to access intimate relationships as they begin everyday life anew.

As feminist philosopher Margaret Urban Walker wrote:

> Not everyone is allowed or enabled to tell just any life (or other) story. The stuff of lives to be told, the discursive means available for telling them, and the credibility of storytellers are apt to differ along familiar lines of class, gender, and race, perhaps along other lines, even rather local ones as well. Life stories, including moral histories, will take shape in response to specific constraints, and for some people may be shaped as much for them as by them depending on their "socially recognized credibility."[59]

• • •

Establishing moral agency is difficult for any young person. Add to this the disadvantage of being a person of a minoritized status and the experience of a mental breakdown, and the task of establishing moral agency can become extremely challenging. In fact, some of the very means that our culture offers to enhance moral agency are particularly dangerous to those who need it the most.

For example, many of the young people my team interviewed were encouraged by American culture to both work hard and play hard, and so they worked hard but also engaged in substance use. For young people in our study, substance use—and misuse—often led to entanglements with authorities. This led to losing moral agency with other adults—landlords, teachers, parents—and sometimes friends. It also contributed to treatment delays as families and young persons confused psychotic symptoms with substance misuse.[60] As with Corrina, who used cannabis and LSD to relax and fit in, young people in our study struggled to meet the expectation that they could play hard while also struggling with the onset of highly disorienting psychotic symptoms. This is the topic of chapter 1, "Work Hard, Play Hard."

Nearly all the young people in our study also began to craft personal myths as explanations for their symptoms, narratives that typically made sense to the young people in crisis but not to others. For others, it signaled a break with reality—a phenomenon I unpack in chapter 2, "Into the Mythos." It is hard to accept someone as an angel or Jesus or a superhero. When a young person tried to claim these identities, others questioned their ability to become a responsible and independent adult. Their moral agency was starting to break down, but the young person could not yet see it.

For most of the youths in our study, there was often a catalytic event—a person had to become dangerous to themselves or others (but not violent per se, as I explain)—before someone decided to call for help. In chapter 3, "Dangerous,"

I explore this phenomenon further. Once a family reached out for help, the people who typically responded to emergencies—especially mental health emergencies—were the police. For persons from ethnoracially minoritized groups, interactions with the police can cause psychological distress.[61] Even so, most of the young adults my team interviewed came to the hospital by police escort because Texas law (and the law of many other states) requires that, to be hospitalized involuntarily, a person who is over 18 who is not under a legal guardianship must be admitted into the hospital from the custody of a "peace officer," or someone who works in law enforcement.[62]

Here again, the US mental health system is failing our youths. Being in police custody and then hospitalized involuntarily, I argue, led to the further loss of autobiographical power and the social bases of self-respect for the young persons in my study. It altered how they thought of themselves and how their loved ones thought of them. Even the handful of my study participants who initially went to the hospital voluntarily described how it affected their ability to be perceived as a good person later.

At most mental health emergency facilities, as discussed in chapter 4, "Disorientations," the first few days after intake focused on controlling the person's risk to self and others with sedation and restraints, assigning a diagnosis for medical insurance billing purposes, and deciding where a young person should go next—often determined by their insurance status, it seemed. The youths in my study were then often released with little continuity of care, no clear directions for next steps, and little to no family, educational, vocational, therapeutic, peer, or substance use supports. This means that peopled opportunities were often thin: most intimate others were now seriously questioning the young person's credibility as the moral understandings between them and their loved ones broke down.

Families had little support in processing with others what had happened or in navigating what followed. For those limited to public insurance, the extended hospitalizations seemingly required by Medicaid or Medicare rules resulted in lost opportunities at work and school as employers, friends, and teachers had ample time to notice that something was terribly wrong. This typical response to psychosis, by both the medical community and the community at large, again diminished our interlocutors' moral agency, thereby complicating their ability to continue their efforts to become valued adults. This also diminished their interest in continuing mental health treatment.

It does not have to be this way.

Far from being passive victims of a failed mental health system who could not think for themselves, the young people in our study, as this book illustrates, worked diligently to restore the moral agency they were losing even as they were losing it. They sought connection and recognition as a "good" person even in their most vulnerable and disorienting moments. More than half refused care, but it was not an irrational decision. Their decisions about whether to use or refuse mental health care were grounded in their ideas about whether using that care was going to help them restore their moral agency and "get back to normal."

In many cases when young people refused services, for example, their family did not support the idea of pursuing care. Some families wanted to rely on religious supports for healing. Others had such a strong bias against people who were "crazy" that their children moved away from the label as much as possible by rejecting care. Young people needed the moral and material support of their families to move forward, and many worked hard to not lose that support even if it meant refusing medical treatment. This book shares their stories.

On the other hand, half of the young people that completed the study did accept services: these were the service users. Often, they did so because their families encouraged or required them to do so in order to receive material and moral support. I share their stories, too. Chapter 5, "Users and Refusers," focuses on young persons' decision-making processes about using or refusing mental health care during the critical period. I also explore, in chapter 6, "Homecoming," the struggles of families to support their loved ones and one another and move forward.

While Americans debate effective ways to reduce costly social problems associated with unaddressed mental illness, such as homelessness, violence, substance abuse, fatal police shootings, and rising suicide rates, the number of young adults reporting increasing amounts of serious emotional distress is rising.[63] There are services (though not yet widely enough available) that can help young people have better outcomes. But, no matter how widely available those services are, no one can force young people to use them outside a crisis situation.

The experience of psychosis does not happen in a cultural vacuum. Attention to American culture and how it complicates the transition to adulthood for all youths, and even more so for young adults experiencing symptoms of psychosis, is at the heart of this book. The mental health system in the United States is failing young people in crisis, and we must consider what can be done to address this crisis in terms of moral agency. Understanding how young people decide when to use or refuse services and the relationship between those choices and moral agency in the context of making a transition to valued adulthood is crucial.

Many young people experience symptoms of psychosis, but with stronger material, medical, and moral supports, they can move forward. Having a psychotic break need not permanently rob a young person of their moral agency; it can be a turning point toward a positive outcome instead. While focusing on the stories and decisions of young people and their families, I argue that attending to young people's moral agency during this period of incredible vulnerability and potential is at least as important as medical treatment, because young people will not seek out supports that they perceive to be—or that are—misaligned with their moral lives and therefore socially harmful for them.

Throughout the book I indicate multiple breaking points when things could be done differently to prevent or alleviate the crisis. In chapter 7, "Turning Points,"

I present what we can do to change things for the better. Mental health care can protect and replenish moral agency and so better engage young people in much-needed early material, medical, and moral support. This book shows all of us how, whether we are persons experiencing psychosis, intimate others, health care workers, advocates, policy makers, or academics. Together, we can work toward constructing a pathway *through* care for young persons with early psychosis— one that doesn't just bring them to the hospital emergency room but guides their families and them through the care process and back into everyday life.[64] First, however, we as a society need to develop a radically compassionate understanding of the challenges young people and their families face when they encounter the breaking point of psychosis so that we can instead transform this moment of crisis into a turning point for the better—a moment when the right supports are provided to a young person who needs that extra support to become a moral agent living out their full potential.

1

Work Hard, Play Hard

I used to smoke weed, but I stopped it. Like, God doesn't want me to do it and I'm doing His will. So I've been three months without weed. I haven't drank since my last birthday. I'm 21. I should be barhopping like all the rest of the kids, but that's not me. I just want to do something with my life. Get somewhere, but that's kinda hard, when you're places like this.

—AMIR, SHADY ELMS PSYCHIATRIC EMERGENCY ROOM, DAY 2

In pictures posted on Facebook, James was often impeccably dressed, his curly dark hair carefully styled. Raised in a leafy suburb, he had well-educated parents and a gainfully employed father. Both of his parents were South Asian, born and educated outside the United States. They came to Texas for work before James was born. James, his mother, Mala, said during an interview, was "a friendly, playful kid." Growing up, she thought James was "totally fine," because he was "always invited to parties and had so many girlfriends."

I first met James at a Starbucks near his parents' house, where he was living, two months after his initial hospitalization. I liked him right away. He was funny, sensitive, and charismatic. He weaved in and out of talking about things anyone who has been a young adult can understand—such as experimenting with substances and looking for love.

> JAMES: I did weed since tenth grade, and I did acid [LSD] since like eleventh grade. So, [I have used substances] for a pretty long time.
>
> NEELY: Why did you start?
>
> JAMES: Because my friends did it. I was like—okay, if they're doing it, it must be fine because they seem normal.
>
> NEELY: Right. So, you were goofing around?
>
> JAMES: Yeah, pretty much. And then, after a while, it got addictive. [. . .]¹ The weed made me feel calmer. The acid I did for fun because it showed me cool visuals, and I like the head trips because it made me think that I was learning about the world.

I was not surprised to hear James talk about these experiences. The college students in my medical and psychological anthropology classes over the past decade freely discuss their experimentation with sex and substance use. James's generation, like many generations before his, enjoyed drinking alcohol, smoking pot, trying psychedelics, and listening to music or hanging out with friends, romantic partners, or potential hook-ups in a relatively safe space. After all, sexual experimentation and substance use can bring people closer together at times, enhancing much-needed social bonds.[2] And engaging in risky behaviors that I call playing hard—often exemplified in sexual pursuit and substance use exploration—is a key part of coming of age in American culture for young adults.

James worried me, though. Even though we were in public, in a Starbucks with an affluent crowd, James looked disheveled. His black shirt was speckled with dandruff and his hair was greasy. He smelled like rotting food, as though he had not showered for a while. He spoke quickly and tangentially, and he had a thousand thoughts that poured out in bursts, which made him hard to follow but fun to speak with overall.

James thought of himself as an aspiring hip-hop artist and regularly posted his music on internet sites, though he had not been discovered—yet. On social media, he tried to attract the "celebrities" he followed, posting pictures of himself partying or rapping, hoping they would notice him and want to be his friend. This seemed like typical adolescent behavior until James added that the celebrities frequently came to his house to get him but his parents kept blocking them from seeing him. For example, he told me, when Jay-Z came to the door, they told him that he wasn't home, but he was just in his room sleeping. Jay-Z then left a public post on Instagram letting James know what had happened using code words James knew were for him. James felt frustrated by his parents' refusal to let him be famous. He thought maybe they did not approve of all the drugs the celebrities used—they definitely did not like his own drug use—but James thought that was ridiculous and old-fashioned. His parents did not grow up in America, he explained, so they did not understand.

James told me that he tried to stay awake to meet the celebrities when they came to the door, but he had to sleep eventually. Sometimes he wandered outside the local airport arrival doors, smoking, pretending to be an Uber driver. He hoped to spot the celebrities who came to visit him before his parents could send them away. The celebrities were making this all clear to him on their Instagram feeds—leaving coded messages to let him know they were coming, which he appreciated. James was sure he was going to be famous.

I left the interview feeling uneasy.

Interviewed separately a few weeks later, Mala, James's mother, did not talk about the celebrities or her son's substance use. Her attention was focused on "the girl." After James's fifth psychiatric hospitalization in a few months—his first hospitalizations ever—Mala thought James was suffering from a broken heart. His whole life, Mala explained, she had let the pediatrician talk to James about "sexual health," but she never thought to warn him to "guard your heart" or "watch for those emotions."

"I never thought of that," she said, her voice cracking.

The pediatrician told her that it was normal for people to take their first romantic relationship too seriously. So Mala told James to take it easy with "the girl stuff." She added, "He was always playful, but in college he got attached to this girl, so . . ." She sighed.

When James was arrested for "an incident with this girl" that landed him in the psychiatric emergency room for the first time, Mala recalled, the pediatrician reminded her again that young people often take their first relationship too seriously. James was just too serious.

Mala advised James, "That is a good heart you've got. You're not like one of those playboys. You're actually valuing the girl, and if it hurts you, she's not worth it." Perhaps, she thought hopefully, he would learn his lesson and grow stronger. What his mother did not mention was that James's behavior had driven his first love away.

In a different interview, James explained how he had forced his way into his ex-girlfriend's car after she refused to see him anymore and told him she was with someone else. Once he was in her car:

> I put my hands on her. She was screaming at me. I think I was in my psychosis state even then. I was doing a lot of marijuana, and that can induce psychosis. I was probably smoking cocaine that was laced with marijuana. Did a lot of acid [LSD]. I think she just got fed up with me doing drugs all the time, so she finally cheated on me—to push me away. But I got in her car, and she was not fine with it, so she told me to get out. Then I put my hands on her by accident. Like, on her wrist—not even harshly. I just grabbed them, and then I got out of her car, and I saw some guy pull up to her car, and I was like, "Is this the guy?" And then she drives to my work. So she tells the work people, gets me fired from over there, and then tells the police I was stalking her. So the cops come to my house. They said I wasn't getting arrested, the charges were still pending, so they just took me to the mental hospital. That was the first time I had ever been to Shady Elms. I was there for about like a week, and they put me on antipsychotic drugs . . . for depression.

After this incident, James lost his job and was expelled from college. He could not enroll again for at least one year. In our early interviews, he blamed "the girl" more than anything. She cheated on him. End of story.

However, over time, his perspective shifted. He thought that the challenges he faced might be attributed in part to his heavy substance use and the power that it had over him. In a later interview, he reflected:

> If I wasn't on so many drugs, maybe I'd not have even got in her car. Maybe I'd have thought more rationally. Maybe I'd have called her up and said, "Hey, we're done."

That would've been the manliest thing to do [. . .] I was looking for, like, the truth in life, and just to help me to make choices in life and stuff. But, honestly, it was just putting me into this psychosis state that was just feeding me false lies—like false truths, actually. So it was pretty much just lying to me.

It took time, but eventually James could see the clear connection between his behavior and the "incident" with the girl that seriously diminished his moral agency with many of his intimate others. It was hard for others to see someone who used so many substances in irresponsible ways and then assaulted their girlfriend as a "good" person. First, his old friends no longer wanted to spend time with him. His girlfriend rejected him romantically. His workplace no longer saw him as a valued employee. The school administrators no longer respected him, and he lost his enrollment privileges. Not having a girlfriend or a job and not being in college amounted to a serious loss of the social bases of self-respect in James's local moral world. He also lost many peopled opportunities in this fall from grace as his intimate others became reluctant to maintain their affiliation or give him another chance to try to be a good person. His substance misuse—which began, at least in part, as a socially acceptable way to fit in with his high school friends and be invited to lots of parties and have lots of girlfriends—became a key part of his loss of moral agency in college as it fueled—and was perhaps fueled by—his emerging psychosis.

· · ·

At first glance, James's and Corrina's stories are not that different from the experiences that have defined young Americans' transition to adulthood for generations. Both graduated from high school, tried to break away from their parents by pursuing higher education, had a taste of the freedom of youth, experimented with substances, searched for love. This is how American adolescents acquire moral agency and become valued adults. They must leave home, work hard, play hard, and prove they can be "fun" while maintaining self-control, attracting a life partner, finding a new community, and becoming financially independent. American culture encourages young people to experiment with risky behaviors and fringe identities but has a narrow window of tolerance for what is ultimately acceptable. American adults who have successfully made this transition may view this time of experimentation as an important and expected part of their own youthful "glory days." But for young people with early psychosis, this way of transitioning to adulthood is often perilous. For the youth in our study, this American-style rite of passage lacked the involvement of wise elders, relied on individual skill, and lured youths with mental health concerns into at times dangerous and isolating excesses with long-term consequences.[3]

Tapping into cross-cultural perspectives on adolescent development and moral agency, this chapter explores how American culture is especially toxic for young people with early psychosis. Some of the very ways that American culture encourages young people to acquire moral agency and become valued adults—breaking away from family, acting independently, working hard, and playing hard—are uniquely dangerous to those who are highly vulnerable to stress and developing symptoms of psychosis. Unfortunately, what can be "fun" and promote social bonding for others can be disastrous for them. In our social media–fueled world, these disasters can be witnessed by more people than ever before. Online social interactions can be easily misread, and misunderstandings and missteps made online are hard to take back. James thought the celebrities on his Instagram feed were communicating with him, and for Corrina, her life was a lie, she was really an angel, and her parents were demons sent to harm her—a "truth" that she also posted on social media.

This book shows many others making these same kinds of mistakes. As psychosis emerges, it reverberates throughout a person's life. By thinking through what it means to be a young American coming of age today, we can see how this environment can be especially toxic for young persons with early psychosis. Once we understand that environment, those of us who could serve as wise elders or supportive friends and family can show more compassion for how challenging it can be, better anticipate how to guide people through it, and offer more guardrails and course corrections along the way.

So, what is it like to be a young adult in the United States today? Modern neuroscience suggests that adolescents transitioning to adulthood are developing new cognitive, socio-emotional, and skill domains, including romantic emotions and sexual behavior, an increase in independence and risk-taking behavior, and shifts in orientation to self and others.[4] And what developmental psychologist Erik Erikson observed in the 1960s—that young adulthood may be characterized as an "identity crisis," or a period of heightened vulnerability and potential—seems to hold true today.[5] During this transition, young Americans are sent off to live independently in the "social jungle of human existence," which Erikson thought was the American version of a "rite of passage."[6] This could include leaving home to go to college, moving out of the house to take on a new job or start a family, joining the military, or attending a trade school.[7]

However, Erikson was no anthropologist, and his proposed American rite of passage falls far short of what some cultures offer adolescents to help them transition. *Initiation rites,* or rites of passage that help a young person transition from a now-devalued childhood identity to a valued adult social role, can be curated, well-directed experiences that help a young person know how to acquire moral agency (the ability to be seen as a good person) in their own culture. Arnold van Gennep, a French ethnographer and folklorist working at the turn of the twentieth century, first detailed such passages cross-culturally. Van Gennep and anthropologist Victor Turner argued that initiation rites found across many cultures guided young persons into their meaningful adult social roles.[8] These rites essentially laid out local ideas about moral agency: what would it mean to become a valued adult worthy of intimate connections with others in this particular social context? Initiation rites thus offered a specific set of directions that made sense in their local social context. In our culture, young people must invent themselves—edit their lives, secure the social bases of self-respect, and find peopled opportunities. In some cultures, young people were instead assigned their future role as moral agents, which channeled and eased the psychological stress of changing roles, encouraged young people to develop locally "prized virtues" like courage and resilience, and helped young people appreciate and respect life's mysteries.

Initiation rites also often involved an "ordeal" and so helped young people learn how to face discomfort and pain gracefully with the guidance of trusted elders.[9] For example, some young Maasai men undergoing initiation rites (usually between the ages of 9 and 15) spend a few months in a special camp being guided by elders to learn about social traditions and life skills. As part of the experience, they are circumcised and then leave their village, not speaking to their loved ones (they are considered to be ghosts) while living outside the village for months with only one another to rely on. Upon their return, ideally after killing a lion (which is no longer possible in most places), they are welcomed back as "junior warriors," a new social role for young men that is both celebrated and defined.[10]

In contrast, in the United States, society affords only limited support for the transition to adulthood. Yes, there are days of celebration such as graduation ceremonies, debutante balls, bar mitzvahs, and quinceañeras, but many of these celebrations require some degree of wealth, do not cut across the population (the whole community typically does not participate), and do not necessarily help young people bond with their peer group and elders in the wider social world of American life. Notably, these American ceremonies also do not involve enduring any kind of ordeal with peers or the guidance of elders, but often instead climax with a party. After the party is over, young people still must reenter mainstream society and reestablish themselves as a moral agent more broadly—and largely on their own.

Thus, instead of being guided through a structured, guided, time-limited rite of passage that helps one to know one's place, American youths are taught to leave home, work hard, and play hard—on their own and in their own way. Most young Americans typically begin this transition between the ages of 16 and 18, when they gain legal privileges such as a driver's license and the right to vote. Learning to drive, graduating from high school, and turning 21 so you can legally purchase alcohol are all loosely referred to as rites of passage in American life.

Any of these may be like an initiation rite in that the young persons have separated from their parents and "village" and are, as Turner would say, "betwixt and between" social identities and roles,[11] but for cultures with formal initiation rites, this phase was typically held outside everyday life. It was guided by trusted elders, close kin, neighbors, and healers all of whom helped young people through the more difficult or challenging aspects.[12] Youths undergoing initiation rites thus had an opportunity to experiment with forgetting their childhood and trying and failing in a socially sanctioned way that brought them closer to their peers and select elders. This was a structured way to display one's competence in cultural values, be tested for that competence, accept one's role in life, and receive social recognition for that role.

In the American version, by contrast, young people must leave their home communities and prove themselves to be worthy and responsible adults with little more than the help of their peers—and, typically, not the peers who were their childhood friends. One would hope that spiritual, educational, or vocational mentors would be in place to reach out to young adults who struggled to find their "tribe" and to help them transition.[13] But wise and humble elders are not something American culture particularly values or helps young persons find. As a result, often there is no one to notice if a youth is struggling with mental health or to support them. Those that knew American youths as children—teachers, clergy, neighbors, pediatricians, even friends' parents—are often no longer in contact except perhaps on social media. Very few of the youths we talked to mentioned having much guidance from someone outside their family or friends when asked about supportive others.

Also, unlike traditional initiation rites, the American version is not time limited and gives young people few clear exit ramps to mark the point when they can consider themselves to be valued adult members of the community or what that role means. In traditional initiation rites, the end is marked by a celebration, a return from social exclusion and isolation, or the acquisition of new names, social roles, and bodily markings like a shaving, piercing, or tattoo that are then recognized and celebrated with the young person's loved ones. Transitioned youths are welcomed back into the community with a new and valued social role, secure in their place in the community and clearly separated from their parents and their childhoods but incorporated into the larger social world.

In the United States, it is not clear when one has arrived at adulthood. There is no official marking of one's arrival, and those who have arrived are not sure how or when it happened.[14] Was I an adult when I graduated from college? Had my first job? Got married? Had a child? Bought a home? What if I moved back in with my parents? And in a country where social and economic upheavals have made it unclear at which age a young person will be moving out, getting a job, and starting a family, and with little change in the expectation that one leaves at the age of 18, this whole process is confusing.[15] In fact, the only real set of directions that I have found—in this research, in my own experience, and in the experiences of family, students and friends—is that young Americans are expected to leave home, establish their independence, work hard, and play hard around the age of 18—right around the time that psychosis can begin to emerge.

· · ·

Pulitzer Prize winner James Truslow Adams wrote that all Americans share "that dream of a land in which life should be better and richer and fuller for every man [*sic*], with opportunity for each according to his ability or achievement."[16] The social expectation is that with hard work and an independent spirit anyone can achieve their dreams. As then-president Barack Obama stated, "If you work hard and meet your responsibilities, you can get ahead, no matter where you come from, what you look like, or who you love."[17] Then-president Donald Trump also said, "The American Dream is freedom, prosperity, peace—and liberty and justice for all. That's a big dream. It's not always easy to achieve, but that's the ideal. More than any country in history we've made gains toward a democracy that is enviable throughout the world. Dreams require perseverance if they are to be realized, and fortunately we're a hard-working country and people."[18]

Anthropologist Margaret Mead wrote in the 1920s that this "myth of endless opportunity" stemmed from a very American notion that the United States is a meritocracy and success is anyone's for the taking, and that this could leave Americans with little peace with their station in life.[19] Immigrants, in particular, Mead noted, were under pressure to exceed the potential of their parents. More recent studies, for example in sociology, have also shown that the American Dream is alive and well and that many Americans think of education as a key pathway to success.[20] In the United States, then, the key to living a "good" life is communicated as becoming a person who works hard.[21] Americans are taught this core cultural virtue from childhood, and the ability to be productive through work is the moral foundation of the American social contract, as well as one of the few clear ways to enhance moral agency and social belonging.[22]

The youths in our study heard this message loud and clear. Corrina's mother wanted her to go to college. James's parents expected no less. Corrina and James had tried, but it was not working out. As wonderful as aspiring to endless opportunity and independence sounds, it comes with a price: an overwhelming array of emotionally charged choices in the absence of clear or practical standards. The expectation of autobiographical power, or the need to be at least the editor of one's own life in order to be seen as a good person, puts a lot of pressure on young people to craft a self-story that others might accept but provides them with few guidelines for what is acceptable. The endless demands of making choices that risk some important relationships in favor of others in order to establish independence can cost young people the very relationships they need for support. While most young people are given opportunities to try and fail by their loved ones, there are so many choices that it can be hard to make sense of the best path. Nor do the pressures and choices stop when one works hard, because in America we also play hard.

For example, James was caught between two differing standards for the social bases of self-respect. He had a desire to fit in with the "celebrities" and his friends who enjoyed substance use, but his girlfriend, his parents, the police, and his school administrators and employers disapproved. The more his substance use amplified, the less time his old friends spent with him. He started hanging out more with what he would later describe as the "wrong crowd." As time went on, James started to lose his ability to be the editor of his own life.

Working hard and playing hard in American culture means that a young person must be able to work hard enough to earn the ability to "have fun," and to spend their time and money consuming whatever they deem fulfilling at the time. Life's purpose can at times revolve around the consumption this cycle perpetuates. In 2012, two years before my study started, American rapper Wiz Khalifa captured this American cultural ethos in a popular song called "Work Hard, Play Hard" about smoking good weed, drinking champagne, and having "so much money I should start a bank."[23] Chances are, James knew this song, which went double platinum, but Khalifa hardly invented the concept. As biologist Lonnie Anderson explained in a *Forbes* article in 2016, the "work hard, play hard manifesto has been around for a long time."[24] In his survey of fourteen hundred Canadian undergraduates, he found that one correlation stood out above all others: "an attraction to accomplishment and an attraction to leisure."

Nor has the appeal faded since then. According to a recent BBC article, "Leisure is the prize, right? We work hard, so we want to play hard."[25] In 2022, a popular television show called *Severance* debuted that *The Economist* described this way: "Imagine if your mind could be divided: surgically separated into two selves so that you might better 'work hard' and 'play hard.' That is the premise of this thrilling workplace dystopia."[26] But who needs surgery? A 2015 study among young people in New York City reported that misusing stimulants prescribed for ADHD helped them to work harder and quickly meet "cultural expectations of achievement and productivity," so that they still had time and energy for leisure and socializing.[27]

For young people, leisure and socializing often mean partying. To be seen as a good person by one's peers in young adulthood, and to attract a partner in an Instagram-captured social world, one must appear to be having fun. Having fun for the young people in my study often meant hanging out and using substances. In fact, 80 percent, without being prompted, talked about social substance use. One-third talked about using cannabis, nearly one-fourth talked about alcohol use, about one-fifth reported using methamphetamines, and another one-fifth reported misusing prescription amphetamines. A handful also reported using cocaine or heroin.[28]

This pattern is not that different from most young people in the United States. In 2019, over half of young adults (18 to 25) reported using alcohol, and one-third cannabis, in the past month.[29] Over half had used cannabis sometime in their life. LSD and cocaine use were less common, with around 10 percent of youths under 25 reporting any use. (I am skeptical that young people will answer questions accurately about illegal substance use on a survey administered by the federal government, so these numbers may underestimate reality.)[30] The data are clear, though: many young people are experimenting with and using substances.

Experimentation in general is a given in young adulthood.[31] Experimentation with recreational substances and alcohol, as James and Corrina found, can be fun and facilitate bonding between friends.[32] And, while playing hard begins when one is a young adult and hanging out with peers, it continues into young adulthood and the real world. Many American work-related events—dinners, office parties, happy hours, conferences—involve substance use. The successful social use of alcohol, at least, can be interpreted as an important signal of adulthood.

Note the phrase "successful social use." In the work hard, play hard ethos, young adults are supposed to learn how to have fun *without* overdoing it, getting in trouble, doing poorly in school, or becoming a burden on other people. You must be able to lose control without completely losing control. When I was a young adult in the early 2000s, people who were partying too hard would get "fired" by their friends, meaning they were becoming too much of a liability and had to be shamed into not behaving that way again. If you could not control yourself, your friends would stop hanging out with you.

In this way, substance use has become, paradoxically, both a way to gain moral agency and a way to lose it. You need to be able to use substances responsibly to earn access to the intimate relationships and the social bases of self-respect that come with them. If you overdo it, however, there are consequences—social shame, the loss of educational and vocational opportunities, and legal problems. This is a challenge for all young people, but as I found in my research, for those who are also struggling with emerging symptoms of psychosis and the at-times-amplifying effects of substance use and misuse on those symptoms, these expectations can be downright toxic.

· · ·

I first met Miranda at her parents' home—a large, ranch-style house on a half acre or so where the relentless urban sprawl thinned out and the Texas Blackland Prairie still thrived. Miranda was a pretty girl with shaggy bangs, thick glasses, and a bright smile. She had attended some vocational training and had an associate's degree in health care. Her white mother, Angela, had fought her way up the socioeconomic ladder with a graduate degree in health care. Her father, Roberto, was a first-generation Hispanic migrant with very little education but a strong mind for business. Miranda's parents were financially successful. They expected Miranda to work hard, go to college, have a good job, and start a family of her own. This would fulfill their own American dream—working hard to provide a better life for their children so their children could achieve even more.

When we met, Miranda had finished her degree at a local community college, but she was "taking a break" from work. She was living at home, smoking a lot of cannabis, playing video games, and watching Netflix. She kept detailed journals, enjoyed dancing to music, and tried to imagine her future. She worried: what was she going to do, who was going to love her, and was she attractive enough or smart enough to attract a partner? A lot of her friends from high school had finished college and were working and living independently. Some were even married. Miranda felt a little useless, even though she knew her experiences with an auto-immune disease and depression had slowed her down.

Then, totally out of the blue, a young man she knew in high school, Sean, started calling her and texting her. Miranda was so excited. She had had a crush on Sean when they were younger, but she never told him. But she kept missing his calls, and her phone kept erasing his texts after she read them. Her parents, she decided, must be tampering with her phone, intervening to keep them apart. Sean was white, Miranda self-identified as Hispanic. It was like *West Side Story*, she decided, or *Romeo and Juliet*.

Miranda started texting and calling Sean through Facebook at all hours, but he was not answering. Sean, thousands of miles away, was very confused and had blocked Miranda—whom he could hardly remember from high school—on Facebook messenger.

Angela said that one night Miranda came to her to announce that she was leaving. She needed to grow up, she insisted; her mother needed to let her go. She wanted to visit Sean. They were planning to get married. Her mother was confused. She had no idea who Sean was. How could she miss something so major, she wondered.

Angela later said Miranda was very defiant, saying, "'You don't want to let me go, and blah, blah, blah.' She says, 'I'm going to leave.'"

Angela just wanted the conflict to end. "I said, 'Honey, you can use the [family] van. The van's right there.' She wasn't really—at that time, she probably was manic, but I didn't recognize it. She actually started packing stuff in the van. She took the van and spent the night at my mother's house nearby. I felt good about that because I knew where she was. I didn't want her to just get in the van and leave."

Early the next morning, there was a great deal of confusion. Miranda's grandmother hid the keys to the van while Miranda was sleeping and locked the external garage where the van was parked to prevent her from sneaking off overnight.

However, Miranda *knew* that Sean was waiting for her in the garage, and she realized her grandmother also wanted to keep them apart. She desperately needed to be reunited with him, to run away with him in the van before their parents caught them. She texted and called Sean countless times. Her family, she was sure, must have rigged her phone, because she could not see his answers.

The next morning, without access to the garage, Miranda broke the metal door down. Her family thought her strength was bizarre.

"Superhuman," Roberto said.

Once she was in the garage, Miranda realized she did not have the van keys in her purse. She did, however, have a knife. She threatened her grandmother with it, demanding the keys.

Her grandmother locked herself in the house and called Angela and Roberto for help. Upon arrival, Roberto tried to get Miranda to calm down, and she punched him. She said they were keeping her from Sean. They were so confused: Who was this person? Where was he? Why was he messing with their daughter this way? They realized they had to call the police.

When they told her they had called the police, Miranda laid down on the ground. Her grandmother stayed in the house, and her parents hovered nearby in terror. Roberto was afraid she had stabbed herself. Then, Miranda startled him by sitting up and throwing her purse to him.

"I knew the cops were being called," she said later, "and somehow in my mind, I thought 'Okay, well I can't have a knife on me while the cops come.'" She also tossed him her sunglasses and her shoes. After that, Miranda laid down to wait.

"In my head," she explained later cheerfully, "I thought I was peaceful protesting."

Months later, Angela told me that she may have overprotected Miranda because she herself had a bad childhood. "We coddled them [her children] and everything, and maybe we were too overbearing, but they never had to deal with what I had to deal with. They are both grown now, and I think they are both trying to find their identity, and the step forward for life as an adult. I believe that when [Miranda] had that breakdown, she was kind of freaking out because she couldn't handle all the stuff that adults do."

Like James, Miranda blamed her own substance use. She said that earlier she had been dancing in her room when she was high, and "I don't know if people could see but I got paranoid, and that was probably a week or so before my psychotic break. I kept telling my mom, 'What if somebody's going to come into the house and murder me because they saw me dancing?'" She did not see anyone outside, but she sensed them there.

She said she initially used cannabis to reduce her stress level and treat her pain from her autoimmune disease while tapering off her antidepressant medication. She said her mom—a medical professional—knew about but initially overlooked her cannabis use.

"She doesn't mind; she thinks it's all right," Miranda told me. "I was taking marijuana. I was smoking; I was trying to increase my tolerance, decrease it I guess. I was slowing down on my usage, but it did make me paranoid [. . .] I don't know if it was the different strain."

"Maybe it was stronger?" I asked.

"Yeah, it was strong."

However, Miranda's friends did not experience paranoia, even though they were smoking the same strain. In fact, she explained, one friend who used cannabis, "she's Hispanic like I am, but she can handle stress pretty well. She's a medical assistant at [place-name omitted], so she's kind of an example for me to look up to."

So Miranda kept smoking cannabis to calm herself, but everything just kept getting worse. "I felt like I was planning like one of those Doomsday preppers people," she laughed later. "I was gathering up weapons. I had a canteen and a nice survival handbook I bought from Barnes and Noble."

Angela later said she would have taken Miranda to the hospital right away if she had had any clue as to what was about to happen. Angela was a health professional, but she and her husband "did not recognize this was a mental health issue. We just thought, 'Oh, she's trying to find herself.'" Miranda *was* trying to find herself, experimenting with love and substances in what seemed to her to be low-risk ways, but she was also having emerging symptoms of psychosis, which complicated everything.

. . .

The American social expectation that young adults can find themselves by working hard and playing hard was especially challenging for those in my study to navigate. Miranda, James, and Corrina all struggled to negotiate love, substance abuse, and early psychosis as they tried to make a smooth transition to adulthood. This ethos, put forth as the way for young Americans to reach valued adulthood, set them up to fail. There are several reasons for this common situation, and they all feed into one another.

First, establishing one's independence while working hard and playing hard is stressful. Many youths struggle with their mental health as they attempt to make a successful transition to adulthood, perhaps increasingly so, as the recent numbers about youth mental health suggest. But young adults with early psychosis also struggle with the additional burden of an exaggerated physiological response to stress that can include not just anxiety, panic, and disturbed sleep but also paranoia, hearing voices of people telling them what to do that no one else can hear, or seeing figures that no one else can see.[33] James said the psychosis and substances were "feeding [him] false truths—lies, really." Miranda was paranoid that people were watching and that her parents were tampering with her phone. She heard voices telling her that Sean was in the garage waiting for her. Corrina heard disruptive noises and then later thought that the world of angels and demons was relevant to her everyday life.

If these same people who are more sensitive to stress are leading stressful lives because of social conditions of marginalization or disadvantage or adverse social experiences, even low-level stressors can push them toward experiencing symptoms of psychosis. Beneath the surface of their stories, many of the young persons I worked with had experienced such stressful social conditions and adversities in their childhoods. Corrina, James, and Miranda all were children of immigrants, which seems to elevate one's risk for developing psychosis.[34] Some of the young adults we interviewed had experienced the death of a parent as a child or childhood sexual abuse or witnessed terrible acts of violence and so had significant adverse childhood experiences.

Any young person's ability to handle increased risk-taking behaviors and impulses in responsible and resilient ways is shaped by early life experiences. As anthropologist Carol Worthman has written, adolescence is "where the rubber meets the road as the strengths and vulnerabilities formed in development hit the demands of transitioning into adulthood."[35] For those young people who had lived through stressful conditions, were experiencing symptoms of psychosis, and were sensitive to stress, everyday social expectations that they work hard and play hard could push them to a breaking point.

Both Corrina and James had parents who wanted them to get back to work and school. They felt pressure to live up to their parents' expectations, and to their own. Miranda's parents, on the other hand, seemed to notice that she was not quite ready to be an adult, and they "coddled" her to some extent. She was not under a lot of pressure to go back to work or school when I met her. While all three had psychotic breaks, Miranda seemed to be doing the best of the three, at least when I first met them. I suspect this was in part because she was under the least amount of pressure at home to become independent—in fact, it was not clear that she had ever really tried.

In addition, many of the youths in my study were also trying to meet expectations that as young adults they should play hard. For many, this meant "party hard," and alcohol and cannabis were the substances the young people in my study most commonly used for fun, relaxation, and stress reduction. Miranda, James, and Corrina all used cannabis for exactly these reasons. Studies suggest that all young people living through unstable life transitions such as changes in living arrangements, academic expectations, or employment are developmentally and contextually likely to increase their use of alcohol and substance use at such times.[36] Substance use is also one way that persons from minoritized groups with early psychosis cope with trauma in their lives—historical and everyday trauma, as well as stress, anxiety and stigma.[37]

Some young people, on the other hand, tried to establish their independence with substances as a form of rebellion against cultural rules they thought were too restrictive. Mohammed, a Muslim from West Africa, told me: "Yeah, I took K2, marijuana, kush, corn. I don't want to take crack. I drank a lot, partied . . ."

"Why? Why did you do that?" the interviewer asked.

"Because pussy, money, weed. That was my motto."

Mohammed was trying to play by American cultural rules by breaking free from his parents and finding a sense of belonging in the world as a hip-hop artist. He used cannabis both to play hard and to rebel against his parents' Muslim cultural ideals of sobriety. But the cannabis use altered his personality, allowing a second self to emerge, Chrome, which was reminiscent of Corrina's angel self, Karina. As Chrome, he thought he was fearless, powerful, and independent and had the potential to be successful. Mohammed wanted to keep Chrome around, but he thought that required him to smoke cannabis.

Many Americans have come to see cannabis as not only acceptable but even medicinal. Miranda enjoyed smoking cannabis with her coworker, a health professional peer whom she admired. Her mom, also a health professional, thought it was fine even though cannabis use was—and remains—illegal in Texas. Miranda said she used cannabis to self-medicate for her autoimmune disease and depression. In the United States, understanding cannabis products as medicinal has made them seem less harmful and has led to more favorable youth and community attitudes toward use.[38] Some research suggests that for college students this acceptance has made it harder to refuse than to use when cannabis is on offer.[39]

Jeremy, an African American we interviewed, explained that he did not do "harder drugs" because he was "too scared of all that," but then noted, "Even marijuana can get scary. The paranoia that it gives is—on my end—crazy."

He continued, "I used to smoke every day, so . . . I mean, it just depends on the day. When I have pain, it'll take away some pain. [. . .] It might make me feel better at the moment, but then I go back to upset because it made me overthink."

These trends toward acceptance and wider use of cannabis as a medicine make it harder to understand that it can be both helpful and harmful for some people. Even though Miranda and Jeremy both seemed to know that cannabis was making them more paranoid, they still liked the way it worked on their other symptoms. And, while it is not widely culturally acknowledged or discussed, cannabis use does seem to be a risk factor for psychosis.[40] My own data and other research suggest that using cannabis may be a very bad idea for people who have a family history of psychosis, who may be developing psychosis, or who are experiencing psychosis.

To begin with, studies suggest that young people developing psychosis who try cannabis are more likely to develop a cannabis use disorder than their peers,[41] which means that their cannabis use is more likely to result in worsened performance at work and school and in interpersonal relationships because of misuse, overuse, and the fallout from overuse such as blackouts and accidents. Certainly, James thought that his cannabis use (among other things) was not helping him with his relationship with his girlfriend or with keeping his old friends.

In one study, more than half of Black youths with early psychosis also had a substance use disorder.[42] Multiple reasons likely account for this statistic. The percentage may be high because Black youths referred to treatment for psychosis are then also diagnosed with a substance use disorder after being overpoliced.[43] In addition, Black youths with early psychosis and a cannabis use disorder are more likely to report childhood and physical abuse than are those without cannabis use disorder.[44] Exposure to childhood traumatic events, a history of incarceration, and having dropped out of high school have also been shown to be associated with co-occurring alcohol and cannabis use disorders for all young people with early psychosis.[45] Local culture can also play a role. One study with primarily Black and Latino inner-city youths suggested that access to high-potency cannabis products can "become an important way of gaining status, prestige and popularity among peers."[46] At the same time, some studies suggest that for young people with early psychosis, using higher-potency cannabis more frequently worsens outcomes.[47]

Moreover, studies show that the misuse of cannabis (but not occasional use) can increase one's risk of developing psychosis in the first place.[48] In one study, cannabis misuse or dependence, especially for people with a family history of psychosis, predicted the onset of psychotic symptoms.[49] Another study found that young people who stopped using cannabis after a psychotic break stopped having psychotic episodes,[50] while individuals who continued using cannabis after psychosis onset experienced higher relapse rates, longer hospital admissions, and more severe positive symptoms than individuals who stopped using.[51]

Which came first—the chicken or the egg? The research on substance use and early psychosis specifically is limited, and interventions designed to prevent or support young people in reducing cannabis use are nascent. There is also almost no research on the interactions between "harder" drugs—LSD, cocaine, methamphetamines—and the individual experience of psychosis. With our current retrospective methods and studies, it is impossible to tease apart the exact relationship between cannabis, alcohol, social marginalization, and psychosis, but they do seem to feed into one another.

Some studies also suggest cannabis misuse might be linked to more violent and aggressive behaviors for people experiencing psychosis.[52] James said he was smoking cannabis laced with cocaine when he assaulted his girlfriend: Was it the cocaine, the cannabis, the psychosis, or just James not controlling his anger? It is hard to tell.

What we do know is that James went to community college, made new friends, had a romantic partner for the first time, and intensified his regular cannabis use to smoking marijuana at least twice a day. He progressed to regularly using LSD and smoking cocaine-laced joints. His girlfriend no longer wanted to be with him, but he kept using. He did not know how or when to quit.

Later, James felt that he had botched his own transition to adulthood:

> Sometimes I hold myself down. And even though I don't realize it, it's just a thing I have to accept [. . .] There's all these crossroads that you need to choose, and if you don't choose wisely, you'll go down, and then it's just messed up. But then, maybe other people, like your supporters, will help you. [. . .] Then you can try to go along with them. But even then, sometimes, my self is just like, "Maybe you just deserve to be in the mental institution." But I don't believe I'm mental. [. . .] Basically, the challenge is just to be more organized [. . .] Just seeing the right paths to take. Sometimes I don't, and I regret that I didn't take that path at that time . . . And then you're like, crap, I'm already too far. That's the crossroads.

A few weeks after this conversation, James found another crossroads. He was extremely high at the time—possibly on cannabis and LSD, but he could not recall exactly. He parked his car on the tracks at the railroad crossing to make sure the train would stop. The celebrities were on the train. They told him on Instagram that they were coming to take him to New York City and make him famous. They would meet him at a specific railroad crossing, but how would he stop the train? He decided the best way to stop it was to block it.

Luckily for him, James did not think it was important to stay in the car. He showed me pictures on his phone of a vehicle demolished beside some tracks. After this incident, James was arrested and hospitalized involuntarily for more than a month in the state hospital. When released, he refused further treatment. All his friends used alcohol and illegal substances, he said. Treatment meant sobriety and social isolation, and he really needed to get back to work and hang out with some friends.

James also thought that using cannabis and other substances would make him seem more attractive to the celebrities—and to his less famous friends. Miranda, Corrina, and many other young people in my study saw using cannabis recreationally as a conduit for securing the intimate relationships they needed to thrive. Using cannabis, in a receptive social context, could offer a source of the social bases of self-respect and peopled opportunities. It helped James and Corrina, and many others like them, secure intimate relationships with others. In the long run, though, cannabis misuse—and substance misuse more broadly—also amplified our interlocutors' loss of control over their lives. They began to lose the thread of the life narrative they wanted to promote, or their autobiographical power, as things started to go wrong.

Paradoxically, playing hard—probably for anyone but certainly for young people with early psychosis—can become a way not just to prove to others that one is a competent adult but also to lose others' confidence. Unfortunately, psychosis and substance misuse seem to fuel each other to synergistically compromise a person's moral agency. Who wanted to trust Corrina after she destroyed family memorabilia, or James after he parked his car in front of a train, or Miranda after she broke down her grandmother's garage door?

. . .

James, Miranda, Corrina, Mohammed, and so many others took steps to break away from their parents, to mark a departure from childhood, and to establish themselves as independent adults who could make their own decisions. They worked hard. They pursued higher education, found employment, and tried to live independently. They also played hard using recreational substances to separate themselves from their childhoods, connect with new friends and romantic partners, and have fun, all of which proved precarious for them. We might even say it set them up to fail.

These stories—and those of many other young people told in this book—suggest that navigating the work hard, play hard ethos of young adulthood in the United States can be perilous, particularly for young people who are also struggling with substance misuse, pressures to find their place in the world, and the underlying development of a psychotic disorder. All the young people I engaged with during my study experienced some combination of romantic failures, substance misuse, lost opportunities with school and employment, and lost relationships with family and friends. Emerging symptoms (and the adolescent brain) complicated decision making, which could complicate substance use and romantic decision making, which led to more isolation and loss. Nearly everyone mentioned having the sense that somewhere along the road they had lost their way.

Instead of offering support, American culture encourages young people to be independent and go out on their own with little guidance during a time when there are an overwhelming number of choices to make and when they are neurologically primed to take risks. This sets young people up to sink or swim. Those who learn to swim may thrive. Those who do not may find themselves drowning, especially since American culture in general provides few lifeguards.

We need to understand that young people are struggling with choosing roles, finding a path that is their own, working hard and playing hard in ways that will mark them as no longer children, pleasing those who are important to them, and navigating all of these challenges without the guidance that many other societies provide.[53] This American-style transition to adulthood is difficult for all but is especially so for those experiencing early psychosis. We need to understand how much it complicates their ability to become a moral agent in the broader culture, and why. We need to look at ways this passage to adulthood might be better supported for vulnerable youths living in this work hard, play hard social context.

The work hard, play hard mentality, and expectation that most young people will experiment with sex and substances to prove that they can become independent adults, is likely here to stay. The ways this experimentation plays out ruthlessly on social media are unlikely to change. The perception of cannabis as a panacea is also likely to remain because most people are not going to have a psychotic break after using it. However, by raising awareness of these cultural features, we can see more clearly the social context in which young people with early psychosis are trying to thrive, and we can better understand the pressures they are under and the consequences these pressures can have specifically for them. We can offer more sensitivity and guidance around this transition if we are paying attention. There may be entrenched American traditions around what young people need to go through to prove themselves as valued adults, but we can make a significant difference by better understanding how it makes some young people especially vulnerable so that we can develop stronger supports to promote a smoother rite of passage for all. While I offer thoughts in chapter 7 on how to develop these supports, in chapter 2, I explore how the young people in my study sought to explain and manage their psychosis-related symptoms as they emerged. It is my hope that further exploration can encourage compassion for and understanding of their remarkably challenging situation.

2

Into the Mythos

I thought the whole world was based on Greek mythology and I actually believed all this, and I was like, "Okay, that actually makes sense." Like I had memories from my childhood just coming up and I would connect my crazy thoughts to those. I was like, "Okay, that's why I had that moment in time with my family because we were actually Mary and Jesus or something like that," so I was just thinking, like, a lot of crazy stuff and it was, like, just completely disattached [sic] from reality.

—JAMES, STATE HOSPITAL, WEEK 3

As Amy walked along the narrow shoulder, the bridge vibrated. Cars and trucks zoomed below.

When I fly, they will know I am a superhero.

"Just try it!" the voices in her head were shouting. "You can fly!"

"It just popped into my head," Amy told me later. "I should jump off the bridge to see if it's real." Amy stood there, arms limp, staring down at the blur of traffic.

Can I fly?

Amy had shoulder-length copper hair and moss-green eyes. She self-identified as white. Her brother and sister, Robert and Addison, raised her after their parents died. Instead of finishing high school, she dropped out to take care of Robert's small children. She then worked hard in dead-end jobs, and when she ended up unemployed due to circumstances beyond her control, she wanted a fresh start. So she moved in with Addison's family in a different city until she saved up enough for her own place and found a new job.

However, the new job did not work out. During our early interviews, Amy shared that her new coworkers had been "zapping her in the chest," causing her chest pains. This had troubled her.

"Why would my coworkers want to harm me, right?" she asked me.

Unemployed again, Amy became very depressed. She had no car, no apartment, no friends, and no romantic prospects despite her so-called fresh start. After watching Amy lie around on the couch all day, Addison suggested Amy help watch her children. She had helped Robert, after all, and his kids loved her. Addison could use the savings on the cost of childcare to help cover Amy's room and board.

This arrangement worked for a little while. Amy was attentive and fun with the children, taking them to parks, teaching them about colors and numbers, and making sure they took their naps. However, things started to seem a little off. Amy sometimes said odd things about "brain zaps." When she had a panic attack after not being able to get a refill at the pharmacy, Addison suspected that Amy was misusing her ADHD medication.

Then, one evening, Amy barged into the children's room when Addison and her husband were reading them bedtime stories. She started screaming at Addison and her husband, demanding that they get out of the children's beds, accusing them of molesting their children. It was hard to calm Amy down.

Over the next few weeks, Addison and her husband tried to reassure Amy that they were not abusing the children during bedtime story reading, but Amy became increasingly agitated. She called the children's school nurse to demand that she check the children for sexual abuse. Child Protective Services opened an investigation. It was a nightmare.

Addison and her husband decided that Amy needed to move out. No one could afford a hotel, so they called around until they found a nice women's shelter with an open bed.

When they told Amy that they wanted her to stay at the shelter and look for a new place to live, she became violent. Amy later explained that she thought that if she left, her sister would poison her niece and nephew. She threw their plates and glasses against the wall, taking care to break them all so that the poison could not be administered.

"I didn't mean to be harmful to her or anything," Amy told me sheepishly; "it just happened that way."

Amy's siblings—people who loved her, who felt like her parents in the absence of their own, who wanted the best for her—now found her to be incomprehensible. They could imagine neither where Amy was coming from nor what motivated her to hurt them this way. Amy and her family had no shared sense of reality. Their common ground of familial love and trust—the taken-for-granted mutual moral understandings—were gone. Their shared sense that they were "good" people having a "good" relationship was breaking down. Sadly, this went both ways; Amy also thought her siblings were "bad" people.

. . .

Feminist philosopher Margaret Urban Walker writes that to live responsible and moral lives (whatever that means to us in our own social contexts), we must preserve "moral understandings" with people we want to be in relationships with, and to do so, a kind of story needs to be sustained among everyone. "We need to keep on keeping straight who we are," Walker writes, "and who we have given others to understand we are, in moral terms. We also need to sustain or refurbish our understanding of moral terms themselves, of what it means to talk about kindness, respect, friendship, or obligation."[1] These shared cultural notions of kindness and respect are the glue that binds moral agents together in relationships that matter to them.

In this instance, Amy's story about who she was in relation to others was not shaping up. She was losing her autobiographical power, or her reliability as a storyteller worth listening to. Everyone in Amy's family was caught up in a damaging vortex of toxic interactions, and their responsibilities to one another were collapsing. Amy thought her family should be taking care of her—and their other children. Amy's family thought she should be responsible for contributing to the family's well-being, not undermining it. Amy's ability to be responsive and responsible in ways that were meaningful to her loved ones was gone. Yet in Amy's mind she was being very responsible. In fact, she thought she was a superhero, sent to save her niece and nephew from sexual abuse.

Maybe if I show them I can fly, they will believe me, she would later consider, while standing on the bridge. *What if I can fly?*

When the symptoms of psychosis emerge, it becomes clear to others that a person is experiencing something that is wildly divergent from what most of the people around them perceive as reality. Some people call this nonconsensus reality. People perceive or interpret *consensus reality* together: it's something on which they can mutually agree. Nonconsensus reality is not shared with others.

In anthropologist Sue Estroff's seminal work on Americans with psychiatric disabilities, *Making It Crazy*, she wrote, "Most of what we know to be real is what we share with others."[2] In this case, Amy was outside that shared reality. As she lost consensus with others, Amy began experiencing a "moral breakdown," or the point at which her sense of reality was so incommensurable with others' that her own sister and brother could no longer understand her.[3] Her moral agency was at an all-time low. This was a breaking point.

The manifestation of psychosis is an unmooring enacted in relationship with others. Medical sociologist Essya Nabbali wrote, "With mad people, very specific behaviors transgress cultural mores and it is these behavioral disruptions which become their supposed impairment."[4] In other words, madness is a person's inability at times to share in consensus reality and behave according to the norms, expectations, and responsibilities assigned to them.

However, it's not just the perceptions of a nonconsensus reality that can make things so challenging. In some ways, it is the attempt to *make sense* of nonconsensus realities that can seem so odd. This is one of the terrifying loops of psychosis. Just when Amy thought she was saving the world, she was damaging that world by her actions. Her right to tell her story, to feel the glow of self-respect from the confirmation and support of Addison and Robert and the children, and the peopled opportunities that having these loving relationships created for a place to feel safe and loved, all were all diminished because she was trying to do what she perceived to be her responsibility and no one else agreed.

How do people who love and care about one another bridge the gap that non-consensus reality creates? To begin, it is important to understand as much as we can about where a person with psychosis is coming from, why they are acting as they are, and what their nonconsensus reality is. It is hard to guide someone back home when no one is using the same map.

From a clinical perspective, most psychiatrists would define Amy's anomalous sensory experiences as symptoms of an emerging psychotic disorder, which is exactly what happened when Amy went to Shady Elms. This is how she qualified for my study. Most of the young people I met were diagnosed initially with "psychosis not otherwise specified" (psychosis NOS), which meant that they had some signs of a psychotic disorder that had seriously disrupted activities in their everyday lives, such as their success in schooling and employment, but not enough time had elapsed to evaluate them thoroughly. A diagnosis of a psychotic disorder takes at least a month; Amy was diagnosed after a short stay in an emergency setting.

The diagnosis of psychosis NOS signaled to other clinicians that Amy was at least experiencing some positive symptoms of psychosis, or possibly both positive and negative symptoms. People are not usually diagnosed based on negative symptoms alone, though. Positive symptoms are conceived as something "extra" added to reality, like hearing voices that no one else hears or seeing things no one else can see. Negative symptoms are understood as signals that a person is lacking something, such as motivation or an ability to experience pleasure or to show emotions.

Many young people use substances recreationally, so the research team sometimes had to wait for substances to clear their systems before their clinician was willing to assign them a diagnosis of psychosis NOS instead of "substance-induced psychosis." Occasionally a young person was brought in a few times for what seemed to be substance-induced psychosis before they received the more formal diagnosis of psychosis NOS. Substance misuse sometimes leads to psychotic reactions, but clinicians thought that a person was unlikely to have a psychotic reaction multiple times in a row if there was not some underlying psychiatric disorder.

We also know a little about what can cause psychosis. Substances are not necessarily a direct cause. As mentioned in chapter 1, cannabis use may elevate the risk of developing psychosis in vulnerable people or lead to development of psychosis at a younger age than the person may have otherwise, but it is only one small piece of the architecture of risk.[5] Many other social factors also elevate risk, and most of them are related to stress. Adverse life events and cumulative social disadvantage raise a person's stress level and their risk of developing psychosis—a risk that seems to rise exponentially as those factors accumulate.[6]

Some people live with psychosis symptoms and do not seek psychiatric care: they are known as people with nonclinical psychosis or psychotic-like experiences. It could be that their lives are less stressful, or that they have better ways of managing stress or their symptoms than those who struggle and seek—or are forced into—clinical support. People who do not struggle with their symptoms also report having more positive experiences of voices and visions such as hearing Gods or angels—as opposed to negative voices like demons—and experience them less frequently.[7]

Others do struggle—and suffer.[8] Amy had persistent symptoms that severely disrupted her everyday life. Her zaps and voices made it hard for her to work, and her ideas about the world—that her sister and brother-in-law molested their children—completely isolated her from her family. She did not have any romantic partners or friends and was not employed or in school.

To better understand Amy's experiences, we can turn to several sources beyond the clinical literature. One includes the narratives of those who self-identify as persons with lived experience of psychosis. There are many: psychologist Gail Hornstein maintains a list of more than one thousand such narratives, dating back to the fifteenth century.[9] Another source is research led by people with lived experiences of psychosis, sometimes called service user research, survivor-led research, or user-survivor research.[10] People with lived experiences of psychosis bring their own experience to the table as they design studies and collect and analyze data in interdisciplinary ways.[11] Their perspectives can usefully complement and contradict clinical perspectives.[12]

Another resource consists of the results of studies like mine that involve researchers who have presumably not had experiences of psychosis. These studies ask persons who have had psychosis about their anomalous experiences in an intentionally respectful and empowering way. For my interlocutors, psychosis seemed to wash over them in a series of waves, at different rates and speeds, sometimes pushing or pulling in all kinds of directions—sometimes in a peaceful, lulling drift, but often moving them further from the shore of consensus reality. They felt as if they were being coaxed toward the breaking point. When you're playing in the waves, a breaking point occurs when you are knocked down, bowled over, and smothered by sandy water. In the case of a psychotic break, this is the point where you completely lose touch with reality. I think of the breaking point in psychosis as an inundation of perception when an overwhelming amount of sensory input becomes unmanageable. Once you are at the breaking point, if the waves are large, it can be hard to fight your way back to shore.

To demonstrate to my students how it might feel to be caught in the breaking point, I start by asking them what happens when they experience stress. For example, how do they feel when they must give a presentation to the class? We then discuss the inevitable answers—sweaty palms, accelerated heartbeat, dry mouth, a churning belly. Next, I ask: *What if your reaction to stress was to hear sounds or voices that other people cannot hear or see things other people cannot see?* Looks of concern all around.

After this, I have them listen to an audio track called the Hearing Voices Simulation, developed by clinical psychologist Patricia Deegan,[13] who herself hears distressing voices and has been diagnosed with schizophrenia. The audio begins gradually with random noises—scratching, bells, and voices speaking random words—"jerk . . . alert." It continues with "You smell" or "You're a piece of shit."

Next, we watch a YouTube clip of the television journalist Anderson Cooper listening to the same simulation.[14] He puts on headphones, plays the audio track (which lasts ninety minutes), and tries to do simple tasks like crossing the street and ordering coffee. He is quite distressed. Anderson also takes a battery of cognitive tests before listening to the simulation and then takes them again while listening to the simulation. His scores drop significantly when Deegan's soundtrack is playing.

This exercise offers my students a sense of how distracting and stressful psychotic symptoms can be. They are almost impossible to ignore. Some go home and try to do work or check their email while playing the voice simulation through their earbuds to see how it goes. I tried out this exercise personally in graduate school, though in my case I was listening to a tape on a Walkman. I found the experience disturbing. It was hard to order a coffee. Hard to cross the street. Hard to think my own thoughts. Impossible to have a coherent conversation. I have never met anyone who enjoyed the simulation.

Most students tell me that, after this experience, they became more empathic toward people who hear distressing voices. Some tell me they will never forget it. Others worry that this might happen to them. I cannot promise them that it will not.

How difficult would it be, I ask them, if this happened often and the voices were interactive and personalized—saying things that matched one's life in some way? Would they start to believe the voices or be compelled to act on their suggestions?

· · ·

Markus, a 21-year-old Black man, was clinically stable when the treatment team recommended him to my study, but it seemed he was still struggling with the waves of psychosis. Despite his confusion, Markus tried to help those around him see him as a good person, but his symptoms seemed to make interpersonal connection challenging.

INTERVIEWER: Tell me about your life's goals. What are your goals in the future?
    MARKUS: I want to be the best that I can be.
INTERVIEWER: That's great.
    MARKUS: I want to prove that I'm one of the best to do it. That's what I want to prove. I won't stop until I prove it. I won't stop till I prove—
    [Long silence.]

INTERVIEWER: How are you going to prove it? What are you going to do?

MARKUS: Keep working with the people I need to work with so that I can have my business at all times. Stay focused.

[Another long pause. Too long for the interviewer.]

INTERVIEWER: How are you doing, Markus?

MARKUS: I'm doing good.

INTERVIEWER: Yeah?

MARKUS: Mm-hmm. *[Affirmative.]*

INTERVIEWER: You seem like you're really distracted.

MARKUS: Little bit. Little bit.

INTERVIEWER: You are distracted, right?

MARKUS: Yup.

INTERVIEWER: Are you distracted by somebody outside [the glassed-in cube]?

MARKUS: Mm-hmm. *[Affirmative.]*

INTERVIEWER: Who is it?

MARKUS: Somebody who guides me.

INTERVIEWER: Somebody who—?

MARKUS: Somebody who guides me.

INTERVIEWER: Guides you? Yeah?

MARKUS: Yeah.

Markus tried to express himself in terms the interviewer could understand. He explained that he knew what he was supposed to do as a young adult—be the best, work cooperatively to have his business, stay focused. Yet Markus could barely pay attention to the interview because he was experiencing a hallucination that was both auditory and visual. The seasoned interviewer could tell it was not a good time and arranged to come back later. Markus's "guide" in the nonconsensus reality was compelling—so compelling that he brought it up to explain his confusion.

Psychologist Eleanor Longden described in her TED Talk how the voices drew her in slowly.[15] They started with seemingly benign, third-person observations about her, such as "She is opening the door." The voices were friendly and didn't worry her, until she told a friend, who was horrified, and Eleanor started to believe that something was seriously wrong with her. When she sought help, her general practitioner referred her to a psychiatrist who, in her perception, viewed everything she said "through a lens of latent insanity" and hospitalized her involuntarily. As Eleanor's fear of the voices grew, the voices turned into multiple, negative, persecutory voices that "were both my persecutors and my only perceived companions."

User- or survivor-led research, conducted by persons with lived experience of psychosis, claims that when people focus on listening to their voices, those voices often take on even more voice-like qualities, which can be overwhelming.[16] According to our consultant, psychologist Nev Jones, whose work is deeply informed by direct experience of mental health services and engagement with the user-survivor movement,[17] if someone experiencing psychosis thought that people at a cocktail party were talking about them (when they were not), the more they tried to listen, the more they would hear, and what they heard would become more disturbing and more specific. This psychosis-confirming thought loop is disorienting and dangerous. The Hearing Voices Simulation demonstrates how cognitively disorienting a soundtrack of random, nonpersonalized voices can be. What does one do when the voices become personal and interactive?

In one of his interviews with me, James, the young man introduced in chapter 1, described how paying attention to the voices made them seem more real. He told me that he heard two voices, a reality voice and an alternative reality voice. Both talked in James's voice (it sounded like him to him), but the alternative reality one was "the crazy one, telling me I'm Jesus." In contrast, the "reality voice" was "calming" and said things like, "'No, you're just normal. You're still not broken, yet. You're not slipping away too much.'" He also called the reality voice "just pretty much the voice of silence," whereas the alternative reality voice was "just thoughts always just running through my head. Constant thoughts."

"Just like a stream of consciousness?" I asked.

"Yeah," he responded, "like if you're reading a book, you're hearing that voice?"

"Sure," I nodded.

"Like your reading voice, so if you're thinking about something seriously, like consciously, you'll hear a voice, right? "

"Right," I said.

"But, for you, it's not like just like a voice that's just involuntarily going and going . . . So that's the worst part is that voice sounds believable, so we start believing it and since you're in that psychosis—you're already psychotic—so you just believe it anyways without a doubt because it's your mind, so you're like—you just believe your own mind, you know?"

"Right, well, yeah—who do you trust if not your own self?"

"Yeah, right! *It's your own mind.*"

James looked pleased that I understood, but I didn't really. I could never understand what it feels like to have an audible, negative voice persistently presenting me with a compelling alternative explanation for reality that no one else shared beyond the voice and me.

But voices and visions are only part of some people's experiences of psychosis. Some people had sensory experiences like being "zapped"—an experience Amy mentioned, as well. Jones and colleagues have written that participants in one of their studies of the phenomenology of early psychotic symptoms discussed their symptoms in "richly embodied ways."[18] These included sensations of anxiety that were not "in the mind," such as a feeling that one was being watched, followed, or "invaded." The entire body was involved in this "knowing"—not just the brain. One's entire neural network could be engaged.

Like Markus, Corinna also found it hard to attend to consensus reality when she experienced symptoms, and even her description was full of contradictions, which she recognized as she tried to describe them retrospectively:

> It feels like your brain is kind of like a puddle. Like it doesn't have any shape to it. It's an amoeba that's just floating around. This doesn't make sense [. . .] It just feels like there's too much going on, but not in the same sense where if you're in a room and there's a lot of noise. It's not the same. It's like a sensory thing, where you're sensing too much, not too much noise, but there's just too much of everything going on [. . . And] you're just so focused on what you're feeling, that you can't really focus on what's actually going on. And you're not feeling anything. I mean, there is anxiety with it, but it's not focused on anxiety, where if you had a panic attack or if you had anxiety, you'd know, like, "Okay, this is all about anxiety." This one, you can tell the anxiety is coming from it and also from the fear of, like, "Okay, what's about to happen? I don't know what's happening." So it's just spacey. It feels spacey and it feels like you're detaching, like you're being pulled away from what is really reality.

Corrina's retrospective description of her experiences makes a few things clear—the symptoms were compelling, they were overwhelming, and she felt that they pulled her away from "what is really reality." It became "too much."

Anthropologist Luke Kernan beautifully described his own experience of psychosis in terms of an intense, holistic way of knowing and being, calling it the "seduction of psychosis":

> The way it peels one's being to rawness, induces an electric excitement anguished by and of its overabundant sensory connectivity—the capacity itself starts with a subtle motion. The vibrancy of the world comes into attunement, onsets with a hypersensitivity that commissions the sensuous. *The way a flush of colors flock before the eyes—so blue its waters become palpable triples of an Australian rainfall, so green its glow reminds you of the emerald irises of your first kiss—those moments with all their affective rage sculpting the body.* These currents of non-normative consciousness flow inward, spark outward—to alter the grammar of what each sensory unit collects and, thereby, to render reality *as* otherwise.[19]

Kernan's sensory flooding was so intense as to become consuming, compelling, even appealing. And it made participation in consensus reality extremely challenging.

As mentioned earlier, Nev Jones and her colleagues and Eleanor Longden both argued that the more one pays attention to experiences of psychosis, the more compelling they become.[20] Psychosis thus confirms itself in a looping effect. The messages start off vague and amorphous—"you're being zapped"—and then gradually entice you a bit further in: Are your coworkers zapping you?

People who have experienced this looping tell me that the psychosis seems to have an agency of its own. It speaks to them and over time that speech becomes

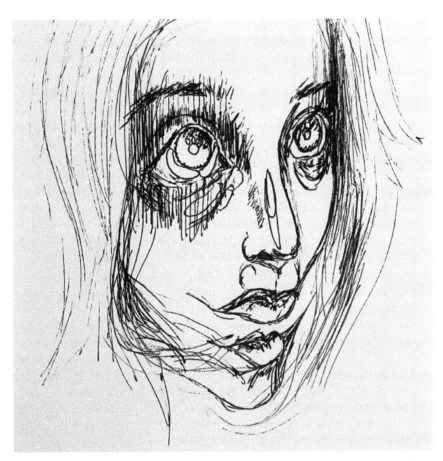

FIGURE 2. "Identity" by Lauren Ann Villarreal. In an email, the artist wrote to the author: "It's about how I fully lost my grip on my reality, myself. I felt like I was desperately trying to hold on to fragments of myself and trying to piece them together hoping I would look like myself again. This piece is also about trying to keep my eyes focused and open, because I felt like they were the only part of me that hadn't fully unraveled yet." *Reproduced with permission of the artist.*

more personalized. The loop, then, seems to follow this logic: the more you pay attention to your psychotic experiences, the more personalized they become; or the more you pay attention to psychosis, the more attention psychosis pays to you, almost like interacting with an artificial intelligence focused on strengthening your belief in an alternate, nonconsensus reality that is also always already your own.

It is difficult to know just how much control people with psychosis have over this cycle—whether, in some ways, they actively and deliberately engage in or perpetuate the loop. While many people think that psychotic symptoms are not within a person's control, our interlocutors felt that sometimes they were. And, according to the literature, this occasional control only made them feel worse—as if maybe they were more responsible for what had happened to them than others thought. Nev Jones and colleagues argue that this engagement can later lead people to feel shame as they question whether they had agentivally, actively "pushed themselves over the edge."[21]

Jones and colleagues' interview participants—young people who had experienced early psychosis—described having some agentival control over their symptoms. Sometimes, they claimed, they could ignore them and actively push them away or choose to engage with them further. Corrina mentioned something similar in her interviews.

"You can tell when it's coming," she said. "And sometimes you can fight it and sometimes you can't. Like sometimes I've been able to be like, 'Just ignore it. Focus on what you're doing and just don't think about it and it'll just go away on its own.'"

Overwhelmed by experiences that had no acceptable place in our culture but that looped around to confirm themselves as real when attended to, the young people we engaged tried to keep pace with these very real experiences that were not part of others' consensus realities. At the same time, they struggled to know, as Corinna and James asked, What is really reality?

When a person gets lost in this process of hyperreflexivity, they typically disengage from the shared common sense about what we can assume and how we can act that is typically the "taken-for-granted foundation of organized action and experience."[22] We can certainly see this happening for Markus, James, Amy, and Corrina. As their senses became overwhelmed, they had trouble connecting their very real psychotic experiences to others' shared everyday consensus realities. In addition, the more they paid attention to nonconsensus realities, the stronger the presence of those alternatives became. The more they looped, the deeper the groove became: the harder it was to find their way out of its rut. They were disengaging with the world and engaging more with their psychosis. As one friend who has experienced psychosis told me, "It was interacting with me, and I knew it was coming from me, but it was not me."

Social isolation only magnifies the experience. A clinical psychologist with lived experience of psychosis, Rufus May, reflected in a recent piece that "a magical child emerged from my psyche to protect me from the loss of roles and relationships."[23]

Sometimes, as with Markus when he was following something with his eyes beyond the glass, people can observe a person experiencing psychosis interacting with their nonconsensus reality—waving away spirits, punching a demon, trying to block incoming sonic assaults, whispering to someone no one else can see. These visible signals of psychosis can make other people feel uncomfortable. It is hard to watch someone struggle against something you cannot see. It is scary to see that someone is experiencing a perceptual field that you cannot access and that is so potent for them that they are responding to it physically. It is not always clear what this means for your relationship with them or even your personal safety.

Legal scholar Elyn Saks described her own strange bodily movements: "As I grew steadily more isolated, I began to mutter and gesticulate to myself, something

I had never done on my worst days. [. . .] When I heard the sounds I was making, I felt neither disturbed nor surprised; for some reason, it helped me feel calmer. It seemed to provide an arm's length distance between me and the people who were walking past me. Oddly, it was soothing, much like clutching a well-worn blanket."[24] Even so, making unusual movements with one's body that break cultural norms for adults contributes to social isolation.

As Corrina's psychosis strengthened its relationship with her, her social relationships with other people wilted. Or maybe it was vice versa: as others took a step back from her and her unusual behaviors, the psychosis replaced them. Corrina's social life in consensus reality was hard to maintain. She explained:

> It makes you really stressed, because at the same time, since you can't control it, it's like you don't want to be suddenly out of the conversation or be gone, but it's like you literally can't pull yourself out of it. And then you can't function. I wouldn't be able to sit here and talk to you guys. I would just kind of be like this, or listening, or just leaning back and trying to figure out what's going on, because I know that that's what happens. Like I usually withdraw. I can't be social. It's not that I don't want to. It's that—you can't.

This withdrawal also happened to James and Amy. Their symptoms isolated them. They became confused. The hallucinations and delusions reinforced one another. The more compelling the psychosis became, the stronger its pull became and the harder it was to escape. They actively withdrew from social life, trying to sort things out on their own.

Psychiatrist and anthropologist Ellen Corin and psychiatrist Gilles Lauzon characterized this behavior as "positive withdrawal," which they identified as a strategy their patients with long-term schizophrenia used to feel better.[25] For their patients, positive withdrawal created a buffer zone between their own inner, lived world and the world of others—a boundary that often blurred when they tried to engage fully and became overwhelmed with sensory input. Positive withdrawal helped them cope with and process sensory input at a distance, giving them time to form clearer ideas about what was real and not real, self and other, and thereby strengthen their sense of consensus reality before they tried to interact with anyone. Corin and Lauzon found their patients kept social interactions very brief and casual so as to enjoy human interaction but avoid rejection.

Corinna was quite withdrawn when she changed from Karina back to Corinna, having spent several weeks in her mother's home without visiting anyone. She made it clear that it was difficult for her to be alone, especially as a young person who was supposed to be finding her romantic partner, occupation, and urban tribe. Instead, she needed to stay away from people to avoid seeming strange, though her need to withdraw also made her stand out, resulting in further negative experiences and rejection.

"And then you feel awkward," she said, "because obviously you're the only person who really knows what's going on with you and everybody else is just going on with whatever they're doing. And then a few notice [. . .] you stand out 'cause something's wrong with you. [. . .] It feels like you've taken a drug, and you didn't, but you can't control it anymore [. . .] And then you get scared, 'cause you can't control it and you're just like, 'This sucks.'"

Corinna looked at me and gestured to all the things—my research assistant and me, my tape recorder, her mother, and her mother's dim living room, where she had spent the past several months afraid to leave the house.

"This sucks."

We all started laughing, laughing in that way that feels a little hysterical, a little like survival. A quote from Emily Saliers of the Indigo Girls crossed my mind: "You have to laugh at yourself because you'd cry your eyes out if you didn't."[26] I felt like crying, too.

Corrina continued: "But, yeah, you don't know how long it's gonna last; you can't necessarily control your body. You just can't function. Like you can't do anything really. All you can do is just sit there and try not to freak out."

She laughed again, but the rest of us did not.

"You have to laugh because it just sucks," she said. "That's why you have to laugh."

Young people like Corrina and James cannot afford to withdraw positively or otherwise. They are at a time in their lives when they are under pressure to make a successful transition to adulthood, when it is more important than ever for them to engage socially. They need to find their place, their people, their purpose, a sense of belonging. And they felt that they really were not supposed to be at home with their families. As Corrina said, being at home sucked.

So even as they experienced overwhelming sensory inputs and became more ashamed and isolated, they tried to make sense of their experiences alone so that they could reengage with the world. One strategy they used was to mobilize culturally available stories, or mythos, to make sense of their symptoms. As Rufus May wrote of his magical child that protected his psyche from the loss of roles and relationships: "To be immersed in a world of espionage and magical connections made me feel valued and gave me a sense of purpose."[27] Amy was a superhero. James was most often a celebrity but sometimes also Jesus. Markus had a guide. Corrina was an angel.

David was a prophet.

. . .

David, a tall, well-dressed African American youth with a bright smile and hipster glasses, strolled cheerfully around the airport terminal, wheeling his carry-on bag. He could not wait to see his mom. It had been a long time, and he wanted to tell her the good news: his head was booming with the voice of God.

"I am a prophet, and God loves you!" he told the cashier at a snack kiosk.

"God wants me to tell you that you are sinners and you need to repent!" he shouted into the air as he made a stop in the bathroom.

"God said to tell you that you will die soon," he told the young woman behind him on the boarding ramp.

She did not look up from her phone. David felt hurt.

"Did you hear me?" He asked her again.

She continued to ignore him.

"Hey!" he said. "You need to repent before you die! Why won't you listen to me?"

People around him were not sure what to do.

"God is telling me that you are all sinners!" he shouted in the middle of the jetway. "You are all going to burn in Hell for your sins! Repent!"

David's urgent call to evangelize was overwhelming him. Noticing that people looked uncomfortable, he attempted to calm himself. He wanted to get home to his mother, and to do that, he needed to be on this plane. He fiddled with his bag and tapped his feet, but he was fighting a great battle.

"Stop it! Stop it!"

Did I say that out loud?

The flight attendant looked at his ticket. She took his bag. "I am going to need to gate check that for you," she said and then reached for the phone.

David rolled his eyes and proceeded down the aisle. He tucked into his seat and closed his eyes to rest while God prattled on. He did not notice that no one else was boarding. He did not even notice the men approaching him.

"Are you okay, young man?" one of them asked. He showed him a badge.

David felt so irritated. Why were the police always hassling him?

"Oh, right, so why don't you just check my bag for a bomb already?" David shouted. "America is the land of the free. And I am free," he stood up, his anger overwhelming him, "to SPEAK in public!"

The officers acted so quickly, he was not sure what happened next, but he quickly found himself in the airport security office, handcuffed and waiting for his dad to come pick him up. Security had confiscated his suitcase and his phone.

When David's father arrived a few hours later, airport security released him. David did not have bombs or anything threatening in his bag. He seemed exhausted and disoriented but had been quiet after they took him off the plane.

David's father told security that he was sorry. He explained that David was having some mental problems, and the family was just trying to get him back to his mother in another state for a visit. They had not realized he was too unstable to fly.

On the way home, David tried to explain to his father what happened; they argued. David knew he was God's prophet. He refused to back down. His father needed to understand how important it was to repent.

His father was heartbroken. What had happened to his son? How could David believe that God had told him to behave in a way that would make him terribly unsafe, that drew the attention of the police, that got him arrested at the airport? David became so upset at his father's rejection of his prophetic skills that he tried to jump out of the car. His father knew something had to be done. He had to keep his son safe.

When he stopped for gas, David's father called 911 while David went to the bathroom. They told him to stay put. He pretended he could not find his wallet to pay for the gas until the police arrived to collect David from the gas station parking lot. A few days later, my team met up at Shady Elms, and he shared more about his experiences.

David described himself as "a military brat with divorced parents who suffers from low self-esteem." When he was 10 years old and his parents divorced, David stayed with his father, but it was hard not having his mother there. To cope, he started smoking cannabis when he was about 13, served some time in juvenile detention, and then tried methamphetamines around age 15.

"I simply got into weed by being a cool person," he said. "But I didn't know I was cool already."

By the time a member of my team interviewed David, he had been in and out of several court-ordered substance abuse rehabilitation programs. He had been homeless. He had been to college. A new church community he had recently joined had helped David get sober for a few months.

His father, David said, did not understand why he was a "bad kid," but David knew it was his father's fault. "The Bible says, 'A bad seed produces a bad seed. A dying tree is not going to produce good fruit,'" David said. "They [his parents] don't understand because they don't hear the same voice I hear."

David had been hearing God speak to him for about a year. "It's like having a positive conscience. I don't think about stealing, lying. [. . .] I know to listen to the voice because the Bible says, 'We are servants unto God before anything else.'"

David knew that he had been a liar and a thief and an addict because he had a rough childhood, but when he found God he felt transformed.

"I am a very mature young man," he thought.

He felt bad for everyone else because they were "mixed up because seeing something spiritually doesn't mean that somebody's crazy all the time."

David had no plans to take medication. He thought that taking medications would limit his ability to see Satan:

> I think it gives room for Satan to come because you cannot see him. I can now, but not a scary figure somewhere. I can see people's eyes change and stuff like that. I don't like talking about it because I know that people who do not believe what I can see because they can't see because the first thing they say is something like, "He needs to get his brain checked and be healthy." If they don't believe, they just don't believe. That's why I don't like to talk about it with people. Even my dad, who is a Christian, does not believe me, and it hurts. If I was a preacher or a prophet or if I was walking on water like Jesus, then everybody would be like, "Okay!" Some people would be like, "Oh, he's doing magic or something."

To avoid staying in the hospital again, David said, he would handle his dad differently, maybe not try to tell so many strangers about his gift of prophesy, and "maybe then [my dad] will see that there's something special in me."

David felt strongly that he was on a mission. "I'm just a man on the road destined to become a preacher, which is harder living spiritually." He sighed. "My family just doesn't understand the spiritual change that I'm going through. That's it."

David very much wanted to impress the judge who was going to rule on whether he could leave the hospital, which meant he had to prove he was no longer a danger to himself or others. He wanted to be released because, "that way, they won't keep moving me towards mental illness because that's depressing enough."

When asked if he had anything to add, David said he wished he could walk on water. "If I was to do that, the whole spiritual thing would go crazy. People would want to come see me." Even so, he added, "I think I can go far. There are famous people across the world who do things for God. They can heal people." David wanted very much to be a healer.

. . .

Many people with psychosis talk about supernatural content, and "hyperreligiosity" is on the list of "positive" symptoms of psychosis. One study found that 39 percent of people with a psychotic disorder discussed spiritual concerns with their clinicians.[28] I suspect the percentage of people experiencing spiritual concerns is even higher, since many may have already learned not to discuss their angels and demons with their clinicians or did not feel invited to do so in the first place. As a philosopher with lived experience of psychosis, Wouter Kusters writes that madness is "the socially awkward expression of a desire for infinity in a world that defines itself as finite. . . . The mad world abounds with Jesus characters, Mary visitations, revelations, prophecies, Gods and demons."[29] People need their psychotic experiences—which are real to them—to make sense, to matter.

Kusters, who has experienced two psychotic episodes in the past twenty years, argues that mad experiences are often philosophically and medically ascribed to the "mentally defective" and so treated as "out of bounds as a nadir of meaninglessness." Kusters thinks that nothing could be further from the truth. Instead, he argues, mad people have been "seized by themes of vital importance" that also "animate the ideas of philosophers, mystics, poets, shamans, absurdists, magical realists, and many others."[30]

This struck me as true for the young people I engaged, as well. Their thoughts were animated by a sense of great importance for themselves and others. Some had destroyed their lives as they knew them based on that conviction. Sascha DuBrul, a person with lived experience of psychosis, recalled his reaction when he could not make sense of his own experiences of psychosis: "I started reading too much meaning into everything. . . . Whatever was going on, it was obvious I was the only one who could see it because no one knew what the hell I was talking about!"[31]

This effort to make sense of nonconsensual reality was confusing, exhausting, and self-defeating. Young people lost moral agency by trying to tell other people about their experiences. Then, they attempted to replenish their moral agency by trying to take on a role that others might see as significant, such as a superhero, angel, prophet, or Jesus. If others did not agree, young people typically tried harder to convince others that their spiritual explanations were real, which only diminished their moral agency.

In their article on experiences of people with psychosis whose interviews highlighted spiritual content, Nev Jones, Timothy Kelly, and Mona Shattell explored how individuals used culture and at times religion to describe, interpret, and make matter the "raw" psychotic alterations of perception and cognition.[32] They asked people to describe what had happened to them since they had begun experiencing unusual mental events. One of their interlocutors, Levi, a secular Jew, told them that he had made sense of his psychotic experiences through Christian discourses. When he posted his experiences on Christian social media and websites, he received validation from other Christians using those sites. Thus, Levi was able to mobilize Christian dogma to successfully translate his otherwise inexplicable—and often pathologized—experiences into events that were instead "consistent with what's been going on in Christianity for millennia," even though, as a secular Jew, he did not believe those events were true.[33] This "double bookkeeping" empowered him to make sense of his unusual mental events in an online community with others where the stakes were perhaps lower than among his everyday friends and family.[34]

Anthropologist Tanya Luhrmann argues that religion and spirituality constitute "cultural invitations" that can open the door to alternative interpretations of anomalous experiences.[35] A person can choose to accept or ignore these invitations. Using Jones, Kelly, and Shattell's example, we could say that Levi had tapped into Christian America's cultural invitation to engage in a realm of happenings that is neither purely imaginary (there is at least a historical Jesus) nor part of everyday consensus reality. By the time Levi was interviewed for Jones and colleagues' study he was living well in the world and had a mythos that worked for him. He had successfully used culturally available invitations from the mythical realm of spirits, Gods, and heroes to make sense of experiences that would otherwise be thought of as signs of mental illness.

David had also tried to use the local cultural mythos, albeit not as successfully. As a Black American, David had no doubt received numerous cultural invitations to seek out and verbalize religious experiences. According to the Pew Research Center, Black and Latino Americans nationwide are more likely than white adults—Black even more so than Latino—to say religion is important in their life, to attend religious services, to pray at least daily, to participate in religious education, to meditate, to feel spiritual peace, to read and interpret scripture, and to believe in Heaven and Hell.[36] Thus, Black and Latino Americans are likely to live in social contexts that offer many cultural invitations to use religion or other culturally available mythos to explain events in everyday life. One fine arts scholar, Charles Rhodes, for example, has found that self-taught African American artists often have "visionary experiences" and that "mystical or metaphysical explanations" are common in their descriptions of creative inspiration and methods, most often the Christian God or "some spiritual presence or force directing things."[37]

Corrina talked about how her own cultural spiritual experience could amplify her paranoia or be soothing in one of her later interviews:

> [T]hat was kind of like the bridge that gapped me being paranoid to me just accepting now that life isn't out to get you. I spun it into something that was positive where it's like, okay, that's God trying to communicate with you, but not literally where you're hearing the voice of God but just that's a connection with some kind of spirituality trying to reach out to you. [. . .] At the same time it's like you have to either try and stay in reality or culturally spiritual. Where, you know, Hispanic people are spiritual, and they believe in stuff like that. So, if I'm gonna believe in stuff like that, I have to stay within the confines of that, and know that—okay, according to this culture and this religion in particular you can claim that you have power over the demons or whatever [. . .] you can also talk yourself out of it if you do get afraid. [. . .] I usually don't get to that point. I usually stay within the stereotypical Hispanic way of seeing it: it's like you can just pray and you'll be okay.

Furthermore, David, as well as the others we engaged, lived in a religious part of the United States. Most Black and Latino persons in Texas report being Christians.[38] Perhaps this is one reason why four out of five young people in my study, most of whom were nonwhite, offered my team spiritual or religious explanations around the time of their hospitalization, even though we did not ask them explicitly about religious experiences. By "spiritual" or "religious," I mean their explanation for their experiences relied on the presence of God, Satan, angels, demons, or the like.

Thinking of themselves as superheroes—secular or religious—helped young people preserve their moral agency at a moment when many other elements of their lives were in upheaval. David's father may have been sending him to his mother's house in another state for better care and psychiatric evaluation, but David knew he was "God's prophet" called to save the world. Amy's family was sending her to a women's shelter, but Amy knew she was really a superhero who could fly. They both developed a way to make sense of what was happening to them at a time when no one else was providing an answer.

Psychologist Jerome Bruner proposed that different cultural contexts offer narrative-based "cultural toolkits" for making sense of the events of everyday life.[39] The Western cultural toolkit, he argued, often falls woefully short when used to examine unusual mental events not detectable, measurable, or trackable with the tools of science. As Corrina said, "On the flip side of it, I'm white in this American culture, and we live in 2014 where it's, like, you kind of can separate—I don't want to say it's not real, but you can tell yourself that's a–you can't see it, you can't measure it, it's not empirical at all." So how to make meaning of experiences like religion, spirituality, and psychosis?

Luke Kernan claims that when there are no cultural containers for experiences of psychosis, a person begins to move away from consensus reality and create alternate realities in their own mind.[40] Psychiatrist Hans Prinzhorn collected the art of persons who had never been trained in artistic methods but began to make art during a period of unmedicated psychosis. One fine arts scholar has argued that the resulting Prinzhorn Collection "boasts a large number of creators who produced highly individual, alternative world-systems and paranoid 'autobiographies' that are often highly sophisticated," such as in the works of Joseph Grebing (1879–1940) and Jacob Mohr (1884–1940).[41]

The youths we interviewed also mobilized culturally recognized mythos, or common recurring narrative themes or plot structures from their own local moral worlds, to relocate their diminishing sense of self in some shared moral understanding or "common sense." This helped them create a sense of belonging, and—while often having the opposite result—signaled their effort to reestablish a sense of trust between themselves and others. Using a cultural mythos as a container for their experiences demonstrated that they were serving a spiritual or heroic purpose, which they hoped might help restore moral understandings about their responsibility and trustworthiness with their loved ones.

But this strategy for restoring moral agency rarely resonated with their loved ones ensconced in consensus reality. Rather, it crystallized others' sense, and typically served as clinical evidence, that the person had indeed made a complete break with consensus reality, that is, experienced a psychotic break. At the time, Corrina, Amy, and David could not understand why their loved ones did not admire their supernatural identities. When their narratives were not validated, things could get dangerous. Corrina destroyed family memorabilia. James parked his car in front of a train. David was arrested in the airport. Amy nearly jumped off a bridge.

User-survivor Sascha DuBrul explained how he used the mythic realm as a coping mechanism for feeling that life has meaning: "It's my protective shell." However, he also pointed out its precarity: "The shaman swims in the waters the schizophrenic drowns in," he wrote in a memoir.[42] When the waves of psychosis pulled him out too far, "I stop being able to tell what's me and what's everyone else. I start thinking I'm the entire universe—the center of everything. It's so beautiful and glorious until it turns really ugly." It "turns really ugly" when instead of being accepted, the person becomes increasingly isolated by the synergies between their nonconsensus realities and psychosis symptoms.

· · ·

So, what if we had a better cultural toolkit, and instead of discrediting people, we used the mythos that was meaningful for them to help support them in crafting a

cultural container that could help them "make sense" of their nonconsensus realities while not discrediting them and this excluding them further from consensus
reality? Scattered through the literature about psychosis and psychosis-like experiences are several examples of such options.

In South India, where World Health Organization studies across 30 years found
the highest rates of social recovery from schizophrenia,[43] Corin, Rangaswami
Thara, and Ramachandran Padmavati found that explaining psychotic symptoms
was less important for patients and their families than "a more fundamental quest
for meaning."[44] They argued that as patients' symptoms came to a head, all concerned were looking for significance in the experience rather than worrying about
the label. Meanings around psychotic symptoms were often highly personal but
were also often driven by religious signifiers. The flexible use of religious frames
helped patients and families in this context shift an alienating experience into a
larger, shared frame of reference that transcended the individual by providing
"stable reference points" that they could share with others.[45] This not only "gave
direction to people's lives" but also helped them find a shared ethical quality in
the experience.

For example, one man in Corin and colleagues' study (known only as S2 in
their article) had a vision that a man who looked like Moses was near him when
he was attacked by a bright light. S2 thought his suffering might be due to his lack
of a similar bright light, and he realized that he was being invited by his visions
to find one. He thought, I might be "a special person, a saint or something like
that."[46] He thus began a deeper inquiry into the meaning of his existence. When
he shared his experiences with his family, instead of questioning him, his father
introduced him to a religious person who became his confidant and adviser.
When necessary, S2 withdrew and slept more, so that he could think less and
was allowed to do so. The support of his family and the use of culturally salient
religious explanations and support from religious leaders had a kind of "reintegra-
tive potential" while also creating a kind of "protective web" around him.[47] Religious frames helped, and the chosen mythos worked in this situation—thanks,
at least in part, to the support of intimate others such as family and respected
religious healers.

Another example of a cultural container that seems to help persons with experiences of psychosis symptoms comes from Vilundlela, a low-resource, rural Zulu
area in KwaZulu-Natal, South Africa. Here, people diagnosed with psychosis, even
by biomedical practitioners, are sent to train as traditional healers.[48] In this context, unusual perceptual experiences over which sufferers had little control, such as
the distressing voices found in early psychosis, are sometimes thought to represent
a call by one's ancestors to become a traditional healer. For those with this calling,
special training to become a traditional healer is the only cure. This training, called
ukuthwasa, is offered by a female "mother guide." The training involves using traditional medicines (which have as yet not been researched pharmacologically),
as well as lessons and rituals (dancing, drumming) that connect one's unusual

perceptions to the presence of one's ancestors and train one in how to control those perceptions.

Ukuthwasa is regarded as a cure, and initiates anticipate a full recovery and a future social role as a traditional healer. Thus, in this social context, psychosis symptoms become a gift that only increases one's value as a moral agent in a place where those symptoms can be channeled culturally into a life-affirming, socially integrated, and financially lucrative social role. Research suggests that this tradition works for most people: even those who met criteria for a psychotic disorder were able to work as healers and manage their psychotic symptoms in this supportive social context.

Egan Bidois, a Maori healer from New Zealand who was diagnosed with psychosis, argues that interacting with "non-apparent stimuli" is a key feature of traditional healers in his culture—a skill that is passed down through families and must be managed properly for a person to be well.[49] Bidois manages these anomalous experiences by seeing them as normal and understanding the rules, rituals, and methods that his culture employs to maintain wellness and safety within that experience. He thus works as a mental health counselor and a healer who can cleanse or bless houses and facilitate healing and recovery from spiritual and physical ailments. "That is the role. The function. . . . It is through understanding and accepting that role that strength is provided . . . and I feel much comfort."[50]

Mad activist Sascha DuBrul designed a kind of cultural container in the United States. He and his friends started the Icarus Project (using the myth of Icarus, who perished after flying too close to the sun), a radical mental health community that promoted face-to-face networks and online spaces for connection.[51] The group also offered "superhero training" to help one another manage what they call the "dangerous gifts" of madness.[52] Some advice was quite simple, such as limiting cannabis use. Other recommendations were more complex, such as tracking potential warning signs like not getting enough sleep that can signal the approach of unusual sensory episodes; or devising a plan when you are well to help yourself manage symptoms when you are not. Some members of the Icarus Project (now the Fireweed Collective) were committed to avoiding psychiatric medication, while others believed that medications were helpful. Fundamentally, though, the Icarus Project mobilized mutual support groups of people experiencing madness who were willing to help and hold one another accountable.[53]

Another recent suggestion from the United States is that clairaudients, or psychics who use voices they hear in their heads to give readings—voices they typically attribute to the dead—are comparable to persons with psychosis. One study compared four groups that included both clairaudients who were not receiving treatment for psychosis and persons who heard voices and were receiving treatment for psychosis.[54] The study found that the two groups were similar in terms of what they experienced phenomenologically and in their performance on psychometric tests. The difference, psychiatric researchers Albert Powers, Megan Kelley, and Philip Corlett argued, was that for psychics the voices were friendly, could be controlled, and were seen as a gift rather than a burden. In addition, the psychic group's voices seemed to start at a younger age than among the group receiving treatment. In addition, the psychic voice hearers also generally had a positive experience of telling others about their voices—unlike so many in my study. Psychic voice hearers also tended to be less religious and so were not inclined to think they were hearing gods, which may have protected them from developing a more grandiose sense of their purpose. It is striking to me that they were also using the voice-hearing experience as a source of income when they offered psychic "readings" to others for money. At least one person in the study was even becoming a licensed counselor. It does seem that finding a real purpose for the voices is therapeutic. More research is being done in this area as well.

Overall, cultural toolkits can offer a person a sense of meaning, a chance to think positively and value their voice-hearing experience (even if the experience itself was negative), positive connections to others who either share in or value that experience, training in how to manage their experience, and at times the ability to earn income by using their experience. Most young Americans likely don't have these types of cultural toolkits available to them, though, and so they try to make their own mythical meaning without any rituals, training, wise and experienced guides, structure, or mutual support communities. It is then that one's personal mythos—an attempt to exercise autobiographical power and replenish moral agency—can become toxic and isolating. At this point, as Jones, Kelly, Kernan, Kusters, and DuBrul have all warned, psychosis starts to take on its own agency and push people toward more pathological behaviors, as the mythos reinforces socially impairing ideas. Without a cultural container of shared meanings, exercising autobiographical power—in this case, around supernatural explanations—leads people away from the social bases of self-respect and peopled opportunities that they so desperately need to thrive.

Cultural containers help channel the transformative potential of psychosis. When these meaning-making practices lack shared understandings and norms, what could be transformative is instead detrimental to one's relationships. As Margaret Urban Walker wrote, "Lack of shared normative ground means that our expectations are not aligned . . . what you expect from me may no longer be what I expect from myself. . . . In this state of affairs, trust is impossible or is destined to be disappointed."[55]

At a breaking point, a person with psychosis has such depleted moral agency that they may not even be able to connect with their own mother. Unlike the Indian father in Corin and colleagues' study who helped his son make meaning with religious signifiers and social support and so turned a breaking point into a turning point, most young Americans lack such an option. The American spiritual teacher and Franciscan priest Father Richard Rohr wrote, "If we don't learn to mythologize our lives, inevitably we will pathologize them."[56] The youths in my study seemed to mythologize in order to belong, but instead became increasingly isolated. As psychologist Rufus May observed of his own experience, "People's wariness toward me seems associated with a fear and suspicion, often prevalent in [Western] culture, toward mental confusion and distress . . . some of my friends were too scared to visit me during hospitalizations."[57]

Psychologist Stanislov Grof once suggested that a mental health crisis may be seen alternatively as an opportunity to "emerge," or rise to a higher level of physical and spiritual awareness.[58] Some social contexts around the world seem to encourage just this conception for some people who are having psychotic symptoms. As psychiatrist R. D. Laing argued, it may be about more than just the mental breakdown; madness may also signal a mental breakthrough.[59] Put a little differently, and more agentivally, we might see it as a turning point—an idea discussed further throughout the book, especially in chapter 7.

In countries dominated by Western psychiatric approaches, though, many accounts of psychotic symptoms focus on what has been lost—sanity, common ground, consensus reality, shared understandings, trust, responsibility, safety, employment, admiration—the list goes on. Perhaps the loss would not be so traumatic, and the wave of psychosis not overwhelm one quite so much, if we worked with people earlier on to prevent those losses, focus on the positive, and offer cultural toolkits and containers that empowered them to reorient to consensus reality with others rather than struggling alone. As Corrina, James, David, Markus, and Amy have taught us, it is when people get scared and isolated that the real difficulties begin.

We know that early symptoms of psychosis are both surreal and compelling. In the absence of support, they leave a young person feeling self-absorbed, confused, and distracted. They flood the senses with unusual information and unmoor the person from consensus reality. They are self-confirming and disorienting. They create internal loops of ideas and experiences that are both impossible to ignore and difficult to share with others in the absence of culturally meaningful ways to interpret them. This leaves young people with a deep sense of self-consciousness. All of this happens at an age when people are painfully aware of how others perceive them and when they are constantly comparing themselves to their peers.

These experiences strain the moral relationships between young people and their loved ones. Stepping further into nonconsensus reality damages trust between a young person and others. The families of Amy, David, Markus, James, and Corrina were not sure when—or if—they could trust them to be reliable and responsible, which eroded their status as moral agents. But is it possible that early interventions that build on locally available mythos could make a difference if people were trained in culturally meaningful ways to help? Opportunities to intervene can be lost if young persons stop trusting others, stop sharing their experiences, and withdraw further into their psychosis.

Unfortunately, what young Americans with anomalous experiences are offered next are not cultural toolkits for self-understanding and mutual connection, but instead police intervention, hospitalization, and forced entry into a fragmented and inadequate mental health care system (a not-so-accurate label[60])—which does little to help anyone restore moral agency and social belonging. This is the topic of the following chapter.

3
_____

Dangerous

They want to wait for something to happen, not like proactive. Maybe some-thing happens and then you have to bring him back to the hospital; then we can try whatever [the psychiatrist] said, some acute care or something.

—MALA (JAMES'S MOTHER), PHONE INTERVIEW, WEEK 12

Michael and his family came to the United States from West Africa when he was young. His family felt welcome in the large African immigrant community in North Texas. In high school, Michael was a star basketball player. "Everyone loved everything I posted on Facebook," he recalled wistfully. After graduation, Michael enrolled in community college to save money on tuition and housing and began studying to be a medical professional. Life seemed good. However, behind closed doors, things started to unravel.

His older sister, Liza, noticed that Michael seemed a little off during his senior year of high school. For example, when she came home from college for Christmas, Michael had stopped shaving. It seemed a small thing, but for her it was a red flag. "He always shaved. He was always [well] dressed. So I was like—he wasn't dressed?"

While visiting home again the following summer, Liza noticed a change in his speech patterns and focus on school. He kept changing his mind about what he wanted to study, but, she explained, "I thought—well, I didn't know what I wanted to do. So he doesn't know what he wants to do! But then, I noticed more when he'd talk to me—it wasn't a structured talk. It was like, he'll talk, and he'll go from one subject to the next subject, and then he won't remember what the last subject was."

Around this time, Michael began spending more time alone in his room. He also started smoking a lot of cannabis. He had smoked recreationally before, but Liza thought this seemed different.

"It was like this whole bunch of things on his mind that he couldn't really get out. He won't talk to anybody, but there's so much stuff that it was . . . a lot to understand. Conversation was hard to follow because it was so much . . . We didn't think it was . . . Nobody in our family we know has . . ."

Liza's voice kept trailing off. She could not even say it: no one in their family had mental illness.

Michael started community college but dropped out after his first semester. He began a job and then quit. Everyone was concerned, but his mom especially so. She valued educational achievement. She kept asking Michael what his reason was for not going back to college, but he did not have one.

"It made [Mom] really sad . . . ," Liza said, "like, depressed, because she didn't know how to help him."

As one year in his room doing nothing turned into two and then three, Liza said the family witnessed a real deterioration in his condition. Liza felt that Michael had been isolated for too long. She explained:

> I know the last year was the worst. The first two years were just, like, you know, but the last year was just the worst. You're isolated for so long, you have twenty-four hours a day to think about just, like, you're—it's not safe to be alone with your thoughts twenty-four hours a day. It's, it's just not safe or healthy [. . .] when you have that much time, you overthink something, and it's really, really unhealthy for you and your mind, and, like, I feel like, for your heart. I feel like your soul and everything, just, not physically, but spiritually, too . . . 'Cause he thought that we were, like, poisoning him."

Michael stayed in his room for the better part of three years. He stopped eating much. "Every day," Liza said, "without fail, [Mom] would go to his room, bring him food, and like make sure that he was eating and that . . . It was just really sad; you just didn't know what to do. Like you didn't even know what was wrong." She continued:

> He got really skinny. He would self-diagnose himself and say he was allergic to this and that. My mom was like, "I've been feeding you like this since you were little. Like, the doctors would've . . . something would have happened to you, if you were allergic to this, when you were little. You're 20 years now, and how did you all of a sudden become allergic to milk?" She's like, "That's what I'm not understanding: why would your own mom poison you?" And Michael thought we were just, like, believing in the devil and stuff.

Michael later said: "I would think my family was trying to kill me, and they were like devil worshippers, and people could read my mind. I don't know. I was thinking I was Jesus. I don't know."

His family felt helpless.

"A lot of the things he did," Liza said, "like unpredictable behaviors, like, feeling . . . we're possessed with the devil, or we're poisoning him, all these really off-the-wall thoughts . . ."

Liza struggled to get the words out. No one offered a lot of detail about what came next, but his family eventually called the police when Michael hit a breaking point and tried to attack Liza's toddler. He thought she was a demon.

. . .

Many families and young persons facing early psychosis do not seek mental health care except as a last resort. Researchers call this "delayed help seeking." Delayed help seeking occurs in many conditions, including cancer, pregnancy, and diabetes, and is caused by many different factors. But in terms of mental health help-seeking delays, one main factor is that the family does not know much about mental illness or that it terrifies them to consider it. Michael's sister, Liza, could not even say the words—psychosis, schizophrenia (his eventual diagnosis), mental illness—even though Michael and the family had been struggling with it for years. Studies suggest that for Black youths, the average period between the onset of psychotic symptoms and treatment is nearly a year and a half.[1] For Michael, it sounded like at least three years.

As part of our research project, my team also conducted interviews with thirteen mental health providers in North Texas who both identified as and worked with individuals from ethnoracially minoritized groups to ask them what helped or hindered people in seeking mental health care. The groups discussed were most commonly African American, Black African, and Hispanic-identifying persons, and one of the providers also talked about the Asian community. Nearly all thought persons from these minoritized groups lacked both knowledge specifically about mental health and mental illness and resources to support mental health.

"I think education is the first step. I don't think it's the only step," one provider said. "I think what's really difficult when it comes to mental health is trying to change the culture. One, you have to speak up about it. Two, you have to educate people about it. And, three, you have to be willing to stand up and have these really tough conversations."

Another provider described a cultural context in which people clearly understood that if they had a "physical thing," then you "see a doctor that can touch you and see what's going on and you can get an X-ray . . . When it comes to mental health, you're just like, 'Oh, just change your thinking and everyone will be okay.' Or, 'Pray more and it's going to be okay.'"

Most of the families I worked with offered some plausible explanation for the young person's behavior that had little to do with psychosis. Amy's family thought she was abusing her ADHD medications. David's father and Michael's sister thought it might be substance use. James's mom thought he had a broken heart. Mental illness is not something people think of first, in part because of the societal stigma against it in the United States, a stigma that affects both family members and the young person in need of help.[2]

In general, widespread stigma discourages people from seeking care and presents mental illness in a negative light.[3] This may be especially true for persons from ethnoracially minoritized groups. Nearly all the providers my team interviewed mentioned their concerns about stigma in the groups they served. Research supports this pattern. Persons who identify as Black, Asian, or Latino are more likely than whites to express higher levels of stigma against persons with mental illnesses.[4] This makes sense: a person with an already-diminished sense of moral agency as a member of a minoritized group begins with less capacity and fewer resources to manage the threat to moral agency that mental illness presents for the young person and their family. Black, Asian, and Latino persons with mental illness may conceal their symptoms to protect their family's resources or reputations or because they fear being perceived as a burden.[5]

Providers held the position that there were also cultural reasons that discouraged families and individuals from seeking mental health support. One of our providers who worked with Asian refugees mentioned that in some Asian communities whose religious beliefs included reincarnation, seeking mental health care meant that you were "not accepting your fate. You're not accepting the fact that something has happened to you because of something you did in your past life that predetermined that you are going to suffer." Seeking mental health help was "anathema" to the culture, the provider said. In some Asian cultures in which reincarnation is a possibility, people saw suffering in this life as a gift—an opportunity to atone for the mistakes of a past life and earn merit for the next one.[6]

Another provider who worked primarily with individuals who identified as Black said that "mental health is . . . considered taboo or something. People who have mental health problems, they are ostracized . . . They are considered evil, or witches and wizards, and it's not very good . . . They're not embraced. People who have mental health problems, they are just left to wander around and deteriorate mostly."

Research suggests that for Black Americans, who for hundreds of years have as a group embodied resilience despite the historical atrocities of slavery and current ongoing racism and discrimination, mental illness may be seen as a weakness, and so people avoid disclosing that illness to avoid judgment.[7] Anthropologist Tanya Luhrmann documented similar perspectives on being labeled as "crazy" among homeless African American women living on the streets of Chicago, for whom it signaled a vulnerability that could invite victimization, such as theft or sexual assault.[8]

Referencing the Hispanic population, a provider from a Spanish-speaking clinic in Dallas explained: "They know the family member needs help, but they . . . are not inclined to look for help because they think—'no loco, they're not crazy, and if not, then why would you be going to that place for crazy people?'"

One of my consultants on the project, Maggie Caballero, a bilingual self-identified Latina who had lived experience of serious mental illness and led her own peer treatment program, told me that there was no gray area—either you were crazy (*loco*) or you were not (*no loco*) in Spanish-speaking cultures—and you wanted to do everything you could to avoid being perceived as *loco*. *Loco* was reserved for people who could not be helped such as addicts and people who could not be cured. Maggie and several other Latinas in the study also told me that they feared *chismes*, or people gossiping about their lives and mental health status. If they were *loco* and became the subject of shameful *chismes*, they worried that the people they cared about might give up on them.

Anthropologists such as Kristin Yarris have suggested that gender affects social norms, roles, and expectations in the Latino community broadly, and also explored how individuals and their families perceive, explain, and handle a psychotic disorder as family caregiving arrangements shift in response to symptoms.[9] In addition, our consultant and providers told me that for Latino men, the Hispanic cultural tradition of machismo required them to maintain an image of strength. Having a mental illness could compromise that image. As one provider explained, "Hispanic men have the machismo thing, and they would be very stigmatized and perceived to be weak within that context."[10]

This is not to say that the stigma of mental illness does not apply to persons from groups that are not minoritized. Many people in American society writ large consider any individual with mental illness, especially psychosis, to be defective, unpredictable, and dangerous.[11] No one wants to be *that* person or have their child labeled as such. Protecting themselves or their children from culturally fueled stigmatizing ideas about mental illness is only one reason to delay seeking help, though.

As mentioned earlier, many of the mental health providers we interviewed claimed that young persons and families delayed help seeking because they had limited knowledge about mental illness. Researchers write about this phenomenon as "low mental health literacy."[12] Health literacy research assesses whether individuals can read health information and understand numerical claims. Mental health literacy researchers argue that this construct, often measured quantitatively via knowledge assessment tests, demonstrates how well individuals understand what mental illness is, how to recognize the warning signs, and how to successfully seek out treatment. They then compare individual scores between different cultural groups. In general, researchers have found that persons from minoritized groups in the United States have lower mental health literacy than their white counterparts. This has, in turn, been associated with the persistent underuse of mental health services and higher caregiver burden.[13]

Surprisingly, I could find little critique of the construct or its measurement to question what—and whose—ideas, knowledges, priorities, and practices were being used to determine what constituted "high" or "low" health literacy. However, I did find literature suggesting that discriminatory practices in health care perpetuate poor health literacy by denying better information and education about health care to groups with lower general literacy levels, which only reinforces power imbalances between professionals and patients and further justifies unequal treatment.[14] Thus, mental health literacy is often promoted to prevent and fight medical discrimination, which seems reasonable.

On the other hand, labeling minoritized persons as having "low mental health literacy" seems to place the onus of reform on the individual—they need to know better by educating themselves; if we educate them, that will fix the problem—while potentially distracting us from the upstream structural barriers that also need to be addressed. For example, the reluctance to seek help may also be fueled by a learned lack of trust in medical settings and practitioners that leads individuals to feel as though they have few options for help in the first place.[15] Medical mistrust is considerably more elevated in Hispanic and Black adults than in white adults, particularly when the former perceive they have been discriminated against by health care professionals, and even more so when they believe that discrimination was due to income or insurance status.[16] Such mistrust can be a survival strategy.

Other structural and social determinants of mental health, such as the segregation of neighborhoods through structural racism, can lead to the unequal distribution of mental health resources for individuals from minoritized groups and also affects families trying to navigate institutional pathways to care.[17] In 2016, the providers we interviewed claimed that there were no 24-hour mental health facilities available south of the Trinity River (and Interstate 30) where the vast majority of Black and Hispanic families lived. More than one-third of these families lived below the poverty line, a fact that can be attributed largely to redlining and other documented racist practices of residential and financial segregation in Dallas—practices that have also affected persons from minoritized groups elsewhere in the United States.[18] Other structural factors like health insurance and treatment costs pose additional barriers to mental health service utilization.[19] Lack of mental health insurance, lack of affordable mental health services, inflexible appointment times, insufficient scheduling procedures, and the long process to initiate treatment have been found to prolong help seeking for Black individuals and their family members.[20]

For immigrants, the stakes are also high. "There's a lot of barriers," one provider explained. "First, these people, they are scared, especially—some of them don't have papers. The fear of coming out, that, 'Oh, I don't have health insurance. What am I doing? Nobody is going to care for me, and I don't know anyone.'" Anthropologists have described both the fear of seeking care for undocumented persons and the mental health distress caused by living as an undocumented person in the United States—two structural situations that feed into each other to delay health help seeking.[21]

Several providers also thought that financial concerns were at the root of the problem. One explained:

> Socioeconomically, I think their chances of being at a higher income level and to be able to afford the necessities of life, the chances of that decreases. And due to that, they are not given the proper education. They are not given the proper care that they need at home because mom or whoever is taking care of them is working two to three jobs to be able to support [her children]. So given all those reasons and

putting that together, they don't get the appropriate care at the appropriate time, which leads to a delay in diagnosing them or taking a violent episode that may end up putting them in a jail initially because they have not ever been diagnosed with a mental health issue. Then from there, you start the cycle of: How do you get them to an evaluation process? How do you get them to a mental health facility like ours? So they go through some traumatic episodes before they get to this point—to some care. There was never somebody looking at them and just saying, "I think there's something going on with this kid," which delays their care.

All these barriers can prevent help seeking despite a strong potential need stemming from high levels of adverse life experiences for minoritized youths, which can heighten one's risk of developing psychosis. Nearly half of the providers mentioned the role of traumatic experiences as affecting the lives of the young persons with whom they worked. For Black youths in particular, research suggests that traumatic experiences include higher levels of childhood adversities such as residential instability and parental unemployment, incarceration, substance use, and exposure to violence than for white children.[22] Hispanic youths are also exposed to more violence than their white counterparts.[23]

One provider explained what they meant by *trauma*: "When I say the word *trauma*, a lot of people go to like, 'Oh, you hit your head,' or some major disaster, that trauma. But trauma can be that you saw your mom get hit by your dad. Or trauma can be that your sister abused drugs and you saw her do it. And so there's a lot of stuff that can come from trauma and how it can affect the brain and affect a teenager in general."

Trauma can also stem from living in foster homes or a single-parent household. As one provider said, "Anything that's in our past that has to do with adverse childhood experiences—there's a lot that has been contributing and it's not talked about." Unaddressed childhood trauma, such as physical and sexual abuse, is also linked to increased substance use as a coping mechanism,[24] which, as we know, can trigger or exacerbate psychotic symptoms. In fact, up to 70 percent of persons experiencing early psychosis also meet criteria for a substance use disorder, defined as problematic substance use that is disrupting one's everyday life.[25]

While the reasons for delayed help-seeking are myriad, all lead to a longer period during which a person receives no mental health support for their symptoms. When those symptoms include psychosis, this period is known in the literature as the duration of untreated psychosis (DUP).[26] Experiencing a longer DUP can have consequences. Research suggests that persons experiencing longer DUPs in the United States and United Kingdom typically have more severe symptoms, are more likely to attempt self-harm, and have lower chances of getting back to "normal" performance in work, school, and self-care.[27] This risk seems to increase the longer a person goes without support. So, for example, a person with a DUP of four weeks has 20 percent or greater severity of symptoms at follow-up relative to a person who had only been experiencing psychosis without treatment for one week. In addition, longer DUPs for young people often place a greater strain on their family.[28]

Of course, all this research highlights how serious it was that Michael had been struggling for three years without care. Researchers argue that, in part because of delays in seeking or accessing care, Black youths with early psychosis typically present with more severe psychotic symptoms and often access care through a "catalytic event" (e.g., accident, arrest) involving emergency services and police involvement.[29] More intense positive symptoms often contribute to unusual or dangerous behaviors that then prompt families to seek and initiate treatment.[30] This was true for Michael, who tried to harm his niece before help was called—and that help was the police. Research on this topic in the United States is limited, but one Canadian study found that "emergency services were most often the contact that helped individuals obtain appropriate treatment for psychosis."[31]

Shortening the duration of untreated psychosis has thus been the focus of many early intervention for psychosis programs around the world, which try to prevent negative consequences such as catalytic events and police involvement by helping young people access care as soon as possible after symptoms begin. However, early recognition of psychosis symptoms requires people in the community—family members, teachers, coaches, pastors—to recognize that a young person is developing a serious mental health issue that requires support as early as possible, and to connect people to those supports quickly before a crisis occurs. Unfortunately, for most of the youths in our study like Michael—and so many others not in my study—a quick connection to mental health support was not part of their story.

. . .

Sofia ultimately got help through emergency services after some long delays— and her early interactions did not initially inspire her to trust or desire more mental health care. Sofia had studied abroad in Latin America during college to improve her medical Spanish but left the program early and returned to the United States after a traumatizing assault at gunpoint. Back at school, she told her roommates what happened to her, and they were not supportive. According to Sofia, they gossiped about her (the dreaded *chismes*) and told others that she was crazy. Sofia thought they were racist. Her mother, Maria, who was born in Mexico, agreed.

Sofia's conflicts with her roommates eventually became so significant that she had to move into a new apartment. "But she is not aggressive," her mother added hurriedly. "She has never hurt anyone." Maria said that everybody at school loved Sofia and repeatedly gave examples of how her daughter was so nice, so passive, and never bothered anyone. Maria thought Sofia had just chosen the wrong friends.

Sofia shared her thoughts: "I think it started gradually because there were little things that were happening in my life that I couldn't control. And I couldn't go to sleep. I was thinking that I was . . . I had the problems with my roommates. And then I couldn't go to sleep." When Maria visited Sofia at college to cook for her, she

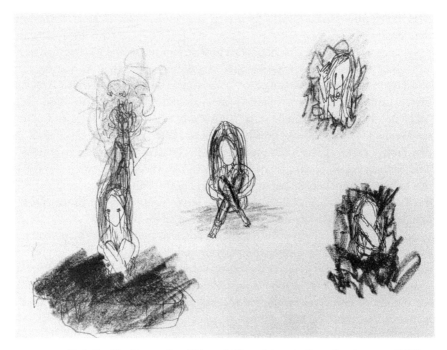

FIGURE 3. "Spiraling" by Lauren Ann Villarreal. The artist wrote the author in an email: "It's about the dark thoughts that flood my brain, seemingly from somewhere else, and I can't stop them. I drown in them, and they consume me. The dark thoughts made me feel small, trapped, I couldn't escape. I couldn't control the thoughts that would come to me. They became me." *Reproduced with permission of the artist.*

found some teas in her room to help her sleep. Maria took her for a walk in the park and tried to help her, "Okay, you look very tired," she told her.

That school term, Sofia failed several of her exams. She had always been an excellent student, and Maria started to really worry, "because she's not sleeping . . . She's very tired, and then she's studying. And it's just a lot of work in the school . . . I think it's too much for her."

Then one night someone at the college called Maria and told her that Sofia was refusing to sleep inside. It was not clear why she would want to stay outside at night. Concerned, Maria picked Sofia up from college to take her to the hospital to get some help for her "nerves." "Nerves" or "nervous breakdown" or "*ataque de nervios*" is a common term for mental distress among Spanish speakers that often signals depression, anxiety, or panic rather than psychosis.[32] Anthropologist Janis H. Jenkins has argued that *nervios* is used strategically by Mexican American families when describing a family member with a psychotic disorder as an explanation that invites less stigma and encourages more family support for the person who is struggling.[33]

Maria initially took Sofia to the emergency room because she did not have any insurance, so that was the only option. At the county hospital, Sofia was given medication for her "nerves" and released. Sofia did not like the experience, and she did not like the way the medication made her feel so fuzzy-headed.

"She came home and she's okay," Maria recalled later. "But then she was reading the Bible. And she—later, she had a lot of nerves."

Things became worse. "I wasn't feeling good, and I just wanted to be outside," Sofia explained. She refused to take more medication or stay inside.

Maria was very distressed. "If she takes the medicine, she's okay. Because when the doctor gave her the medicine at the hospital, she's okay. She comes home, she's okay. But she don't want to take the medicine the next day."

Sofia would not come inside that night. Maria stayed with her, afraid to leave her outside alone. She was terrified Sofia would be assaulted again. She begged her to please go to the hospital with her to talk to "a friend." Sofia refused.

Maria cleaned houses during the day—a form of employment that is difficult to take a day off from for family emergencies. So she worked through the day and watched Maria at night, but it was not a sustainable solution. Not knowing what else to do, she called the police. Maria cried as she explained, "She don't want to go. And then police—he helped me take her because she don't want to go. Because I don't want to leave her outside. I'm very tired. Because I don't sleep two days because [at night] I'm staying at the hospital and then outside with her. And then I'm very tired. I was very scared. I want to take care of my daughter, but this is not a good condition."

The officers took Sofia into custody to transport her to Shady Elms. Sofia admitted herself voluntarily, though later she had no recollection of doing so. Possibly because she was on public insurance, within 24 hours of her arrival at Shady Elms she was transferred to a state hospital for a minimum of twenty-eight days.

In retrospect, there were signs that Sofia was in serious trouble: self-isolation, deteriorating relationships, difficulties with sleeping, a precipitous drop in her performance at school. Yet all these symptoms could be explained away by her traumatic assault, her roommates' lack of kindness, and having to move out. As we have seen, families delay care for a whole host of reasons. But when people delay seeking help, at some point things become unmanageable—a breaking point. The young person becomes incomprehensible in their words and actions even to their own parents—a sign that they are having both a mental and a moral breakdown. Even the most advantaged people can end up in a dangerous situation when they are in crisis. Add in a whole host of social disadvantages, and it can be disastrous.

Without any intervention, people with psychosis can and often do become dangerous to themselves or others. Dangerous, it is important to note, does not necessarily mean violent, though the behavior can involve aggressiveness.[34] It was dangerous for Sofia to stay outside at night in a high-crime urban area. Sofia did not harm anyone, but she did physically resist the police when they tried to take her to the hospital. One Canadian study found that around half of young people were physically or verbally aggressive leading up to their admission to an early-psychosis program.[35]

In these studies, factors related to more severe kinds of aggression included young age, lack of education, prior offending, and substance use—all well-known risk factors for violent behavior in general—as well as a longer DUP. Violence was also more likely in the period after initial treatment if a person was treated involuntarily, indicating that powerlessness in the treatment encounter may contribute to later aggression. Of course, these studies have their limitations, and more research is needed. Notably, however, a recent review of data from fifteen countries found that among persons with schizophrenia spectrum disorders, the odds that a person would engage in violence toward another person was less than 1 in 20 for women and less than 1 in 4 for men over a thirty-five-year period of their lives.[36] Obviously, the associations are complicated, and violence is hard to predict. Clearly, poverty, substance use, education level, and the experience of unchecked psychosis play a role. However, we must use this information to support people rather than stigmatize them.

Caution is all the more important since persons with serious mental illness are also at high risk of becoming victims of violence, especially if they are experiencing homelessness, substance use or abuse, or severe symptoms of psychosis or are engaging in criminal activity.[37] Sofia might have been seriously harmed if her mother had not guarded her during her nighttime wanderings. In addition, young people in the United States with early psychosis are at a heightened risk of mortality: they are 24 times more likely than their age-matched peers to die within twelve months of their diagnosis.[38]

And so, even though people with psychosis are more likely to be *victims* of violence or to die early, the media often highlight stories that vilify those who have engaged in extreme violence. The young people in our study were aware of these stories, too, and it frightened them. For example, while I was engaged in this research, Thomas Johnson, a 21-year-old Black Dallas native and former Texas A&M football wide receiver randomly attacked a local runner, 53-year-old Dave Stevens, with a machete early in the morning on a public trail. Johnson then stopped the next cyclist approaching, asked for a phone, and called 911 to let them know he had just killed someone. Later, at Johnson's trial in 2019, his aunt said, "He kept telling people that he was hearing voices and he needed help. And all they saw was his athletic abilities and no one would listen to him."[39]

Amy heard this story, too. She mentioned "the machete killer" about six weeks after her first admission. It had been on her mind:

> There shouldn't be such a stigma around it, and it should be easier for people to obtain mental health care. Hearing stories like that guy who took a machete to that guy, that runner. Did you hear about that? I guess this young guy, maybe 20 years

old, who had mental problems, and his mom [her voice trembles] knew that he had all sorts of mental problems. I guess he went up to a runner at random and macheted him to death. Then the wife [of the runner] just committed suicide because she was disenfranchised by it. Things like that I feel like shouldn't happen. There should be more of a responsibility of people around and people in mental health care.

Such stories perpetuate the vicious cycle of stigma that makes it harder for people to seek help and thus more likely that they will engage in dangerous behavior when they become confused. My own research unearthed many distressing stories. Some of the people I engaged with tried to harm themselves or behaved in ways that could result in bodily harm. Corrina locked herself in an extremely hot car. James parked his car in front of a train. Amy nearly jumped off a bridge onto a busy interstate. David tried to jump out of his father's moving car. Sofia insisted on sleeping outside. The list goes on.

At other times young people were at risk of harming—or did harm—others. James assaulted his girlfriend. Michael tried to harm his sister's child. Miranda punched her father. The following chapters contain many more examples. A dangerous crisis was often what prompted the young person to connect with a mental health care provider, most often via the police. It was difficult to connect a young person with care in the absence of medical insurance or easy access to mental health support.

The availability of mental health services and the laws that govern admittance to these services differ from state to state. However, each state system has similarities to the Texas system, and all present significant challenges to those who need help. One of the few avenues available for people in crisis, especially after hours, was to call the police. If someone was not deemed dangerous by the police, they could be treated in an emergency room and were often released quickly, as when Sofia visited the county hospital.

A medical facility might also place an "emergency hold" or "psychiatric detention" on someone for observation prior to release if they have been admitted to the facility for psychiatric reasons. Rules vary about the duration of emergency holds, who can initiate an emergency hold, the extent of judicial oversight, and the rights of patients during the hold.[40] In most states—and in multiple other countries, including Australia and South Korea—a person can be held involuntarily for up to 72 hours for observation. In Texas, to extend an involuntary commitment beyond 72 hours, a court overseen by a magistrate or justice of the peace can rule that person to pose so substantial a risk of harm to self or others that they cannot remain at liberty.[41] This was typically determined by review of a medical certificate issued by a physician and testimony from the patient and their family members. If a judge ruled that a person remained potentially dangerous, and if that person refused to be admitted to the hospital voluntarily, they were involuntarily committed.

A person could also voluntarily admit themselves to Shady Elms if they had symptoms of mental illness that could "benefit" from inpatient services, if a payment plan was agreed upon, and if they had been informed of their rights as a voluntary patient. A person 16 years or older could request voluntary admission from hospital administrators; their parent or guardian could also make such a request if the person being admitted was under 18 years of age even without their consent.[42] Moreover, as soon as a person was admitted voluntarily, they could easily be shifted to involuntary commitment status if they refused treatment or asked to be discharged. They could then be held for a longer period. Sofia was brought to Shady Elms by police, admitted herself voluntarily, and then was shifted to involuntary status when she asked to be discharged. Notably, whether voluntarily or involuntarily, most of the people in my study landed at Shady Elms through police involvement.

. . .

People make initial contact with mental health care via what are called pathways to care. The pathway to care begins the moment a young person starts having symptoms and run to their first point of contact with someone who offers mental health support. This care can be as simple as a visit to a general or family practitioner who offers them counseling or psychiatric medication, or as traumatic as a 911 call that results in armed police forcibly taking someone into custody for an involuntary psychiatric hospital visit.

There were three common pathways to care at Shady Elms. These routes emerged when members of my research team analyzed the stories of the thirty-eight young people who offered in-depth answers to our question, "Tell me how you came to be in the hospital." James, David, Miranda, Corrina, and Michael all came into the mental health care system because they seemed dangerous to themselves or others, and someone in proximity called the police, who brought them to the hospital. Nearly half of the young people entered care this way.

At that time, most people in the seven-county radius surrounding Dallas who had a psychiatric crisis and needed to be held for observation, or who were uninsured and so needed to enroll in the regional public mental health care plan, were sent to Shady Elms. In 2014, during an orientation to the facility, I learned that Shady Elms had served 26,000 patients representing about 80 percent of the annual psychiatric "patient population" in the region. Seventy percent of those had arrived in handcuffs.

For persons who are Black, their pathway to care is more likely to involve contact with law enforcement than for other racial or ethnic groups.[43] Black individuals are also less likely to seek mental health care from a primary physician than are individuals from other ethnic groups.[44] One study reported that pathways to care for African Americans were "often less desirable . . . with higher rates of involuntary civil commitment and police involvement."[45]

For most of the young people in my study, the police were involved in their introduction to mental health care. In most states, police are mental health crisis first responders and, thus, frontline providers of "care." Thirty-eight states allow police to take a person into custody without a warrant for an emergency psychiatric admission, and police officers are often explicitly in charge of initiating the short-term emergency commitment process.[46] Thus, to get help when someone will not do so voluntarily, the police must be involved.

But police interactions can be toxic. In my study, where most of the participants were Black and Latino, about two-thirds claimed to have been arrested before, and one-fifth had been arrested four or more times.[47] Some argue that criminal injustice falls along a racial gradient, with Black youths being treated worse than Latino youths, who are treated worse than white youths.[48] This may be due to the structural racism baked into policing practices around Black youths.[49] For example, by the age of 24, Black youths have nine times more interactions with police than their white counterparts, are more likely to experience force in those encounters, and are five times more likely to be injured.[50]

Police exposure is also associated with adverse mental health and substance use for Black youths.[51] Black Americans who have had a police interaction are twice as likely to report experiencing poor mental health as those with no police interaction.[52] While it is possible that individuals with poor mental health report more negative police interactions, some of these cited studies found a positive association between police stops and police victimization on one hand and psychological distress, psychotic experiences, depression, suicidal attempts, and suicidal ideation on the other, even when controlling for a prior history of mental health diagnosis.

Interactions between those with mental health problems and armed law enforcement are also common, can be dangerous, and can deter future help seeking. The risk of being approached or stopped by law enforcement is sixteen times higher for individuals with untreated mental illness than for other civilians. Data collected in 2020 and 2021 show that one-fifth of fatal police shootings involved persons with mental illness.[53] Being African American (instead of non-Hispanic white) and having a mental illness were strongly associated with those fatalities.[54] Fatal police shootings of persons with mental illness are more likely to take place in small and midsized areas, but there are plenty of examples from communities of all sizes across the United States.[55] Fatal police encounters for persons experiencing mental illness are also more common among those who are armed with a knife and at home.

James was at home when his parents called the police for help. Since he had come home from Shady Elms, things had taken a turn for the worse after he stopped taking his medications and intensified his substance use to more frequently include LSD and a homemade kind of methamphetamine made in the tailpipe of a car. He had been out of school, unemployed, and refusing to see any kind of mental health provider, his mother told us later when she called us for a phone interview. She hoped his story might help prevent the same thing from happening to someone else.

His father told the police that he was hiding in their house with his knife. They never imagined how badly things could go. In retrospect, his mother said, she was not even sure he had a knife. She thought he had something in his hand, and anyway, a person had to be dangerous to themselves or others to get the police to come to the house and help.

James did not go to the police voluntarily. He tweeted threats and racial slurs to the police. As a result, James was taken to jail instead of Shady Elms; it took weeks in jail for him to access mental health treatment. He had two surgeries for injuries he sustained. His mother's home was ruined. However, given that he allegedly had a knife, was at home, and had taunted the police, he was lucky to be alive.

The second most common pathway to care for people in my study involved members of a person's family or church—or both—bringing them in for emergency care. If the young person went to the local emergency room, they were often then escorted by police from that hospital to Shady Elms for the 72-hour hold. The police seemed to be the main form of transportation between facilities rather than an ambulance, likely for safety reasons. Staff and patients at Shady Elms noted that police arrivals came in the "back door." Sofia was one such arrival when she was transferred from the county hospital after her second crisis.

A few did arrive at Shady Elms with their family (and no police) through the "front door"—a sliding glass door that opened into a small reception area with a TV, a couple of couches, and a welcome desk. From there, they were escorted through the first locked door into an intake room with a cot, a computer station, and a chair. Here, young people could be processed for a voluntary admission.

Gideon was a voluntary admission. When I first met him in the hospital, I was struck by his charm. He was a long, lean, first-generation African immigrant. He had moved to the United States about five years prior. He looked completely put together, and I wondered what he was doing at Shady Elms. He shared that he was attending community college and living with his family.

He accentuated that he was a strong Christian and he thought people would understand him better if he could go back to the place of his birth, because he felt Africans were more spiritual than Americans and more likely to believe in the demons that Gideon could see everywhere. Months later, I asked Gideon's brother, Jacob, if he agreed that Gideon was just a more spiritually sensitive person living in the wrong culture. He responded, "I'd say no. It's mental." He emphasized that no one agreed with those beliefs here in the United States and that people in their home country, as well, would think he had both a spiritual and psychological problem.

Because of his faith, Gideon had never used drugs or alcohol. He also said he did not have a lot of friends because he spent most of his time praying. He told me, "I pray a little bit and pretty much speak in angelic tongues. I pray for the salvation of the United States. I might walk up and just, say no. 'In the name of Jesus Christ, we know the rapture is coming.' I used to think that at my age, I'll probably just write a book about things that will happen at that time."

Gideon tried talking to others about his faith, "telling people about the Gospel, preaching and stuff," but in later interviews he acknowledged that his dad did not like it. The other church members did not like it. They convinced him to go to Shady Elms voluntarily. They told him he was just going to the hospital to get a test, so he agreed to go. "I was supposed to get the prophet testing," he told me. He thought "the test" would prove he was a prophet.

However, after his dad and his pastor left him at Shady Elms, he was forcibly strapped to a bed and injected with medications that made him feel horrible for days. Gideon thought that approach had to be against his rights as an American.

Gideon expressed his frustration: "Some people are supernatural beings, you know? I guess those who don't understand, they think, 'Oh you're really nuts or something to see into the supernatural.' You can hear the talking of God and demons and stuff yourself . . . You can do everything, but just relax, you know? Relax and try to block them out. You don't want to be called nuts or anything; that's exactly what has come to pass."

Veronica, too, said that the first time she went to the hospital was somewhat voluntary. Veronica, a young woman who self-identified as African American, went in with her sister. "I was actually good," she explained, "until they put me all by myself. When I went there, I was like, 'Okay, my family's here; we're good. I'm just going to calm down or try to figure out what the heck is going on and then everything will be back to normal.' My sister was in and out of the door. She was on the phone. I think she was telling them, 'She's crazy, low-key crazy, but don't let her go out.'"

Since she was younger, Veronica felt that her older sister had more credibility. "If they follow you and are like, 'Hey, she has schizophrenia—don't let her leave. She's going to try to leave.' Then why wouldn't they try to keep you there, to make sure that you're fine and that you're okay to leave? I understand that aspect of it. They're doing their job! They were. Yeah. Now I hate hospitals."

This pathway to care was hard on young people. It often involved some type of manipulation from families or other trusted community members, and a betrayal of trust. Knowing their family has left them in the facility because they think they have a serious mental problem, having their stories dismissed or discredited, being locked into a hospital that they cannot leave without permission—all is difficult to process on one's own.

The third way a young person found themselves in contact with mental health support was to ask the police for help. This was unusual—only one in six of the young people in my study reported this—but it did happen. These young people just walked up to the police on the street or called 911. In my study, the people who directly contacted the police included one white woman, two white men, one Hispanic woman, and two Hispanic men. All had a history of arrest, and one had been arrested more than four times. Even so, they seemed to trust the police.

Amy was one of these people. As mentioned, she stepped away from the ledge of the bridge and asked for help. Another young Hispanic woman, Elba, was struggling with postpartum psychosis and called the police to keep her safe from intruders. When they arrived, they thought she seemed paranoid and took her to the hospital. Similarly, Josue, a young Hispanic man, asked the police for help when he was drunk. He was hoping for a ride home or a booking into the jail so he could sleep off his buzz. Instead, they took him to Shady Elms.

Tyler, a tall, blond white man with sharp grey eyes, had a history of treatment for methamphetamine use. One day, Tyler explained, he walked to a local donut shop where he convinced the workers to let him use the phone. He then called the police and told the dispatcher they had better come get him because "I am 110% crazy." Then he called them again. "They weren't coming fast enough," he continued,

> and then I kept going and going and going. And then I threatened to break a window. And then, then the Hispanic workers walked out, and the police came with their big guns. You know, ready to shoot to kill. And I surrendered. Peacefully. And then I went to the cop car. And then down the road we go, and down the road we go, and down the road we go. And I ended up here. In my cage.

Tyler made it all seem so simple, like any other day. In all these instances, police were contacted for a variety of reasons and ended up assessing that the young person needed help with their mental health.

None of the young people who told me that they called the police for help were Black. While Black family members did call police when there was an emergency, the Black youths we interviewed did not. Yet, even though these young people did not call them directly, studies suggest that Black people with psychotic disorders interact with the police more often than white people and are more likely to be admitted involuntarily.[56] And, based on the research cited earlier, they are also more likely to have a fatal encounter with police.

And while we can—and should—critically parse the differences among persons from minoritized groups in their pathways to care, the fact remains that no pathway is ideal. Most involve police intervention and, too often, a crisis. The system—if there ever was one—is broken. There are better ways of caring for our young people.

. . .

Families from ethnoracially minoritized groups delay seeking help even when a young person is showing multiple signs of potential extreme mental distress. The young person—regardless of background—may be doing poorly at work, school, and relationships. They may increase substance use, hole up in their room, sleep less, and express paranoid thoughts. However, it often takes a catalytic event or crisis for people to seek out care.

In this chapter I discuss some of the reasons revealed in the research literature as to why this may be so, including overall mistrust of medical providers, cultural stigma against having a mental illness, aversion to being labeled a person who is mentally ill, and low mental health literacy. I also describe structural barriers, such as the accessibility of mental health services, their availability for people who do not have mental health insurance, police involvement that seems to criminalize people in distress as "bad," and the threat of police violence.

The pathway to care that emerges from this situation—waiting to seek help until a catalytic event has occurred and a person has become a danger to themselves or others—requires police intervention. This typical scenario fails everyone: the young person needing care, their key supporters, and society at large. Entering the world of mental health care through an arrest and forced admission to treatment can be dangerous physically and mentally and has profound impact on a person's moral agency. Even those who are brought by families or trusted community members directly to an emergency room have often had interactions with the police before they received care. The police were sometimes seen as allies—and they can be—but police involvement in the pathway to care through emergency services can be distressing and even dangerous.

What would mental health care look like if we did not wait until people become dangerous before we got them help? We need to change the rules of engagement, and chapter 7 offers additional ideas for how to achieve this change. In chapter 4, we turn to what does happen to people when they finally arrive at the psychiatric emergency hospital—in this case, Shady Elms. Everything that has happened so far has led them to this point, but what kind of care will they receive?

4

Disorientations

When my ex told me to go get a prescription, he's like, "You have schizophrenia. Go get a prescription for schizophrenia." Which I've never been diagnosed with it, but he told me to go get a prescription and then they end up omitting me—is that the word? Omitting me in the hospital.

—VERONICA, SHADY ELMS HOSPITAL, DAY 3

Flashes. They remember it in flashes. Bright lights, loud sounds, rough handling, confusion, a lack of information, forced separation from family for up to 72 hours, the possibility of unwanted injections or being placed in restraints. The experience is like no emergency room arrival they ever imagined, and it is the hardest part to remember—the intake.

On top of that, they were experiencing psychosis.

Take Amy, for example. We know Amy. She asked for help from the police instead of stepping off the overpass. When I first met Amy at Shady Elms, she had been admitted a few days earlier. She haltingly pieced together what happened upon her arrival.

> AMY: Of, of course, they admitted me. I was going crazy . . .
>
> NEELY: Mm-hmm. *[Affirmative.]*
>
> *[Pause.]*
>
> AMY: I—they had a camera where they had to take a picture.
>
> NEELY: Mm-hmm. *[Affirmative.]*
>
> AMY: And I guess it set me off and I tried to smash it, and they had to put me in four-point restraints.
>
> NEELY: Oh.
>
> AMY: Yeah.
>
> *[Pause.]*
>
> NEELY: That must have been really tough.
>
> AMY: Um, not as tough as what was going on with me.
>
> NEELY: Right.

> AMY: Like it all needed to happen in order for me to find out. Because for some reason all these bizarre things can happen . . .
>
> NEELY: Mm-hmm. *[Affirmative.]*
>
> AMY: And you can still feel like you can normalize.
>
> NEELY: Right. So, how do you—how do you feel now?
>
> AMY: Um, it's pretty humiliating.
>
> NEELY: Yeah.
>
> AMY: I get nervous because I can hear some things that I could misconstrue and it makes me fearful I could start hearing those voices again. [. . .] I feel like I've forgotten a lot, but I think it's just from being in here, whatever it is . . . It is making me forget and I didn't consent to any of this.
>
> NEELY: What could your brother and sister do next time? What would they do differently?
>
> AMY: They could talk to me. They didn't even talk to me about anything.

Amy had trouble remembering the details of her intake, but she remembered being humiliated. She tried to avoid having her picture taken because she did not look very nice after traveling by bus and wandering the streets and this was not an image she wanted on any record. She said she overreacted, and they strapped her to a table—spread eagle—against her will. Amy was angry with her family, confused by her own behaviors—fighting with her sister, trying to smash a camera, forgetting things that had happened—afraid of having more symptoms, and dismayed that she was now being held at Shady Elms involuntarily. Later, she reflected on her experience:

> AMY: One thing that does frustrate me is the whole time I was going through all of that, they never told me what was going on.
>
> NEELY: Right.
>
> AMY: I don't know why they do that.
>
> NEELY: Do you think if they told you, you'd have been able to comprehend? Would it have helped to know?
>
> AMY: No. I really don't know that it would've.

But how could she know? She never had the chance to find out.

After her intake experience, Amy struggled to accept further mental health treatment. Even though she was admitted voluntarily, when she refused medications and wanted to leave, the doctor and judge changed her status to involuntary. She tried to throw herself out of her brother's moving vehicle to avoid a follow-up visit.

In the end, however, she accepted care because she needed housing. She did not want to be homeless again. That is what got her into this mess in the first place. Her brother would not let her stay with him unless she took her antipsychotic medications and went to her follow-up appointments, and so she did.

Miranda's intake experience was similar. She did not give me the details of her hospital arrival until a few months into our interviews. When the time came, her story, like Amy's, began with a point of humiliation, as though these humiliations anchored people's fragmented memories.

> *MIRANDA:* It was just scary. The "squat and cough"—that was scary. I felt that, you know, I felt like I didn't own my body, like my body wasn't mine.
>
> *NEELY:* Okay . . . were they doing that with every person that was brought in?
>
> *MIRANDA:* I don't know. I mean, I only experienced mine, I don't know if they did it for everybody. But they did it for me, you know? And I understand that they have to do that for safety reasons. But, ideally, they would trust you. [. . .] Because what happened was, I didn't really even know what was going on the whole time. So, if somebody let you know, "You're here because of this" or "You're here because of . . . you're going to have this happen to you because . . ." You know? Because the whole time I was like, "Oh, I don't know what's happening . . ." It was really disorienting.

Later in the interview, I asked Miranda if she thought people's hospitalization experiences influenced their treatment decisions.

> *NEELY:* Do you think the kind of treatment that, you know, you received upon getting to a hospital influences a lot of people's decisions about whether to go back or not?
>
> *MIRANDA:* Oh, yeah. Definitely. I was brought to Shady Elms by cops . . . I wanted to go to therapy . . . I don't like authority figures and I think a lot of people don't like authority figures, period. I think that added to my hostility that I was brought by cops. And I think that I wouldn't have sought psychiatrists; I would have sought out therapy. Because I almost was at the breaking point where—well, I *was* at the breaking point where I needed help. And I think that I, if I didn't go through my manic phase, I would have gone to therapy. But I don't know if I would have gone to a hospital.
>
> *NEELY:* Right. So, in an ideal universe, definitely that's not the treatment you get.
>
> *[Miranda and Neely laughing.]*
>
> *MIRANDA:* No. No, yeah.

Intake was much the same for everyone in our study. A young person came to the hospital through the front or back door and then was separated from the world as well as their families. Once inside, they were escorted to a room by police who searched them, photographed them, and took their personal belongings—phones, valuables, clothes. If they resisted, they were put in four-point leather restraints used to strap their wrists and ankles to a gurney or chair.

Most were given a liquid concoction to calm down—a "Shady Elms cocktail" as the local police called it—of liquid Haldol (an antipsychotic), Benadryl, and Ativan (an anxiolytic). A nurse told me that the cocktail enabled the patients to sleep off whatever had brought them in. Those who resisted the paper cup typically received an injection.

As the sedatives took effect, the patients were laid on dark-blue plastic recliners in a room the size of a junior high school gymnasium. When they awoke, typically quite groggy, they continued the intake process by going into a small, dim, windowless room for an in-depth interview with a social worker who typed notes furiously into a computer. People like to compare mental health concerns to having diabetes or a broken bone, but this was not anyone's typical visit to the emergency room. The psychiatric emergency visit is unlike anything else.

I am not saying that Amy and Miranda did not need help. They did need help and they knew it at the time, and they knew it when I talked to them after their intake, whether that was days or months later. What I am saying is that they—and many others—did not get the help they were seeking. Instead, their experiences in the hospital were harmful to their moral agency. They had been treated like a "bad" person—police escort, handcuffs, mugshot-type photos, squatting and coughing to check for drugs, put in four-point restraints, not informed of their situation, forced to take medication—which was dehumanizing and had a lasting impact on their perception of care. And even beyond the hospital, being a person who had experienced a psychiatric hospitalization threatened their perception— and others' perceptions—that they were good people. Damage control was not an option. It was almost impossible for them to edit this part of their life stories. Their initial hospitalizations constituted a rupture in their life narratives that would be difficult to repair.[1]

. . .

At Shady Elms, I was able to watch most of this happening from what I came to think of as "Central Control." Central Control was a panopticon designed to render all patients visible while protecting staff from danger. The staff enclosure was bright, but the patient area was dark—lit by eerie, dim, blue lights. Beyond the glass, up to eighty people at a time lay prone on rolling plastic royal-blue recliners. Men rested on one side, women on the other, but the two sides had no barrier between them. The people I saw lying there represented a range of ages, socioeconomic backgrounds, and cultural orientations. Most were asleep—sedated—under a thin blanket.

The staff area was segregated, enclosed by a wall of bulletproof glass with little windows the nurses could slide up and down a few inches to talk to patients. Overhead, several large, soundless, closed-circuit television screens flashed images of often-handcuffed new admissions undergoing those first interactions—police searches, intake photos, restraints, injections. Phones rang while staff tapped away at a dozen or so computers, looking up patients' records. Doctors in white coats flipped through patients' paper charts in binders. The more frequently a person visited, the larger their chart. The youths in my study usually had near-empty binders waiting to be filled.

A few weeks after his arrest for trying to "bless" people in line at Starbuck's, Gideon offered a few thoughts about his experience. "The funny thing was the police arrested me and took me to Shady Elms and told me to lay down on a rest table, tried to calm me down or whatever. I know, 'Why you put a handcuff on me and tell me you're not arresting me? What kind of sick joke is that?' 'It's okay, I'm punching you, but you don't feel anything.' [. . .] I was like, 'No.' I just kept quiet."

Keeping quiet and not resisting, Gideon had learned, helped keep him safe.

Sometimes people woke up agitated and started causing trouble. The psychiatric technicians—dressed in distinctive black scrubs—would handle them as quickly as possible, but occasionally, workers were punched or bitten, or patients were knocked over by other patients. It was a tense environment. I feared for my own well-being more than once. This was hard, unpredictable, and dangerous work. I understood why many staff hardened themselves against empathizing much with their patients; they always had to be on guard for the unexpected. The other patients, especially the young ones I worked with, had no idea how to interpret or navigate this volatile environment. For them, it was incredibly scary.

One morning early on in my fieldwork, I had just used my badge to open the first of two sets of doors that led to the outside courtyard when a patient burst through the second door. I was supposed to pull the door closed behind me to keep anyone from getting out, but I was so startled and frightened that I did not think to close myself into a small space with a large, frantic man in paper-thin scrubs. I flattened myself out of the way as he burst past me across the enclosed courtyard and tried to climb the only wall that provided any access to the outside. Of course, it was too tall for anyone to climb, and even if he made it over the wall, the police parking bay was on the other side. I watched as two psychiatric technicians—large men dressed in black scrubs—pulled him off the wall and enacted what they called a "takedown," which meant restraining him until an injection of sedatives could be administered.

Shaken, I considered going home for the day. However, this was early in my fieldwork, and I had a feeling this experience was like falling off a horse. If I left, I might not be able to get over the fear. So, instead, I took a deep breath and reentered. It reminded me, though, that patients saw these kinds of things all the time—an agitated person, a threatening encounter—but unlike me, they could not choose to go home. They had to stay. While I could hide behind the nurses' desk or move from one ward to another, quickly putting a locked door or some bulletproof glass between myself and a stranger who rushed at me, the patients had no such luxury. They were constantly exposed to the possibility of danger.

Miranda talked to me about this. She said that at one point she felt like Winona Ryder in the movie *Girl, Interrupted* when she realized she was at a mental institution, but she did not know why.[2]

> That was really scary. I mean, anybody—you don't know what's wrong with them. Or, you know, they could have done something more severe than what I'd done. I'd threatened my dad. But it's just the fact that everybody was in there and you don't know what they did. You know? It was just kind of like—they didn't have a— I don't know, *screening* or something. But I guess in an ideal world, people with violent tendencies would be separated from the ones who don't have violent tendencies. I mean, but, you know, I threatened my dad, so I could have been put in with people who had violent tendencies. I mean, all I did was threaten him. Well, that sounds— that almost sounds like I'm dismissing it, but . . . you know?

Miranda wanted to be separated from the "bad" people, and she was struggling to distinguish herself from them. We can see her moral agency coming into question. Is she one of the people that others need to avoid? Of course, she also wanted to avoid dangerous people—who wouldn't?

Miranda's mother, Angela, told me that something happened to Miranda in Shady Elms. The first night she talked to her, Miranda said some strange things.

"It was just a big mess," Angela sighed. She demanded that they transfer Miranda to a private hospital, using her mother's insurance. Angela was allowed to watch her exit from the ambulance at her new location, because she had a medical license, and she could see that she had a hickey on her neck.

"That just baffled me," she said. "I just couldn't believe what was happening." Angela could not imagine why medical professionals would put Miranda on suicide and homicide watch in a room with other people who could take advantage of her vulnerable state.

During another visit, I stood listening to a nurse talk to patients who came up to the Central Control window. She gave them psychiatric medications in a little paper cup to help them stay calm while they waited. She told me that the initial intake area was hardest on the "first-timers" because they woke up in a room of people and had no clue where they were. They always looked the most freaked out.

"Look!" She smiled. "Here comes one now."

A young, white man whom I came to know as Jack shuffled up to the window. Jack was the first first-timer I met, and it was heartbreaking. He was crying, wiping his tears on his sleeve as he approached. The nurse slid the window open, and his voice cracked as he asked, "Did I die? Am I dead? Am I in Hell?"

"No, you are not dead. You are in a hospital, and you need to go lay back down on your chair and wait," the nurse responded.

"Please! What happened?" He begged. As mentioned before, Jack could not remember. A lot of young people could not remember: they had some amnesia about events surrounding their psychotic break. It was not clear to me if it was the Shady Elms cocktail or the effect of potential dissociation during their episode for psychological protection or something else entirely, but it was common all the same. Sometimes their memories came back, and sometimes they did not.

Jack and the nurse went back and forth a few more times, him hobbling up to the nurse's station, her telling him to sit back down. Finally, she placed another pill in a paper cup and pushed it through the slot.

"We will wake you up when the doctor comes," she insisted. Jack nodded and sobbed.

"Can I go and sit with him if that's okay with him?" I asked.

The nurse agreed and asked me to take him away from the recliners and talk to him in a chair on the perimeter so that we did not disrupt the other patients.

Jack was eager to talk.

I explained that we were at a psychiatric emergency room called Shady Elms where the doctors would see him and help him know the next best steps to help him manage his mental health. We looked over the patients' bill of rights posted on the wall behind us.

He had many questions.

"What time is it? What day is it? Where am I in Texas?"

Jack was not from Dallas. I showed him our location on Google Maps on my phone.

He then asked to use my phone, and I regretfully said I did not think that was an option. Later staff confirmed that patients should not be allowed to use my phone, and near the end of our study they banned cell phone use around the patients completely to protect confidentiality, though in general we had only been using them to record interviews.

Jack asked me where his phone went, and I told him I did not know, but I was sure he would get it back when he was discharged. We asked the nurse if he could make a phone call, and she pointed to an unmarked gray phone on one of the walls for local calls. But the extra pill made Jack sleepy. Maybe he would wait until he woke up again, he said. He had stopped crying, and I offered to tuck him into his chair. He nodded and lay down on the blue recliner and I placed his blanket over him. He tucked it under his chin and smiled.

"Thank you," he said, reminding me of a child.

Jack went on to accept medication and needed very little further mental health treatment. He was one of the few young people in my study who was hospitalized only once, to my knowledge. But Jack had a large family who loved him and a lot of resources. They circled around him and helped preserve his moral agency through this difficult time while also making sure he followed medical advice.

Amy, Corrina, and Miranda also eventually accepted mental health care for various reasons—housing, familial pressures, a way to move forward. Ariana was different—she refused care. On the day I met Ariana, a nurse told me to look for a first-timer in the "secondary" emergency room. This was a smaller, very dim, yellow-lit space where people who had been through the intake interview and thus "processed" then waited for up to 72 hours to see a doctor. At that point, they were either admitted (voluntarily or involuntarily), transferred to another inpatient facility, or discharged. Once there, I paused in another glassed-in nurses' station—a miniature version of the Control Center with a few chairs and a computer—to ask for help identifying Ariana.[3]

"Oh, *her.*" A nurse pointed at a young Latina in another recliner. "Good luck with her. She's not talking. She will just think you're part of 'The Conspiracy.'" A hand gesture of air quotes communicated how silly that idea seemed.

"She looks asleep," I noted.

"Oh, she's not asleep," another nurse said. "She hasn't slept since she came in two days ago. She's been in four-points twice already."

Three months later, Ariana told me how she had ended up being restrained and given injections of sedatives without permission.

> I wouldn't open my eyes. I remember that. I wouldn't open my eyes. And I thought it was the end of the world, blah blah blah, if I opened my eyes they would kill me, blah blah blah. And so they'll sedate me. And, apparently, they sedated me twice. I just remember one time. I was acting crazy. And they're like, "Okay, if you act crazy, they're going to take you up there because you're acting crazy." I know I would never try to hurt nobody, I just—they [her voices] don't want to open my eyes. I'm like, "Don't open my eyes!" I'm like, "Let me go! Let me go!"

When I saw Ariana's eyes flutter open, I scanned my badge again and entered the smaller patient area: here the recliners were packed side by side, and there was no gendered segregation that I could see. The Syfy Channel was playing on all the televisions but was mercifully on mute. Even so, it was showing bizarre scenes of witches and demons. It seemed like an odd choice.

I asked Ariana if I could sit with her, and she nodded yes. As soon as I sat down, though, she leaned in. Our heads were too close. She looked me straight in the eyes, our noses an inch or two apart. I felt uneasy.

A few days later, during a more formal interview, Ariana told the interviewer that she had a language barrier—English was her second language—and a hearing problem that made it hard to advocate for herself. She said:

> *ARIANA:* I don't ask questions because I can't hear, and if I can't hear you, then I'd just rather not. I try to get close, and people take it the wrong way. You have to talk loud enough so I can hear you and I feel intimidated by my hearing.
> *INTERVIEWER:* Right. Have you tried telling people that you can't hear?
> *ARIANA:* I tell them, but it's like they don't listen.

I felt badly when I learned about her communication concerns, because I had misinterpreted her proximity when we met. Her closeness made me uncomfortable. But at the time, I wanted to connect with her, so I forced myself to stay.

"Are you the chaplain?" she asked me.

"No, I am a volunteer here. Would you like to talk?" I showed her my volunteer badge.

Ariana pressed my arm with her hand. "I gave blood three times!"

"Oh, that's nice."

"In high school, like a charity thing."

I nodded.

"And I did pretty well in high school."

I nodded again. Looking back, now I can see that Ariana was trying to express some moral agency and signal to me that she was a "good" person even in this difficult place, but at the time I was too busy worrying about her distress and monitoring our physical proximity to notice. She fidgeted restlessly.

"Stop nodding!" She snapped. "Why are you nodding?"

"I am sorry," I said, confused that my body language had offended her.

She exhaled heavily into my face. "See?" She asked. "It's bad, right? It's bad breath. It's Ebeullah. We are all going to die of Ebeullah, which is in our lungs and it's spread through our bad breath."

I struggled not to nod my head again while Ariana continued exhaling heavily into my face. Her breath was terrible. Had she been offered a toothbrush?

To break our overwhelming proximity, I noted that the clock on the wall had stopped, and I pulled out my phone to check the time. Like Jack, Ariana immediately asked to use my phone.

"I want to know what's happening out there," she said in frustration.

I did not see a phone in the room, but I assured her the outside world was well and told her it was St. Patrick's Day.

"It is?" Another patient called to me across the dim space, suddenly creating a rare sense of community in a space where most people struggled alone.

"Really?" Another asked.

"Yes, it's March 17. St. Patrick's Day."

Ariana was still in her street clothes; she said she felt dirty. She was waiting for a shower, but there was only one, with an attendant who kept watch from the other side of the curtain. She rubbed her arms persistently, which she said ached where she had been restrained and injected with sedatives. She told me she was very tired. I suggested she rest.

Her posture softened. "Will you watch over me?" She whispered. "I am afraid, but I won't be afraid if you stay with me."

"Okay," I said, feeling maternal. "I can't promise I will be here when you wake up, though."

My mind raced. I thought of the late hour, my own young daughters, relieving the nanny, making dinner. But, as with Jack, I also felt her powerful need for someone benevolent to share space with her.

"I will just feel better if you are here," she said. Ariana needed to feel safe. I felt that I could offer this to her, at least.

She reclined her chair and closed her eyes. I tried to relax, but it was pointless. A few minutes later, Ariana was awake again, trying to explain about Ebeullah and how she was going to save the world, all the while exhaling long, warm, foul sighs into my face. She kept rubbing her sore arm, asking me about my religious beliefs, trying to see if we shared ideas about the Book of Revelation. Again, I later realized this may have been an attempt to establish herself as a "good" person and find some kind of common ethical ground, but in the moment, it was just tiring. I tried to be soothing and encourage her to relax, but she moaned, "But relaxing makes the voices louder!"

When the real chaplain came, I was greatly relieved. It is difficult to be present with people in the throes of psychosis. It can go on for days if they cannot sleep. Sofia's mom noted how hard it had been to keep watch over her for days when she could not sleep. I could imagine.

Ariana ended up being admitted to the hospital. Months later, she decided to completely refuse mental health care. I share more of her story in chapter 5, but one piece she reflected on when explaining that decision was this early hospitalization. She explained: "You're so scared. You don't know what's going on because you don't understand what's going on with you. And it's like, What the heck? It feels degrading and aggravating."

· · ·

Once they were processed through intake, patients were either admitted into the hospital with private insurance or—if they lacked coverage and had to use the regionally offered public mental health insurance[4]—it seemed to my team that they were then sent to the local state hospital. We were not able to get a clear answer about this during fieldwork, and when I tried to check retroactively as this book was going to press, no one could recall the policy in effect from 2014 to 2017, and the regional public insurance was no longer offered. However, during our fieldwork, a transfer to the state hospital seemed to happen consistently to people without private insurance and did not seem to happen to those with private coverage.

During our initial interview, only 9 participants claimed to have private insurance out of the 27 who answered the question; 10 had regional insurance, 1 had Medicaid, and 7 had no insurance. Miranda, Jack, and Corrina all had private mental health coverage through their parents. They never went to the state hospital. Amy did not have insurance, but her brother Robert panicked and purchased private insurance when he heard she might be sent to the state hospital if she had only public insurance. His alleged conversation with hospital staff was the closest we got to confirmation of this pattern during the study.

"They're like, 'We're gonna send her to [the state hospital],'" he explained. "That was the breaking point. I said, 'No, I'll pay. I'll pay. She's not . . . she's not going there. She's worth this,' I would tell the doctors. I begged for people to help her to get her out of that ER room." It turned out that Robert and Amy's grandmother had died in a state hospital after being hospitalized for schizophrenia. Robert could not bear to think of the same thing happening to Amy.

Sofia, James, Ariana, Latoya (mentioned below), and Michael all lacked insurance, and all went on to the state hospital about an hour's drive from Shady Elms. It could be that their families authorized it, but that's clear only in Michael's case, which I share below. Sofia's family definitely did not authorize the transfer, but Sofia may have agreed and cannot recall doing so. We don't have access to that information, and people were often confused about what happened. We do know that many people without private insurance went to the state hospital for a nearly month-long or longer stay.

The state hospital, built in 1885 in the old asylum style, consisted of a crumbling set of red-brick buildings with white columns—some boarded up and condemned, others still open for business.[5] One news report described one of the condemned buildings: "The roof leaks, stalactites and stalagmites grow on the second story, and yellow paint is peeling off the walls . . . Young patients [there . . .] walk past the building every day on their way from their dorm to their school."[6]

Every member of my research team, me included, felt haunted by the place. It was just spooky. There was even an old patient cemetery onsite. Visitor check-in, which my research team used regularly to visit young people in the study, was in a portable building. Visitors could meet for an hour or so each day with their loved one at a table there.

The people the team followed who were transferred to the state hospital were typically held for around 30 days total (including their time at Shady Elms) and we could only guess that this was to meet government readmissions requirements designed to "improve health care quality, improve the health of the US population, and reduce the costs of health care."[7] To meet these government standards for medical reimbursement, a patient could not be readmitted to the emergency room within 30 days of their last service. If they were, it counted against the quality metrics being used to evaluate the hospitals for Medicaid and Medicare reimbursement by the federal Centers for Medicare and Medicaid Services. To avoid penalties for the entire hospital in the event of excess readmissions, people who seemed as if they might be readmitted during that time had to be sent somewhere to make sure they were not. They needed to stay "admitted." Shady Elms could not really hold people that long, so they were sent to the state hospital. These rules apply to any psychiatric inpatient program that bills Medicaid or Medicare in the United States, and I have visited psychiatrists who ran psychiatric wards on the East Coast who have shared that their hospitals had similar practices.

However, a 30-day total psychiatric inpatient admission was highly disruptive for a young person. Coworkers, friends, roommates, teachers, and neighbors take notice when a young person is gone for an entire month. For first-timers, or any young person trying to keep their lives on track, this disruption was devastating, and it seemed to disproportionately affect the young people in our study who needed public insurance to cover the cost of mental health care.

Sofia remembered experiences at Shady Elms and then at the state hospital in an interview about four months after the research team met her. Her mom, Maria, had brought her to the county hospital after she noticed her declining college performance, but also, as revealed earlier, because Sofia refused to sleep inside.

> SOFIA: I just remember writing down information, and they wouldn't tell me anything. So I did not like it. I think that if I would have spoken with the doctor there, I wouldn't have gone to [the state hospital]. I think I could have been discharged immediately. I think I wouldn't have to have gone through all that, but I really don't remember what they did to me. I just remember like being at Shady Elms and then the next day just waking up and being at [the state hospital], so I don't remember that.
>
> INTERVIEWER: Really?
>
> SOFIA: I don't remember, that's why I don't know if they gave me some kind of injection and put me down to sleep or what they did. But I was perfectly fine in Shady Elms and then when I got to [the state hospital] I just remember having to speak with an attorney and having to sign the paper, and also signing to be part of a study, and that's all I remember when they took me to [the state hospital] but I don't remember.
>
> MARIA [in Spanish]: Yeah, I talked to the nurse. The nurse she told me, "She's okay, she speaks, she's okay, but she needs to move to [the state hospital]." I said, "Why?" "Because she needs to stay there, because here is only for emergency—for one day, two days."
>
> INTERVIEWER: Did you want her to go there?
>
> MARIA: And then I go see her the next day, but I don't see her. She said, "You need to wait 42 or 72 hours," or something like that [. . .] I had to go to a pastor that was there, I had to wait like three or four hours so that he could go in for me and I could know how my daughter was.
>
> SOFIA: Oh, I remember him talking to me once.
>
> MARIA: Yes, it was him. I had to go. I don't know how I thought about that, but I needed to know, so I saw that there was a pastor. They told me at what time he would be there. I waited for him. So then I went with him, and through him I found out about her.
>
> INTERVIEWER: That she was okay, because that was the only thing you wanted, to know that she was okay . . .

> *MARIA:* In Shady Elms, they wouldn't let me at all. But the good thing was that they took her quickly over there.
>
> *SOFIA:* They took me that same day.
>
> *MARIA:* Yes, 42 hours had to pass before they could tell me anything.
>
> *INTERVIEWER:* Why 42 hours?
>
> *MARIA:* Because they had to do paperwork and I don't know what else, supposedly. I don't know. Very strict.

Luckily, Sofia's mom had permission to ask about her, because Sofia had consented to sharing medical information with her. Maria went to visit her every day despite having to leave her other two daughters, the cost of gas, the long distance from the city, and her two jobs cleaning houses. Unfortunately, because she was at the state hospital for so long, Sofia lost her college scholarship.

"I think they did their best to help me out," Sofia reflected, "but I really wish I wouldn't have stayed there for so long. 'Cause it definitely does—it marks you. Something that's hard to, I don't know, to just kind of get over."

Looking back, Sofia decided to use mental health care because she was very afraid of being sent back to the hospital. Sofia and her mom explained:

> *MARIA [in Spanish]:* Yes, she is still with the fear of "it's going to happen again," and it's not something easy. Just by simply being in the hospital seeing the other patients, because when I would go see her, I would see her well compared to the others, and I myself would become traumatized from being there. From seeing the other people, because there is a lot of sick people. And she was not sick, but she was hearing everything and so she was getting traumatized. She became traumatized there.
>
> *INTERVIEWER:* It like adds on to the fear of going back and having those hard thoughts on top of all that.
>
> *MARIA:* Over everything it was the fear of being there.
>
> *INTERVIEWER:* Wow, how tough. And for you, was it the same fear of being like that?
>
> *SOFIA:* Yes, of going back.
>
> *MARIA:* Because she couldn't sleep, from the noise, because they would curse a lot. They would say a lot of nonsense. It's obvious that it is a hospital, but I think she couldn't be in a hospital like that.

. . .

Others, sometimes because they were confused or angry with their parents, refused to give permission for families to receive information. This may have also prevented family members from advocating for them or stepping in with private insurance as Robert had done for Amy. Miranda's mother, Angela, could not get any information about her, because Miranda had not consented to letting her mother hear more about her.

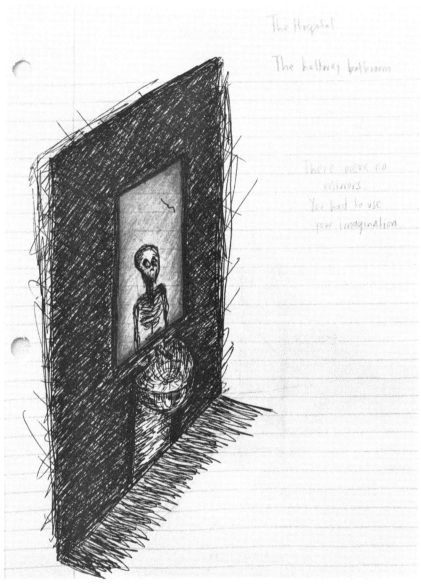

The Hospital

The hallway bathroom

There were no
mirrors.
You had to use
your imagination

FIGURE 4. "The Hospital: The hallway bathroom" by Lauren Ann Villarreal. The artist wrote the author in an email: "It is about my time in the mental hospital. As on the paper, there were no mirrors in the facilities, we had to use our imaginations. While I was there, I saw myself as already dead. The space was so traumatic, I was at the lowest place of my life. Not being able to see my reflection made me feel like I didn't exist anymore. Being there made me feel like the only way out, both from the hospital and my pain, was dying." *Reproduced with permission of the artist.*

"She thought I was the enemy. She wasn't allowing anyone to talk to me. So it was very difficult—very, very difficult. I even tried to get guardianship over her because I didn't know what was going to happen. How can they let her sign papers in this state of mind? How? I mean, I don't understand that."

Michael's family also had difficulty gaining information about his well-being once he was at Shady Elms. They had called the police when Michael tried to harm Liza's daughter, who (as related earlier) he thought was a demon. During an interview six months later with Liza and Michael, they explained what happened.

> *LIZA:* I called up there multiple times, and they wouldn't let me talk to any-
> body, but it was Michael who wouldn't let us know what was going on
> . . . I thought, if he just signed that paper for—what if someone can
> see what they were doing to him in the first place, then we can be like,
> "No, he don't take this [medicine]," but since he did his legal guardian
> himself, and he wasn't well, they could really do whatever they wanted
> to do, because—
>
> *MICHAEL:* I think the court . . . like, the judge, like, ordered it, for me to take it,
> so that's why they forced me to take it.
>
> *INTERVIEWER:* Right.
>
> *MICHAEL:* I don't know.

The judge eventually declared Michael incompetent, admitted him involuntarily, and contacted his mother. He asked her for permission to send Michael to the state hospital. She agreed.

Liza said they regretted it right away. "We thought it was something nice and it will help. We didn't know it was like—what I knew was crazy." She described how they had pictured it: like a place on television, a place to rest and relax, a place with a view and natural beauty. They clearly had no experience with this sort of institution.

Then, Liza confided in a friend.

> *LIZA:* When I said, "You know what, my brother is in [state hospital]," I told
> my friend, and she was like, "Where?" "In [state hospital]." And she is
> like, "Go get him out of that place." She told me, "Go get him out."
>
> *INTERVIEWER:* Wow.
>
> *LIZA:* She was like, "*People*, like—what?" The reaction—it was a negative
> reaction. You know? It was bad.

Unfortunately, Michael's mother had already signed the papers. She had tried to talk to Michael, but he was not making any sense. He had not taken any medications. She thought the hospital would help.

Later, Michael said, "I think you guys kinda got to understand, like, at that time I wasn't in the right mind. I was like thinking my family was like secret organ— organizations."

Michael was confused. His family was confused. People did not have the right information. It was hard to make good decisions about treatment. Options were limited by insurance and the cost of private care.

Other young people were cut off from their families. Some were not clear about where their families were, and their families did not visit them. One Latina who did not follow up with my team after she left the hospital claimed: "The major challenge I am facing is not actually being in my family on a daily basis and saying that they're with me and knowing that I'm not crazy."

Another young Latino shared in Spanish: "I am simply waiting until I finish my imprisonment here and that I can go back to see my brothers. I'm happy to go start a new chapter in my aunt's apartment and begin a new chapter with them without fighting and without lying, getting along well with everybody."

"But have you been comfortable here?" a member of my team asked.

"Kind of. Not very well because I haven't slept. I have not been at peace because I am surrounded with people that are not my family, people who are white, they are Black, I don't know what type of problems they have about my culture. I don't know what kind of problems they have, what else they can add on to my case."

He also wanted to find the staff members in authority: "Because the ones that know about one are the ones that know more: when the time comes for one to leave, to make decisions about going outside, being able to go to the park, being able to go eat lunch, or being able to go anywhere else with their authority. Because without their authority we are just whatever. We are all the same. We are all like mosquitoes."

Patients with their own children faced additional challenges. Among the young people in my study, 10 were parents of small children and 7 of those self-identified as Latino—2 fathers and 5 mothers. The others were 1 African American parent, 1 South Asian parent, and 1 white parent.[8]

One young, hijab-wearing woman I met in the hospital, Haniya, was a first-generation immigrant from South Asia. Haniya missed her mother, whom she had not seen in a couple of years. She was hearing voices and felt that "everyone is reading my mind and I feel very ashamed of it. I think something or I do something, and my body sends a very wrong message." She had told the intake nurses that she heard voices telling her to harm her children and the Department of Family Services had become involved out of concern for her children's welfare. Haniya was pregnant and desperately wanted to see her two young children and husband. She stayed at Shady Elms for three weeks (she had private insurance), but the research team was not able to follow up with her after she was discharged home.

A young African American woman, Latoya, had also been sent from Shady Elms to the state hospital when we followed up with her. Latoya stayed there for at least six months, the length of our follow-up time with her. During one visit, she told the interviewer that she thought her stay had been extended when she became upset at having to leave her daughter at the end of a visit. Latoya lashed out verbally at another patient then shoved her out of her way.

"I was angry 'cause I had to leave, and she [the daughter] was crying and screaming. And I just seen her outside the window. My mom stood there outside the window [holding her daughter]. And I was standing inside and [the nurse] was just standing there. And I was like, Just walk off, just walk off. I was just mad. I was like, 'My baby is leaving and she don't want to go.'" Latoya said she tried to explain her behavior to the doctor, but he said she had to stay at the hospital longer for acting out against others. Latoya felt he had dismissed her pleas.

"They can do anything they want to do to you in a crazy home, am I right?" Latoya observed. "Anything they want. If you say anything, you're crazy." After a six-month stay at the state hospital, Latoya surely knew better than me.

Another young woman, Lucia, had a three-week-old infant whom she was not allowed to see. Her family had found her wandering outside in the middle of the night carrying her naked newborn. She refused to go home or let them take her child. Her mother called the police for help, and she was hospitalized at Shady Elms with postpartum psychosis. Lucia's breasts visibly leaked milk during our early visits, and she was not offered a pump but was instead advised to let her milk dry up since she would not be able to breastfeed due to her medications. She cried for weeks, which did not help her in ending her confinement. It took her weeks to get back to her child. Research shows that incarcerated mothers experience a sense of loss; separation from their children also seemed painful for mothers in long-term inpatient care.[9]

· · ·

Separated from their loved ones, feeling embarrassed and ashamed for events they had trouble remembering, lacking their cell phones, and denied basic information ranging from the time, location, and date to how to use the public phone and what they were even doing in the hospital and for how long, it is no wonder that many young people felt extremely disoriented during their early hospitalization. Ideally, this first exposure to care would be one that helped a person orient to a future of seeking out mental health support for safety, empowerment, and belonging with others who understood them, but most young people I engaged with did not have that experience the first time they accessed mental health care in these emergency circumstances.

Instead, many felt that they had somehow been placed in the wrong environment. Several seemed to be making a concentrated effort to distinguish themselves from the "bad" people around them, such as the people Maria felt had traumatized her and Sofia. The young people the research team talked with emphasized that they were not on drugs, or stupid, or trying to scam the system and get a free place to stay like some of the more experienced mental health service users they met in the hospital. Many also insisted that they were not "crazy."

As Veronica, whose sister dropped her off (chapter 3) said, "There are people here that are supposed to be here. People here who actually have drinking and alcohol and drug problems, and psychos. [. . .] I'm put in here because, not because I'm crazy or because I'm . . . but because I'm different."

Gideon, the young man who tried to heal people in Starbuck's, felt similarly. He had never used alcohol or drugs. Other patients teased him in the Narcotics Anonymous and Alcoholics Anonymous groups he attended at Shady Elms for never having tried anything. "Being brought here is like a worst nightmare. I try my best to always stay clean and always be clean. I have Black friends drinking alcohol and everything. I'd just find an excuse." This frustrated him. "Yeah, that's why I'm angry. [. . .] I have nothing wrong with me. I'm just fine."

"Do you feel fine?" I asked.

"Completely fine, trust me. I'm even better than the so-called normal people out there," Gideon replied.

Sage, a young African American woman whose story is fleshed out more in chapter 6, was an inpatient at Shady Elms for the longest period of anyone in our study—perhaps because she had private insurance through her parents (making her a high-paying client for the hospital) and refused medication. She pointed to her social media feed as evidence of her social worth.

"I have Instagram, and you can just do your research because I know people think I am crazy, but I am really not, and you will see. You will be able to tell how I really am. [. . .] I mean, people judge a book by its cover; people think I don't have a brain, I'm just retarded, and I look funny, but no. I have more of a brain than a lot of people."

Later, she added, "I don't think this facility is logical, because I'm wasting—it's expensive to stay here and I'm wasting my time. I could be doing my college. I am laying in a bed because I don't think I should interact with some of the people because they have—we're on different levels. It's like they actually need help. And, honestly, I don't think I need help."

Markus, the young Black man introduced in chapter 2 who was struggling with psychosis symptoms and who would go on to refuse care, also felt he did not see people who were like him in the hospital.

MARKUS: When I was in that hospital, I didn't really meet people like me; I met people, either they weren't in a school, or they weren't in a university, or they were disadvantaged in some sort of way. I don't know. I felt like there was no one around who had an experience similar to what I went through.

INTERVIEWER: Okay. So it didn't seem like that was the right place for you, or do you think?

MARKUS: Not at all, I didn't think I needed to be there, you know. The workers at the hospital tell me, "I don't think you even need to be here."

The young people were looking for others who looked like them, who had similar experiences, who were getting help and getting better and moving on. Those connections would have helped them make sense of their life stories. Instead, they found themselves mixed in with the people they perceived to be addicts, "psychos," and people who they felt were just trying to "get things for free."

Keep in mind that while my research team was meeting with young people with many things in common, they rarely came across other young first-timers. None of our participants got to know each other (or even met, to our knowledge), in the hospital or elsewhere. They were not being oriented to a new community of supportive young people who had been through similar events. Instead, people who had already been disoriented by the symptoms and the people around them were being persistently further disoriented—from their loved ones, their everyday lives and identities, and their sense that they could be a moral agent—a "good" and competent future adult. Their hospitalizations offered a sustained assault on their sense of personal well-being and potential. This is not unusual: most individuals who use emergency departments for mental health care view their experiences as negative.[10]

This is not to say that people who provide mental health emergency services are bad people. Most were trying hard to understand and serve the people on their caseload. The staff the research team interacted with informally had useful insights into the injustices people experienced in the hospital and the mental health system. However, in this emergency setting, things moved very quickly. Patients were unpredictable. The staff worked amid a continual fear of danger and a sense that their hypervigilance and enforcement of firm social, physical, and emotional boundaries were imperative.

Mental health workers with their own traumatic histories may have been especially triggered by this setting. I know it was highly triggering for my research team, something each of us struggled with and, over time, talked about in team meetings or sometimes on our way to or from our paired research visits. I also advised everyone on the team to see a therapist when they joined the team so they would have a neutral person to talk to, as well—a service partially covered by SMU insurance.

And we were not even feeling responsible for people's care or outcomes. Studies suggest that those who were—nearly half of mental health professionals—experience burnout.[11] This group includes psychiatrists, over half of whom report burnout early in their careers.[12] Specific reasons for burnout may include lack of perceived job control, heavy caseloads, the mental health professional's own mental health history (many are called to this line of work for a reason—personal or familial), and limited or poor supervisory support.[13]

The ways Americans respond to mental health emergencies can no doubt be traumatic, both for staff and the patients they serve. All these findings point to the strong need for more trauma-informed care in inpatient settings. Trauma-informed care focuses on not *re*traumatizing patients with procedures that resemble aspects of past abuse or violence, such as using handcuffs or restraints, forced or threatened medications, involuntary commitment, boundary violations, or police "takedowns" or exposing people to other, extremely sick or frightening patients.[14]

These recommendations are important because many of the young people the research team engaged with had significant trauma histories and so were vulnerable to the possibility of being retraumatized. Previous chapters mention some of the connections between stress and psychosis, but to be clear: two-thirds of our participants had a significant traumatic experience that occurred at some point during their lives such as physical assault, sexual assault, or the death of a parent, and my research team was not asking explicitly about trauma in our interviews, because we were focused more on experiences of care and how that affected treatment decision making. These past events just came up. Many of the traumatic events they shared had happened in childhood. But given that the interview protocol and demographics sheets did not ask explicitly about trauma, we missed the opportunity to document systematically the potential traumatic impact of structural racism, inequality, colonialism, and war on the immigrants and persons from ethnoracially minoritized groups in the study.[15] Future research might delve more specifically into these areas.

The negative mental health impacts of traumatic life experiences make a person more likely to experience a psychiatric hospitalization, which is then often a retraumatizing experience. Research suggests that traumatic stress is at the root of many experiences and behaviors that lead to a psychiatric hospitalization for children and youths.[16] Among adults, 25 percent of men and 40 percent of women in inpatient psychiatric units had a history of interpersonal trauma.[17] In one study, nearly all of the adolescents in an inpatient psychiatric unit reported exposure to at least one traumatic event such as being a witness to or victim of community violence, witnessing family violence, or being the victim of physical or sexual abuse.[18] Evidence also points to a dose-response effect in which the severity of one's clinical symptoms reflects the "dose" of trauma they have experienced.[19]

Not surprisingly, high levels of childhood adversity have also been associated with the presence and persistence of psychotic experiences.[20] Childhood trauma is common for people experiencing psychosis,[21] and individuals with a psychotic disorder are more likely than those without one to have experienced childhood trauma of all kinds (e.g., emotional, physical, sexual).[22] Individuals who experience childhood sexual abuse are more than twice as likely to develop psychosis as those who do not.[23] Moreover, recent evidence suggests that sexual assault or abuse at any point also makes a person more vulnerable to developing psychosis.[24] Lady Gaga's revelation that she experienced psychosis in the aftermath of sexual assault when she was 19 years old is only one of many examples.[25]

The research literature and my data both make plain that young people with early psychosis are likely to have experienced significant trauma. Yet our current forms of care fail to address this likelihood. People experiencing mental health issues have described how the emergency room environment can trigger fears or traumatic memories, which may stop them from seeking support.[26] Harsh lighting, strong smells, high noise levels, and a hectic environment can increase patients' stress, trigger feelings of panic, and have a negative effect on their well-being and ability to cope.[27] Emergency rooms lack private or quiet therapeutic spaces, making people less willing to disclose mental health issues.[28] All of these conditions could definitely be found at Shady Elms.

Moreover, in several studies that explored the experiences of people with mental health issues, patients described emergency department staff's communication with them as "pushy," disrespectful, insensitive, and judgmental.[29] Patients felt dismissed and stigmatized and were unsure whether emergency department staff understood their needs.[30] This may be especially relevant in nonpsychiatric emergency spaces where the focus is not on mental health treatment.

Although Shady Elms *was* dedicated to psychiatric emergencies, there were still traumatizing procedures. Demeaning physical examinations like the "squat and cough" routine that Miranda experienced can also cause unintentional harm to patients.[31] These perceptions can be exacerbated by staff threats of using force or the actual use of force, with patients describing being yelled at, held down, and restrained—all practices that I witnessed during my time there.[32] These staff behaviors and methods can increase the severity of patients' signs and symptoms, heighten their risk of suicide, and reduce their willingness to seek support in the future.[33] Long waiting times before visiting with a medical professional like a psychiatrist—also common at Shady Elms—also contributed to people's concerns about compromised care, exacerbating their hopelessness, disempowerment, anxiety, and fear of being held against their will.[34]

Nor do the problems stop at the emergency room. One rigorous study revealed high rates of reported lifetime trauma occurring in all psychiatric settings, with one-third of patients reporting physical assault, nearly one-tenth reporting sexual assault, and almost two-thirds witnessing traumatic events.[35] Over half were frightened by the dangers posed by other patients. Reported rates of institutional measures of last resort were also high: two-thirds had been handcuffed, more than half reported involuntary restraint, and nearly one-third reported experiencing a "takedown." From start to finish, the current emergency health care system takes an already traumatized and stressed population and subjects them to more trauma and stress. It also offers very little training, supervision, or support for the mental health professionals trying to help them, who themselves are exposed to trauma and suffer from burnout.

· · ·

This chapter indicates some of the many ways that a psychiatric hospitalization can be traumatic: by stripping a person of their identity, their loved ones, and their safe space; by denying them ways to orient in space and time; by making them feel disempowered through subjecting them to strong authority figures who allow them little power or say over what happens to them; by denying them collaborative conversations whereby they work together to plan the next steps of their treatment; by using restraints; by forcing people to take medications against their will—the list goes on.

These sources of possible trauma led me to wonder, Is there an evidence base for how to do trauma-informed work in psychiatric settings? Are there existing practices that can help people with traumatic histories have a less disorienting and traumatizing hospitalization experience? The answer is yes. From my review of the research, I found a lot of good information about what to do and not to do to reduce and address trauma in psychiatric settings. These best (and worst) practices are discussed in chapter 7, but now we turn our attention to what happened to the young persons during the critical period after discharge, when positive outcomes are typically thought to result from continuing treatment. It turns out that many young people do not follow up with any mental health provider. For the persons in our study, we observed how they made decisions about whether using mental health care was going to help them move toward the future they had envisioned for themselves or if they instead refused the care on offer. More important, we wanted to know why they decided one way or the other.

5

Users and Refusers

Basically, they just send you out, and they're like, "Well, looks dismal. Looks gray. They can either recover and figure out how to fix this on their own, or they can just probably off themselves."

—AMY, AT STARBUCKS, WEEK 12

Pedro was an easygoing Hispanic youth with kind, amber eyes who quickly put people at ease. He was the youngest of six boys followed by three more sisters. Pedro said he had moved to the United States when he was six, but that his parents were Tejanos—which he described as the Mexicans who lived in Texas before it became part of the United States.

Though intelligent and dynamic, Pedro had always struggled to belong. In his first interview, he explained: "I was always tired. I didn't want to go to school anymore. It was just a bad time. And people tried to pick on me—bullying, harassment, racial profiling, all of that. I left high school in the eleventh grade and decided that was it. I was already 18. I went and got my home-school diploma."

He tried starting a career without a college degree, but didn't get very far, so he went to community college to start working toward a four-year degree. When my team first met up with him at Shady Elms, he was on mandatory leave from a four-year college that he had transferred to that year.

Pedro said his father served in Vietnam and then later worked for the FBI to help take down the "Cocaine Cowboys," which is also the title of a crime documentary released in 2006 about the police taking out a drug-trafficking ring in Miami in the 1980s.[1] His father had a posttraumatic stress disorder (PTSD) diagnosis from these experiences, Pedro said, adding that he, too, had been diagnosed with PTSD when he was 6 years old. He had also been diagnosed with attention deficit hyperactivity disorder (ADHD).

It is hard to know which parts of Pedro's story are true, but clearly the world of drug traffickers and the potential for violent death had become a sticky place in his mind—a theme that preoccupied him. Pedro lived in a social context where drug trafficking and people being murdered for their involvement was very real. The US "war on drugs" started in 1971 when Richard Nixon declared "drug abuse," or the use of illegal narcotics, to be "public enemy number one."[2] The "war" began with strict laws and harsh penalties that ultimately came down hardest on small-time dealers or people experiencing substance use disorders in the United States, and the policy approach has been criticized for its long-term negative consequences for American communities of color.[3] In countries that were supplying cocaine and heroin to the United States, the war on drugs meant destroying coca and poppy plants and supplying local security forces with arms to take on organized drug lords.[4] These activities seriously impacted countries in Central and Latin America and the Caribbean where organized crime in the form of "cartels" battled with those trying to stop drug trafficking to North America.

The negative effects of the US-backed War on Drugs continue to be seen today.[5] In 2018, Latin America was home to 8 percent of the world's population but had over one-third of its total homicides. While drug trafficking is not entirely to blame, places like El Salvador, where two rival gangs have declared a truce still in effect at this writing, have seen a sharp decline in the murder rate.[6] While some white residents have also been affected by drug-related violence, Latinx US residents are more likely to experience drug war–related trauma than white residents.[7]

It was in this social context that Pedro developed the understanding that he was being stalked by Central American gang members in the guise of women who drank alcohol. He called them the "Liquor Ladies." He thought the Liquor Ladies were trying to murder him for his connections to his father. Pedro knew who they were and what they looked like, but no one else he knew personally had seen them. Pedro saw them all the time before his hospitalization. He saw them when he went to clubs with his fraternity brothers. They left him secret messages on Facebook that vanished after he read them. They appeared on his college campus, too—in the library and in his classroom during exams. They distracted him so much that he failed his classes.

Pedro's college was a few hours away from home, so his family did not realize something was seriously wrong until he began posting comments about these Liquor Ladies on Facebook. He posted pictures of random women consuming alcohol and demanded they leave him alone or he would hurt them. Concerned, his family obtained a warrant from the local magistrate while he was home during a school break, which enabled the police to escort Pedro to Shady Elms for further evaluation without his permission.

Once there, he reported that he was forced to take a medication that made it difficult to breathe. He explained: "The prescriptions . . . I had a hard time breathing so I stopped taking them and I was able to breathe better. I just had a hard time sleeping at night."

Pedro was also dealing with other stressors. Prior to his break, he had been placed on a three-semester forced leave from college for poor performance. Even so, his student loans were still due because he had been dismissed after the deadline for a refund. He needed to work to pay the loans, but the only jobs he could get required hard labor, which he did not enjoy. He had gone to college to avoid these jobs, and now his college loans were forcing him into them.

A couple of weeks after he stopped taking his medication, Pedro decided that if he burned his clothes—a technique he thought might help to get rid of "bad vibes"—he would feel better. Pedro's family understandably saw his effort to burn his clothes as a complete break with reality rather than an attempt to restore things to normal. They asked the magistrate for another warrant.

This time, the police took him to the county hospital, where he stayed overnight while he waited for a bed at Shady Elms. At the county hospital, he claimed, "the doctor laughed at me. He said I was mania, and I was like, 'What the hell?' I go, 'What's so funny?' and I asked him for his license number, and he laughed at me even more. Even his medical student was like, 'What the hell?'"

Pedro thought the medical student also felt this doctor was out of line. The doctor's dismissive attitude triggered something in him. Pedro reflected, "It kind of broke me down and [. . .] the next few days I kind of got myself together. And they transferred me to [the state hospital] . . . So I was pretty much in the hospital for a month." The state hospital, of course: Pedro had no private insurance.

One of my team members asked, "How was that?"

"It was kind of heartbreaking; it was a little bit depressing. But I was able to get myself together and realize what was going on. And then the medication that they gave me originally . . . it would have clogged up my nose. I wasn't able to breathe. So now they've given me a different medication. So now I'm able to breathe and I feel positive about things now."

"That's good."

"With my PTSD, it helps a little bit."

However, while he was open to his new medication—for his PTSD—Pedro was skeptical of the mental health care he had received. Things did not seem quite right to him:

> PEDRO: To me, it's like one of those things that—how can you diagnose that quick?
>
> INTERVIEWER: Yeah, you get ten, fifteen minutes maybe.
>
> PEDRO: Not just that, but you're seeing somebody that you don't know. It's somebody that just walks in and reads the chart and just throws you out to the side, like you're a piece of garbage.
>
> INTERVIEWER: Yeah, is that how you felt?
>
> PEDRO: It just didn't make sense to me, the system that they have.

Pedro thought he had been diagnosed as "mania," which he would later call bipolar disorder, but he described his main challenge as "mostly just my PTSD straining me." He added, "I have ADHD and I'm dyslexic. I'm still able to overcome things when I really want to do them, and my family knows about that. And college is hard, but if I really put my effort in, I am able to overcome everything." Pedro's family knew about PTSD—a diagnosis his father had apparently been given—and that diagnosis was acceptable in their local moral world. For them, PTSD signaled service to one's country—as when Pedro's father helped the FBI and served in Vietnam—something to be proud of.

However, he did not feel he had a chance to discuss his "mania" or "bipolar" diagnosis with his doctor. "I was there for three weeks," he said. "I only saw the doctor twice. That's something that I didn't feel comfortable with. I said, 'What's the whole point of being here if I'm only going to see a doctor once or twice?' Then he sees you in front of six other people so it gives you that uncomfortable feeling where you can't open up. Gives you that feeling where you feel kind of down and you're like, 'Okay.'"

Pedro wanted more privacy—something he said he did not get with the college counseling center, either, because he thought the walls were too thin.

> *PEDRO:* I would say, in general, even for doctors it's hard to diagnose people with . . . It's one of those things that with time and with your life going on—I think, yes and no bipolar exists, but I think there's other ways besides pills and medications . . . I think with time . . . I do think bipolar exists, but I don't think it's as bad. I think some MDs [and] patients kind of exaggerate about it. I think it's something that with working, having a job . . . I think it's one of those things that—yes, it exists, but I just don't think it's as bad as people make it.
>
> *INTERVIEWER:* Do you think that that diagnosis fits your experience, or are you skeptical about it?
>
> *PEDRO:* In general, I think for them to diagnose people with bipolar, I feel like it should be more than just having a brief conversation with a few people. I think it should be something where you're able to, not just that, but you're able to work out, or do this—have more interactions with people for them to diagnose it. I would say it's not just something that you just sit there, and you have your bed in the next room. I think it's something that should be more than just that . . . it's claustrophobic being in the room.

Pedro needed more time and attention from the doctor after receiving a major diagnosis, a diagnosis that put him in "the room" or, as others described it, "in a box." It was disconcerting and suffocating. Pedro could not breathe.

His first doctor at Shady Elms, Pedro recalled, was nice, which was one of the reasons why he was willing to continue to seek help through mental health care. He described the doctor as Hispanic, which helped Pedro feel a connection.[8] When asked to share more about that relationship, he said: "It was just more interaction with the doctor. He would come in and ask me if I was okay. He would at least see me once a day or every other day." This personal attention meant a lot to Pedro.

Pedro thought ideal forms of mental health care would include a half hour per day with the doctor and a few other trusted people, such as other patients and family members, "where you can sit down, or play something, and have a few people hang out with you . . . it makes a big difference." He wanted to have more time engaged with something, "like therapy, where you have different activities, and you can actually express yourself." He needed relationships, interactions, opportunities for self-expression—a shared moral world—in order to heal.

After his discharge from the hospital, Pedro did attend his follow-up appointments, or "med checks," though he—like many others—found them unsatisfying:

> The follow-ups, that's another thing. There's the nurse sitting at the desk; you just go and sit down, and they ask you a few questions that you answer and that's pretty much it. They check your vitals and that's it. It's just a ten-minute walk-in. [. . .] They just ask you the same questions and that's pretty much it. [. . .] I just don't want to go in there, sit down, answer the same questions. She's at the computer typing a yes or no, or I don't know what she's doing. I just feel like it's redundant.

So, why did Pedro continue with care even though he felt misrecognized and misdiagnosed and needed more time and attention? Pedro had decided to apply for "disability," or a US government stipend through Social Security Disability Insurance (SSDI).[9] According to a US government publication, the Social Security Administration "pays benefits to people who can't work because they have a medical condition that's expected to last at least one year or result in death."[10] Pedro's father received disability payments to help support the family financially, because he had PTSD, which made it difficult for him to work. Pedro also said that several "college students" advised him that Social Security helped them not have to work while they were also trying to succeed at school. He accentuated that all "the college students" do it and so he was going to try, as well. In his way, even though he was asking for government support, Pedro was trying to maintain his social bases of self-respect by asking for it in a way that was respected in his local moral world.[11]

About two months after Pedro's first hospitalization, he was adapting to the new medications and applying for disability. He could breathe better on his new medications, but they also initially made him sleep all the time. However, after six weeks or so, he reported, "I'm staying awake more often in the day, so it's still much better."

After about four months, Pedro was confident that the medication was helping and described using medications as essential to his health care. He was also delighted to report that he had been invited to his niece's birthday party. While at the party, Pedro thought the medications made it possible for him to interact with other people and enjoy himself—something he felt had become difficult prior to treatment.

His family did not talk about his illness, though, and they never agreed to meet the research team. "When things change for the better, we don't like to talk about it," he explained. "We just kind of let it go. We just don't like thinking about the past. It's kind of where you're like, 'Yeah, it was a bad scene but blah blah blah.' We kind of blow it off, you know what I mean? We start over and that's pretty much how we work. We don't like to go back unless it's something real important and we need to go back. We'll resist something." For Pedro, his family was a *we*, which was highly meaningful for him.

During his treatment, he continued trying to save money until his school lifted his suspension. He could not afford a gym membership—something he thought would be helpful for young people struggling with mental health issues—so he ran several miles each day in the Texas heat. All the while, he kept his eyes peeled for any sighting of the Liquor Ladies. The local police, he told my team, had promised him that if they came around again they would arrest them and put a restraining order on them. He trusted the police since his Dad had served in law enforcement. Pedro was hopeful that if the Liquor Ladies were arrested, he could finally prove to everyone that it was not all in his head. He especially hoped his school would return his student loans that he lost during the semester when those girls harassed him until he failed his classes.

In his story, we can see how Pedro was slowly securing his moral agency on his own terms with the help of his loved ones. He built up autobiographical power by editing the narrative about his diagnosis and experiences with the support of family.[12] He insisted that he had long-term PTSD like his Dad, that it was nothing new for him, and that his family did not object. The Liquor Ladies were real; the local police were looking for them to arrest them. At the same time, he stopped posting on Facebook about them because he recognized that it was not helping him be seen as a moral agent. Whatever the veracity of these statements, they were helping Pedro heal morally.

With his moral world secure, he accepted medical and material help. He took his medications and applied for social security disability because the cost to his local moral world in doing so was not prohibitively high. The people that mattered to him did not accuse him of being an addict or dependent on the government for accepting these supports. He even claimed that "most college kids were doing it." Once he stopped sleeping all the time and adjusted to the medications, he was grateful that they helped him interact with people. He went to his niece's birthday party and had a good time. These were also signals that he was replenishing his social bases of self-respect and expanding peopled opportunities as his family embraced and included him. By editing his story his own way, Pedro replenished his moral agency, at least with his family, and in the process moved toward feeling better.

Not everyone had Pedro's eventual success navigating the minefields in the post-crisis stages of treatment for psychosis. All struggled with, and at times refused, the care on offer: the diagnosis, the medications, and for some, the possibility of seeking out disability support. Some seemed to strategically use care to replenish their moral agency in those first few months: these were the treatment users.

. . .

Others ultimately refused care. These young people were treatment refusers. Ariana was one of them. Chapter 4 leaves Ariana's story at the point where she had been forcibly restrained and medicated, was terrified that the world was ending, and was waiting for the hospital chaplain. My research team talked to her again about a week later at the state hospital where she had been transferred (again, she had no insurance).

During that interview, and several that followed, Ariana reflected on her time at Shady Elms. She described being discredited multiple times while trying to tell her own story, which she felt the nurses dismissed as evidence of her delusional paranoia. However, as with Pedro, her paranoia likely had some basis in consensual reality. At the state hospital, she shared vivid stories of "war on drugs"–related violence that she had witnessed as a child, including a man pushed to his death from a moving vehicle and the arrest and imprisonment of her father when she was a young teen. She also shared teenage experiences of sexual assault and a recent miscarriage. She said that her recognizably "Cartel" last name made her a target.

This was "the Conspiracy" that the nurses dismissed during my first attempt to visit with her. It is quite possible Ariana's psychotic break had its roots in repeated traumatic life experiences. However, Ariana told my team that her admission notes (which she had requested) stated only that she was delusional and confused.

"I guess the counselor, whoever that is, he really didn't believe what I had to say about my dad," she said. This made Ariana feel isolated, misunderstood, and dismissed, which eroded her sense of moral agency.

Ariana understood that her thoughts were at times unreasonable. "Right now," she said in her interview at Shady Elms, "I am just paranoid, thinking that I connect all the dots and it leads to all the information, that cartel and that. And sometimes not even in . . . I'm connecting dots that are not even there."

"And you say you're connecting dots that are not there?" the interviewer asked.

"Well I kind of do and I kind of don't."

"Okay, what does that mean?"

"I'm hoping that I am just connecting dots that are not there."

And while she understood that her ideas were "stressing her out," she had few opportunities to work through these ideas in the hospital. "I feel that I'm normal," she explained, "and probably everybody else here feels that they're normal. And I just need, they say, to take a chill pill. And just pray more and read more. [. . .] But they're trying to erase my identity. Who I am. That's how I feel." Many of the young people the team talked with felt as if no one was listening to them or taking them seriously. Rather than feeling heard, they felt erased, even "omitted."

That a psychiatric diagnosis is made by mental health professionals based on their own subjective interpretation of what is going on with the patient presents a problem. At Shady Elms, the psychiatrist on call typically spent about ten minutes with each patient during their stay in the emergency room. They glanced over the notes of the intake nurse and then determined a diagnosis to enter into the electronic health record. This diagnosis was used to decide medical treatment and the length of stay, prescribe medications, bill the appropriate insurance, and make recommendations for next steps in care. If involuntary admission was recommended, the doctor signed paperwork for the judge to evaluate on site (as with Michael). It also factored into a person's ability to apply for a psychiatric disability income later. The diagnosis of a psychotic disorder thus had serious legal, financial, and medical implications. For the young person, the diagnosis also had major implications for their sense of self, their relationships with others, and their perceptions of mental health care.

While looking through the Shady Elms electronic health records to screen for participants, my team noticed that the psychiatrists typically labeled first-timers as having a diagnosis of psychosis NOS (not otherwise specified). However, there was no rule of thumb for arriving at this diagnosis. The psychiatrists I asked at Shady Elms and elsewhere all had their own tools and tricks for assessing which diagnosis to offer, making it seem subjective to outsiders, though perhaps not to a psychiatrist who had been through a decade or so of training.

In addition, psychiatrists and other staff were under pressure to meet with patients and produce the necessary paperwork about risk assessment, suicidality, dangerousness to self and others, and so forth, which, as one psychiatrist told me, "has nothing to do with the patient and everything to do with covering the hospital's ass in case of an accident." The pressures of documentation, the chaotic environment of Shady Elms, the endless line of people needing a diagnosis, and the quality and completeness of the notes made by the intake nurse and treatment team all shaped the doctor's decisions.

This perplexed many of the youths who expected their diagnosis and treatment to be based on tangible scientific evidence. In the American imagination, medicine and its biotechnologies have great potential and engender hope for patients who use them.[13] Americans expect technology and science to be part of their health care. Many youths in our study were skeptical because their diagnostic process (from their perspective) had involved no scientific evidence.

Corrina was one of these people. A few months after her diagnosis, she told me, "I think simply because there are no tests, just like with the rest of medicine, you can be like, 'Okay, you have diabetes. I've done the bloodwork. This is what we do for diabetes.' But with this, it's totally different, because nobody knows what's going on inside anyone's head, psychologically or chemically."

Ariana was also a skeptic. She could not understand how her diagnosis had been made in the absence of any technical evidence.

ARIANA: What was it they diagnosed me again? [. . .] Psychosis.

INTERVIEWER: Okay.

ARIANA: And I looked up the dictionary what "psychosis" means, and you don't put reality—that you're living a fantasy life.

INTERVIEWER: Okay.

ARIANA: I'm like, psychosis? I'm here. I'm all here, you know? It's just, yeah, issues with my Dad was affecting me, which I realized what my Dad did doesn't affect me.

INTERVIEWER: Right.

ARIANA: How do you know there's something wrong with my brain when you haven't actually looked at it? That's what I'm saying.

INTERVIEWER: Right. Right. Yeah.

ARIANA: I'm like, "Don't you need to see my brain first to judge it and say there's something wrong with it?"

INTERVIEWER: Right. Right.

ARIANA: That's just my opinion. I'm no doctor . . . But yeah, I didn't like what they diagnosed me with. I guess I'm just going to have to stay with this treatment and prove them wrong. I don't live in no fantasy life. My life is as real as his.

INTERVIEWER: Yeah. So, how did that make you feel when—?

ARIANA: It just, it got me confused. I'm like, really? That's what he thinks? Everybody has their own opinion, and that's his opinion . . . I'm still going to be taking the treatments just to prove them wrong, because how can they know what's wrong with me when they haven't gave me, you know, they haven't gave me a physical or anything like that?

Then the interviewer asked what she thought would be ideal mental health care in the future.

ARIANA: You examine the brain. I'm like, how can you just tell? How can you just say, "Oh, that person's such and such," because of what they speak? And like sometimes you can't express everything you feel. Examine the brain. Look at—you know, I don't know what they do or what's the process to look at an X-ray or check all of—what's wrong with the brain? But like examine the brain first.

Diagnosis literally means "to be known through." Psychosis has no definitive biomarkers like a blood test, and so diagnosis is an interpretive process. With many assumptions being made by the doctor—ideally based on their clinical experience and sensitivity—a diagnosis so made can have a powerful impact on one's sense of identity and moral agency.[14] For many people, being diagnosed with a highly stigmatized and serious illness based on some intake notes and ten minutes of being asked unusual questions seemed arbitrary and often did not

match their own version of events. Pedro was being stalked by his father's ene-
mies. Ariana was just struggling with the situation with her dad. James's parents were denying the celebrities access to him because they did not want him to
become famous. Miranda's parents were keeping her from Sean because they did
not want her to grow up.

Given their convictions about what was going on with them, the seemingly
quick and severe diagnoses they received only seeded their distrust of the mental
health professionals, who they felt did not know them. It was disempowering and
sometimes scary for them to be "known" in a way that had such strong implications based on so little evidence.

Corrina described her thoughts about her diagnosis a few weeks after
her hospitalization:

> *CORRINA:* The one thing that I can say that's really weird is being diagnosed with
> psychosis unspecified disorder, and that freaks me out a little bit.
>
> *NEELY:* Can you tell us a little more about that?
>
> *CORRINA:* Yeah. He said that I have PTSD and unspecified psychosis disorder,
> 'cause he can't figure out necessarily what's wrong. So it's just weird. I
> mean, I don't understand why I feel weird, but at the same time I don't
> feel bad. It's kind of like floaty, but at the same time I feel happy, 'cause
> I'm not depressed chemically, so . . .
>
> *NEELY:* So, what does psychosis mean to you?
>
> *CORRINA:* Oh, just a break with reality, I think.
>
> *NEELY:* Yes.
>
> *CORRINA:* It's kind of scary. I don't want to intimidate people or freak them out. I
> just want to be myself again. I just want to be back to the way I was in
> high school, but that's not—I don't know.

Psychosis is not a word associated with a positive identity in any culture of
which I am aware. Once a person has been so labeled, they feel self-stigma and distress. As with Corrina, it makes them doubt who they are going to be in the future.

Amy was also anxious about receiving a diagnosis during her hospital stay. "I
don't know what they're diagnosing me as or with, though," she said.

"What do you want them to diagnose you with?" I asked.

"I just want them to just let me go and not diagnose me."

A few weeks later, Amy observed that it would be nice if the doctors could treat
a person by using technology of some kind. "It would be nice," she said, "if they
could just hook you up to a machine and see which chemicals are off or what's
misfiring and just correct it somehow. Maybe just give you some happy pills and
send you away."

Over time, Amy replenished her own moral agency by insisting that her
Adderall caused her to have some psychosis symptoms but that she did not have
psychosis. Notably, though, she—along with everyone I spoke with who was on

ADHD meds—desperately wanted the medication back regardless of the possible connection with triggering psychosis. In this way, Amy retained some control over the diagnostic narrative and became a "user" of mental health services. She, like Pedro, decided she did not have to agree with the mental health professionals' version of events. Some might say that this signaled she was sick and lacked insight. I believe that this resistance helped her move toward getting better.

It sustains young people's moral agency to be given more space to shape their diagnoses, especially in the absence of technological ways to "prove" that something is wrong with them. People can experience psychotic symptoms and meet criteria for many psychiatric and organic conditions, including bipolar disorder, major depression, borderline personality disorder, posttraumatic stress disorder, brain tumors, and temporal lobe epilepsy, as well as psychotic disorders. Referring to anyone as a person who *is* psychotic is a culturally loaded term even though it signals a wide range of possible diagnoses. It is not clear that this diagnostic label is at all helpful, given the tremendous societal stigma attached to it. Many people hear "psychosis" or "psychotic," and they think of psychos and psychopaths—two derogatory terms associated with extreme social deviance and violence emblazoned in the American psyche through popular films like Alfred Hitchcock's classic *Psycho* (1960).

The term *schizophrenia* or *schizophrenic* is no better. A diagnosis of schizophrenia in a patient record can lead even health care professionals to exhibit stronger negative attitudes.[15] Many societal stereotypes are associated with schizophrenia, including dangerousness, unpredictability, and incompetence, that lead others to have prejudicial reactions against people so labeled. This public stigma in turn can lead people so diagnosed to lose self-esteem, self-confidence, and self-efficacy.[16] Evidence suggests that this also holds true for people labeled as medically *at risk* for developing psychosis—which only shows how much power these terms exert over people's self-understanding.[17] In addition, public stigma against people with psychosis has gotten worse over time with increasing perceptions that people with schizophrenia are more likely to be violent than those without schizophrenia.[18]

Of the twenty-four people who discussed their diagnosis with my team, six people said they had been diagnosed specifically with schizophrenia. All but one was Black. Only eight Black individuals shared diagnostic information (out of fourteen interviewed), so it is striking that five out of eight had received the diagnosis most associated with dangerousness in the public imagination. Indeed, those who had been given a diagnosis of schizophrenia perceived it as especially persecutory or punitive.

Veronica, the young African American woman whose sister walked her into the hospital to gain access to psychiatric medications (see chapters 3 and 4), viewed her schizophrenia diagnosis as unacceptable. She felt she had been misrecognized and misunderstood:

VERONICA: I do not agree with the fact that they accuse me of having schizophrenia.

INTERVIEWER: Accused you of having, that's how you feel?

VERONICA: It's like you ask for medicine, obviously you may need it. It's like I asked for it because they [her family] told me to go get it, but not because I needed it. I don't talk to myself. Overall, I feel confused about that whole thing. Of all things, you could have said bipolar, you could have said something else, but I have *schizophrenia*.

INTERVIEWER: Do you have any thoughts on why they did that? Do you have any inkling about why?

VERONICA: Why? Because I hear God's voice, but it's not like an audible voice. It's more like I feel what he's saying. I sense bad things. I sense good things. He lets me know. Whenever they said, "Do you hear voices?" I said, "The only voice I hear is the voice of God." I think that's where it rooted from. I just thought about that. When they asked me that in the very, very beginning, they're like, "Do you hear voices that we can't hear?" I said, "Yes." I forgot. I said, "Yeah. You can't hear them apparently because I'm here." That sucks, but yeah, that's the case. Not to be mean or anything. I was upset. My family was supposed to be there, and they weren't. They were there physically at the moment, but they weren't there.

It is not surprising that Veronica was confused, as were many others. She had been answering questions honestly and felt that her answers had been misconstrued. She "forgot" to conceal her relationship with God from others who would not understand. And her family was not there to help.

Over time, Sofia and her mother worked hard to find a doctor willing to shift her diagnosis from what they described as "schizophrenia bipolar" to "nervous breakdown" or *nervios*—an idiom of distress in Latinx culture associated with traumatic experiences that had less negative weight to it.[19]

MARIA: Yes, because we did not agree with the diagnosis that she was given, because what happened to her has to do something with fear and stress. How do they call it?

SOFIA: Like a nervous breakdown.

MARIA [continuing in Spanish]:   It's because the doctor who had seen her before was not there that time. Unfortunately, he did not give the attention, like he didn't really care. So then that is why we were so unhappy. He was like, "Here is the medicine," and he didn't have any kind of conversation with her and wouldn't even look her in the face. And I would be like, "well, this is not a doctor." I was very upset and said I wanted to talk to another doctor, and so much that we had asked God, and that doctor was not at work that day. [. . .] We talked to the new doctor and told her that we wanted to keep seeing her. And, right now, we are seeing [about more care] because she is not receiving the therapy, because she needs therapy to be able.

Maria and Sofia needed a doctor to pay attention and listen to their story before they could accept a diagnosis and treatment. They also needed that diagnosis and treatment to align with their cultural values and what they perceived to be a realistic representation of Sofia's experiences. And they, along with the other youths in our study, needed to know that using the mental health services on offer would put them back on the path toward getting better, not weigh them down with a stigmatizing label for life.[20] These are all examples of the moral dimensions of care that are so important for treatment decision making.

There are places in the world where people have tried to shift the stigma that accompanies psychiatric labels of psychosis and schizophrenia. In India, anthropologist Amy Sousa documented how people diagnosed with schizophrenia were never referred to as "schizophrenic" by their care providers, nor by their families, nor in everyday life. Instead, Indian physicians practice "diagnostic neutrality" to avoid upsetting patients and families, since schizophrenia is a highly stigmatized condition that can bring shame on an entire family for generations. Why use such a label when it makes no difference in treatment and can spoil one's reputation and social recovery processes?[21]

In Japan, the term *schizophrenia* has been abolished. Despite a good deal of controversy, in 2002 the Japanese Society of Psychiatry and Neurology changed the diagnostic label of "mind-split-disease" (*Seishin unretsu Byo*), a term for schizophrenia that many argued was outdated, to "integration disorder" (*Togo Shitcho Sho*).[22] The goal was to decrease stigma.[23] Years later, evidence suggests that the change has worked in reducing societal stigma and the negative effects that this stigma has on people's lives.[24] There was also a significant decrease in negative stereotypes about people with "integration disorder,"[25] and they were less often portrayed in media reports as being dangerous.[26]

The United States has seen no move toward an alternative to *schizophrenia* or *psychosis*, even though the terms are heavily stigmatized, not required to access treatment, have legal implications, and are often upsetting to people and their families who fear their negative connotations. Those burdened with these labels must find their own ways to come to terms with the diagnosis. Everyone in our study struggled; some figured it out. If they did not, they could always refuse the label—and the treatment.

. . .

Latuda. Lexapro. Seroquel. Risperdal. Haldol.

Prescribing antipsychotic medications, like determining diagnoses, is also a socially negotiated process between patients, families, and mental health professionals. Some families don't want their children to use medications, especially families that believe people who use medications regularly are "addicts." Others want to "pray it away." Sometimes, the young people in our study did not want to use medications, and their parents used the threat of losing their housing to achieve compliance. For those who did agree to take medications, questions of which medications, at what dose, and with what side effects had to be continually negotiated with prescribers. The person doing the prescribing changed frequently, especially at the early stages, and was often assigned based on insurance access. Prescribers might include psychiatrists but, outside the hospital, were more often general practitioners, physician's assistants, or nurse practitioners with varying degrees of experience with psychiatric medications.

Many of the young people tried to avoid medication completely when they left the hospital. Some wanted to drink alcohol or not have to take these new medications the rest of their lives. Often, they found the side effects—which could include memory loss, stuffy nose (as Pedro noted), restlessness, itchy skin, excessive daytime sleepiness, sexual dysfunction (such as impotency), excessive hunger, disrupted menstruation, cardiac arrythmia, postural hypotension, sudden cardiac death, or weight gain—to be intolerable.[27] One study suggests that tardive dyskinesia—or the onset of *irreversible* and uncontrollable twitches and tics resulting from antipsychotic medication use—affects around 7 percent of first-episode patients who use older antipsychotics like Haldol and Thorazine, the same medicine that Corrina was using.[28] This proportion is significant among people prescribed these drugs for short-term use. In the same study, the newer antipsychotics caused less incidence of tardive dyskinesia, but still affected 3 percent of first-episode psychosis patients who used them and were also more likely to cause obesity and type 2 diabetes. One starts to wonder why anyone would take these medications.

Pedro had to be hospitalized a second time before he asked for different medications. The first medications made him feel congested and as if he could not breathe. After his second hospitalization, his family supported him by taking him to follow-up med checks with a nurse and helping him pick up the prescriptions at the pharmacy—support that was needed to keep him on the medications until the side effects were manageable.

Other mental health treatment users in my study had medication-oriented support from their loved ones—typically a family member—as they navigated prescriptions and side effects. Corrina, for example, tried six different medications with the help of her mother Sandra's advocacy, insurance, and support. They talked about this support with me during Corrina's first interview at home, though Sandra did all the talking:

> *SANDRA:* Thank God, she's—this is the sixth antipsychotic medication, and this is finally starting to work okay on her. Yeah, we went through six of them.
>
> *NEELY:* That's a lot. It's only been a few weeks.
>
> *SANDRA:* Oh, absolutely. Because she went through one almost every week, every week, every week, and it would get to the point on the weekends I was kind of dreading it because that's when she would just have the reactions and stuff. One of them was so bad, I mean, we thought we were going to have to take her to the emergency room.

NEELY: What kinds of—?

SANDRA: The tremors, the arching . . . almost convulsing and stuff, because these are heavy-duty drugs.

NEELY: They're powerful.

SANDRA: Yes. And so we watched her constantly and stuff, but thank goodness this Haldol that she's taking—and that's the minimum she's taken. I mean, and the doctor said, "I can't increase it anymore because you are so sensitive to it"—

NEELY: To the tardive dyskinesia symptoms?

SANDRA: Mm-hmm. She's highly sensitive to it and stuff. And so it seems to be working okay. She's on a mood stabilizing, the Lamictal, and that seems to be helping her. [. . .] They're all supposed to help you just put your computer back in order, and that's the way I tried to tell Corrina. I said, "Think of it as your brain is the computer and you're going through a major overhaul, and so they had to go ahead and unplug it, and they're having to redo every program in there."

NEELY: She's rebooting.

SANDRA: Yep. Rebooting. Exactly.

At times, Corrina wanted to quit her medications, but Sandra told her she could not live at home unless she took them. In another interview a few weeks later, Corrina shared more:

CORRINA: I think I'm at the point where I've realized I can't refuse any help anymore—it's not an option. If I want to keep my lifestyle that I have now, which is—there is no alternative, so you just have to cooperate.

SANDRA: Well, there is an alternative, you just don't have a place to—you know.

CORRINA: Well, I wouldn't want to go back to how I was. I'd rather just keep going up steadily.

NEELY: Okay, so you're not refusing help you're just—

CORRINA: Yeah, I'm accepting it.

Corrina also received psychotherapy. She told me that she really appreciated the help of her therapist, especially with stress management. "I think probably the therapist being able to tell me, 'This is how you deal, worrying about this problem.' That really helped because that was one of my main problems. I would just get so worked up and so worried about something, that now I have an experience to draw back on and just calm down. It helps to have that person there now, really reassuring you." Given that psychosis has a lot to do with stress, a therapist who can help the person manage their response to stress is a valuable item to have in the toolkit.

Several young people identified therapy as an important piece of care that they were *not* receiving, regrettably, even though therapists present a peopled opportunity that can help a person work through the grief and shame related to their psychotic break to move toward recovery.[29] One Latina named Lola said what she wanted most was to receive "a lot of counseling. I think I really need somebody to talk to so I can express my feelings, cause once I talk about it, I feel better. Somebody heard me, you know? And I need someone that's not gonna judge me or assume things about me." Finding a nonjudgmental space was hard, but it was important to help restore their sense of moral agency while using care.

Yet, while most young people in my study were not being offered therapy, they were being offered powerful medications that had strong side effects, with few directions about how to deal with them except not to drive for six weeks while they adjusted to their medications, and to stay away from alcohol and drugs. Those whose parents were not helping them understand their medications, advocating with them for better medications with their doctors, or requiring them to take their medications regularly to access material supports like housing had trouble seeing how medications were helpful. Experiencing negative side effects such as slowed thinking or speech that limited their ability to work, go to school, and connect with others further challenged their sense that using medications was a good idea.

Michael, for example, struggled a great deal with side effects and ultimately decided not to take any medications. "I don't think [the doctors] know what they're doing," he said. When the interviewer asked why, he gave an example: "One doctor at [the state hospital], he said that I'll be able to function if I take the medicine. And, I don't know, I didn't really, like, feel able to function." He continued:

> I think he said maybe not all the way back to normal or something like that, but I don't know. Like, another doctor was, like, "Yeah, you'll be able to go back to school, and you know"—I don't know, saying I could go back and talk to friends. I don't know, just like it's hard to explain, but it doesn't feel—like I think they think the medicine will take you back to like normal, like how you were before the illness. But me, if I'm watching the *Today Show* or news, I could see the difference in how I perceive things and how the news is, like how reality is. My reality doesn't seem the same as theirs.

Michael understood that he had schizophrenia and that he thought differently than the people around him, but the medications—from his perspective—did help him function better. First of all, they made him impotent, and Michael wanted to have a wife and children.

MICHAEL: It's almost better to have the schizophrenia and still have your body parts working like they should. It's like if something is pros and cons, like, would you still want to have schizophrenia but still have your male organs working like they were.

INTERVIEWER: Feel more like a—

MICHAEL: Like a man. [. . .]

A few weeks later, Michael was still struggling. "It's better, like, 'cause you know now I wouldn't hurt my family or nothin' like that, but it's bad because I don't feel good. [...] I don't feel normal, so that's the bad part. But it did make me, like, more rational . . . At least I can be with my family, but [...] I kinda lost my identity. [...] I lost my personality. Like I don't know who I am really."

Michael's family listened to his concerns. They wanted what was best for him. The doctor told Michael he needed to take his medications for life, but neither he nor his family could imagine a life with the medication's side effects, and no one liked who Michael became after the psychotic break, which they associated with the medications. In the absence of any signs that he might harm them, they decided he could stop taking his medications after five months or so. Michael's family did not seek additional mental health care, and Michael became a treatment refuser. The team did not see him again after that point.

Other young people had doctors who helped them see the value in their care, especially by helping them tinker with their medications—changing, adding, taking away, tapering. This seemed to help people want to stay in care. Four months into the interview process, Gideon mentioned that he continued to use mental health care because he had a good relationship with his prescriber:

> GIDEON: I talk to her, and we talk about my life. What I'd mention is working, what is not working, what is giving me fat . . . For example, the medicine I used to take is getting me all plumped up, a little bit, so she was like, "Let's cut it off." I like her, I like her a lot; she just told us, "Cut it off," because I hated our medicine, makes you sleepy. [...] See, last time you came, I was really sleepy.
>
> NEELY: Yeah, you were really sleepy.
>
> [...]
>
> GIDEON: I'm taking a new one, which doesn't make me feel sleepy, it makes me active and everything. [...]
>
> NEELY: Have you had the same [prescriber] the whole time?
>
> GIDEON: I used to have [a different prescriber], but she wanted us to take things slower because she didn't want to take the meds off. This one, though, she listens to you, she does things fast for you . . . I just like the new one because she listened to me, and she cut off the medicine, and she'll give me a new one. [...] They're just doing their best to try to make me better. I don't feel anything. I actually enjoy going to her now. We can talk, she answers what's going on.

Clearly, an interactive partnership with his prescriber helped Gideon to navigate his side effects and to choose to use treatment. He saw some of the benefits of his medication, but he needed time and a supportive prescriber to really move forward in the process. Gideon was able to find one after his original prescriber "left" (they did not tell him why or where) and he was assigned to a new provider. Gideon had regional insurance.

Ariana refused further mental health care, including medications. It wasn't so much the side effects, though by the third week she was complaining that "the medicine makes me feel like a robot." She knew she should probably go back to the doctor and ask for a lower dose, but no one encouraged her to do so. But what really made her dismiss medications was that her local moral world was not supportive of people who used medications. Her family made fun of her visit to the "crazy house," and a coworker gossiped about her. The stigma at work became so intense, she quit her job. Ariana also worried about developing a substance use disorder like her Dad.

Ariana had originally wanted to prove to the doctors that she was not out of touch with reality by being a "good" patient and taking her medications, but after it had serious social consequences, she decided instead that she wanted instead to prove the people wrong who were gossiping about her. So she quit her job, even though she was finally making enough money to save up for college, stopped taking her medications, and drove to another state to help her brother with his new baby—a fresh start.

Ariana took back some autobiographical power by dissociating herself from mental health care and calling it all a mistake. She found a meaningful social role by caregiving for her nephew, which was also a peopled opportunity. Her family was instrumental in making this happen. They gave her a chance. What is important here is that refusing care made more sense in Ariana's local moral world, as it did in Michael's and in many others. Ariana hoped that family support would be enough to help her get by without medication. For as long as the team was in touch, it was working out.

Other young people in our study also mentioned their fears that using medications was a kind of addiction. Lucia, the young mother who had to stop nursing, quit taking her medications after her husband accused her of "popping pills"—an activity he compared to abusing oxycodone.

Others who had been abusing substances prior to their hospitalization were confused that they had to use more chemicals to get better. As one white woman who had a cocaine use disorder said, "I feel like I'm not really sober to have this to medicate with. But [the doctors] are like, 'No, it's different when you have a prescription!' [The doctor is] like, 'You don't want to hear voices again, do you?' I'm like, 'No.' He's like, 'Then, you have to take this.' Yeah, I've been on that since I got out of the hospital."

Young persons whose families had a negative perception of psychiatric medications or of people who used them typically refused mental health care. Keep in mind that their family is often the only material and moral support young people have when they are discharged from the hospital. Coworkers, roommates, and friends have often disappeared or are gossiping about them—or at least that's how the young people the research team interacted with saw it. If their family did not want the young person to pursue mental health care, then it was not at all clear to them how using medications or seeing additional mental health providers would help them be seen as good people in the only local moral world to which they still had access. Back home was the place where many of them had felt safe before they tried to go off and make their own way in the world. Many needed to feel well received in that context at least.

Some young people who refused treatment had families for whom using medication signaled a lack of religious faith. Markus's parents were divorced. His father was African American, and his mother had immigrated from Africa. Even early on at the hospital, when asked about ideal mental health care, Markus indicated that he was not planning to use medications for his psychosis. "Hmm," he said in an interview, "if mental care was better, maybe if they prescribed less medications and spoke to more people about their issues, I think that would be better. Because some issues can't be solved by medication unless it's like a biological thing."

Over the next several months, Markus's mother, Hazel, also maintained that he was under spiritual attack by a jealous relative who had sent a powerful curse his way. She believed his problems were caused by demonic forces. When asked about whether Markus was using medications, Hazel replied:

> No, [Markus] is not on any meds right now, and really, to be honest with you, he doesn't need any medications, but spiritual intervention is what he needs, and he is getting it. So I may sound naïve to layman Americans. They will be like, "She is crazy—what the hell is she talking about?" But I am in the medical field, and I know what I am talking about, because the root of his problem is not physical. It's not physical.

Hazel explained that she used the hospital strategically as a kind of holding tank—a place to keep her son safe when he seemed dangerous. She dropped him off but did not go with him or visit, because "there is no point pouring water on a stone. Right? If you want to pour water you want it to sit and collect; there is no need discussing it because [the medical professionals] won't understand it. Where will I start? They won't even understand it. So I let them say whatever they want. [. . .] Admit him. Fine. All I needed is shelter, and then I'll go back to my praying place and start praying."

Hazel fasted and prayed for him while he was away. Then, when Markus was discharged from the hospital, she explained,

> they do referral for him to follow up and stuff like that. Then [Markus says], "Oh, mum I'm not going to do it. Mummy, I'm not doing it. I'm not taking these medicines. I'm not going there; I'm not doing this. I'm not." And I don't force him; the reason why I don't force him is because he doesn't need medical intervention. [. . .] I'm into now praying that God should intervene completely, so he can be a normal kid and go back to school, and finish. You know, God is in control.

Markus remained a refuser throughout the study. It made no sense in his local moral world of family and church to do anything besides pray for a total intervention from God to alleviate the intense spiritual attack on him. The one thing his mother thought would be helpful was a life coach—someone could advise him to study and continue to better himself. She thought it might be especially helpful to hear more about people who had experiences like Markus's but were also successful so that he would be encouraged by their stories and learn some strategies for success. This option made sense to Markus, his church, and his family—his local moral world—as a way to boost his moral agency and material resources; medical interventions like accepting psychiatric labels and medications did not.

I hope it has become clear that diagnostic neutrality or flexibility can be helpful for moral agency. Flexibility around pharmaceutical and psychosocial options for treatment is also needed. It is no longer medically true that a person who has psychosis needs absolutely to be on medications the remainder of their life, but this is not always clear to youths. It is not even clear to prescribers, who have varied levels of knowledge about psychosis. The literature itself is confusing and often contradictory. One study on young people experiencing early psychosis found no difference, at a two-year follow-up, between treatments that used antipsychotics and psychosocial interventions together, and treatments that used only psychosocial interventions.[30]

It does seem that being prescribed antipsychotic medications with powerful side effects for the rest of one's life in order to treat a psychotic disorder at times does not support people's moral view of themselves or what it means to be a good person. It uses all the wrong terms and ignores the strategies that young persons and their families employ to remain well morally—which they often choose over medical wellness when they perceived the two as conflicting. Longer-term research with a larger sample is needed, but this work calls into question whether medications are necessary if good moral supports are in place. It also suggests we may need to do more research on who is responsive to psychosocial supports, which ones, and why. I anticipate that the ways those psychosocial supports align with and even enhance what is upheld as good, beautiful, and true in the person's local moral worlds is key.

· · ·

The young people in our study who used care did so because it made sense in their local moral worlds. They needed to restore moral agency by accessing autobiographical power, the social bases of self-respect, and peopled opportunities to work toward living meaningful lives as valued adults. Even if they were often not able to choose their initial diagnosis and treatment, they did want to choose the relationships with people who defined what it meant for them to be a good person, and they wanted to be seen as moral agents in the eyes of loved ones. This

TABLE 1 Frequency of factors that participants identify as key to treatment decision making

Factor	All participants (N = 37)			Young adults (N = 18)			Key supporters (N = 19)		
	Rank	N	%	Rank	N	%	Rank	N	%
Desire to get back to normal	1	36	97.3	1	18	100	1	18	94.7
Care on offer is not enough	2	29	78.4	4	13	72.2	2	16	84.2
Police involvement	3	26	70.3	3	14	77.8	3	12	63.1
Feeling worse	4	25	67.6	3	14	77.8	4	11	57.9
Relationship repair	4	25	67.6	4	13	72.2	3	12	63.1
Paying for care	5	23	62.2	2	15	83.3	6	8	42.1
Living independently	5	23	62.2	3	14	77.8	5	9	47.4
Distrusting diagnoses	5	23	62.2	5	12	66.7	4	11	57.9
Social substance use	5	23	62.2	5	12	66.7	4	11	57.9
Feeling disempowered	6	21	56.8	3	14	77.8	7	7	36.8
Transportation issues	7	20	54.1	5	12	66.7	6	8	42.1

SOURCE: "Table 3: Ranking of factors identified by young adults and key supporters as affecting treatment decision making after the young adult's initial hospitalization for psychosis," in Myers et al., "Decision Making about Pathways through Care," 187.

drove their decisions whether to accept treatment, regardless of whether they were users or refusers.

In fact, contrary to my early expectations, there were not many clear and striking differences between the lived experiences of users and refusers prior to initiating treatment or during their early hospitalization experiences. Both groups had extreme symptoms and serious emergencies leading up to their hospitalizations. Each group had both positive and negative experiences of hospital care. Both questioned the science behind the diagnostic process. Both experienced difficult side effects from psychiatric medications. Both resented and resisted their diagnosis and the stigmas, the stereotypes, and the questioning of their ability to be in touch with reality and their ability to be a good person. Both wanted to reconnect with family, friends, and employment and educational opportunities as quickly as possible. My team analyzed the data from 37 participants—18 young persons and their 19 key supporters—to identify what was most important for them in terms of treatment decision making, separately and overall; table 1 summarizes our findings.

Strikingly, everyone—users and refusers, youths and families—wanted to "get back to normal," however that was defined in their local moral worlds. The difference lay in whether they saw using mental health care as a means to that end. I have previously referred to pathways *to* care—the ways that people first came into contact with the mental health care system. Here, I am referring to the pathway *through* care—a pathway that helps people get back to normal, to their everyday lives, and so move on from the fallout of a psychotic break.[31] In most of my work, pathways through care highlight how we can keep young people engaged in services that they need. But writing this book has made me realize that—for some—this pathway means refusing services.

Refusers needed, more than anything else, care and support from other places—most especially their family. They relied mostly on moral and material, instead of medical, support because either medical support was not necessary to gain access to moral support or because it impeded that access. It is likely that most young people would benefit from all three forms of support, but service providers need young people and their families to be on board morally to make that happen.

Changing how youths and families and society at large perceive medications or diagnoses is not easy. There is not one obvious intervention for all. Change will require following the old social worker adage of "meeting them where they're at," but also knowing where they want to be, and with whom, and how to help them get there in a way that is meaningful to them and the people they want to care about them, gently and over time.

People who used care and came to appreciate it, such as Gideon, Sofia, and Miranda, had prescribers who were more flexible about diagnoses, medications, and dosages. The people who stayed in care often described shopping for a provider until they found one who listened to their concerns. Therapy was also an important component of the care that users found to be helpful, but not all insurance covers it.

As is true for many of the problems I unpack in previous chapters, there are solutions available. Many of the solutions brought up by the youths in my study pointed toward the family offering material and moral support, as well as well-informed medical decision-making encouragement early on. The following chapter takes us out of the hospital and focuses on what happens when young people return home and how challenging efforts at this stage can be for youths and families trying to get back to normal.

6

Homecoming

As a system I think it's very broken, very not helping. [. . .] You don't know when he will do what and you need, like, support. Okay, we will allow this 24-hour person to keep an eye, or for you to—for everything you have to worry about, insurance, for everything you have to worry about.

—MALA (JAMES'S MOTHER), PHONE INTERVIEW, WEEK 12

Sage had been at Shady Elms for nearly a month without being transferred to the state hospital when she was finally sent home. She stayed there longer than anyone else we met. Sage had private insurance, so maybe that made a difference. It struck my team as worse in some ways than the state hospital because Shady Elms was a chaotic, transient environment not set up for longer-term stays. The other patients were coming and going continually and were always in the throes of dealing with the first few days after a crisis since most were discharged or sent somewhere else within a few days of admission. But not Sage.

To get permission to leave Shady Elms, Sage claimed, the doctors wanted her to accept antipsychotic medications. She had arrived against her will and did not want to take anything. She just wanted her Adderall back, but the doctors wanted to detox her from Adderall, which they thought had triggered her psychotic symptoms. When she finally agreed to take what the doctors prescribed, after several weeks of refusing them, she was given a long-acting injection of Abilify, an antipsychotic medication that could last up to thirty days on one dose.[1] After the injection, the hospital discharged her and Sage had nowhere else to go but home.

It was the winter holiday season, one month after her discharge, when my research assistant and I first visited Sage and her parents in their stately, two-story brick home in an upper-middle-class Dallas neighborhood. The neighborhood glowed with holiday lights. Every house had an upscale SUV parked in the driveway. It felt a bit like a movie set.

I was not sure what to expect. In the hospital, Sage shared stories about her parents and how they lied to have her admitted—twice before for depression

126

and this time for psychosis. It was really her parents who were crazy, she said. Since this accusation was troubling, one of the research team members followed up with hospital staff. This was a first break of psychosis, the clinicians caring for Sage insisted. Her former hospitalizations were related to depression. This was different. She had been taking Adderall and her blood work when she was hospitalized showed a high level, which may have triggered a psychotic break. However, the effects of the drug would have worn off in a few days and Sage remained psychotic, according to the staff's clinical assessment.

Whose story to believe? I wondered. I hoped a home visit might bring clarity.

Sage's father, Harvey—a stout African American man with kind eyes—answered the door in a nice oxford shirt and fleece pullover. He struck me as the epitome of a loving, calm father. He welcomed my research assistant and me in and had us sit down.

His wife, Rhonda, who also identified as African American, took longer to appear. She had dyed blonde hair and a smattering of freckles. She had dark circles under her eyes and looked very tired.

Sage appeared last. Her hair was dyed bright red, and she looked very thin. She also had, as I wrote in my notes at the time, "the funny look of psychosis on her face, that sort of wild-eyed energy [. . .]. But it was low-grade, not super intense."

On this visit, my research assistant and I split up and talked to Sage and her parents separately. I visited with Rhonda and Harvey at a wooden circular table in their chef's kitchen. Their little dog was nearby, barking persistently through a baby gate.

Her parents leaned in and spoke in hushed tones, afraid to be overheard. Rhonda said she had initially been worried that Sage was abusing her Adderall, so she hid it while she was out of the house one day. Sage became very angry, threatened her with a broom, and took her mother's car.

Harvey showed me a video Sage had made with her phone while she was in the car that day. He had her phone with him, which made him extra nervous because he was afraid she would come in and see us watching something on her phone. They were pretty sure she had not seen the video herself and had not pointed it out to her. They were not sure how she would react.

In the video, Sage was sitting on the side of a highway. Vehicles flashed by outside the window, which was completely rolled up. She looked very distressed: tears poured down her face, her makeup was badly smeared, and her lip was trembling. On the recording, Sage said that God was moving her car home and so she just needed to sit there and have faith even though she was out of gas. It was clear that the car itself was not moving and that the windows were up. The date on the video indicated that it was filmed in August—inevitably, a hot summer day.

Rhonda had called the police when Sage took the car to report it stolen, so they were looking for Sage. When they found her, the police, basing their decision on her family's story and her behavior, transported her to Shady Elms, where she was admitted involuntarily for being dangerous to herself and others.

Now that she was back home, though, everyone felt the family's living situation was extremely tense. Her parents wanted a family therapist to help them understand how to monitor an adult child living in their house:

HARVEY: So we're trying to figure out, as a grown-up and as an adult, what can we do to help her? I think maybe family therapy with her individually and with us collectively, 'cause the two have to play hand in hand. We need to all be in sync.

NEELY: Yeah.

HARVEY: 'Cause bottom line, she's coming back home for now, and then hopefully, at some point, she can get on her own feet if she wants to live on her own. But we want her to take care of herself properly if she'd choose to do that. For right now, she needs someone to monitor her care.

. . .

In the other room, Sage and my research assistant were talking about Sage's concerns, which were focused on the side effects of Abilify (her long-acting injectable antipsychotic medication), her need for Adderall, and her feeling like an empty hole. She had not really been in touch with friends.

SAGE: They all know—well, some of them know I was in the hospital. It was kind of stupid, you know what I mean? It's just kind of embarrassing, so—

INTERVIEWER: Okay.

SAGE: I just leave it alone and I don't want anyone messing with me.

INTERVIEWER: Okay. What do you mean by messing with you?

SAGE: Oh, I'm sorry. Just thinking it's funny, the fact that I was in the psych ward, because it's not funny, you know?

INTERVIEWER: Yeah. No, it's not funny at all. If anything, it's a tough experience in life.

SAGE: Yeah, it really is.

Sage also did not feel she could talk to her family or siblings. She was afraid she might end up back in the hospital again if they started lying about what she said.

"I really don't have anyone to talk to, that I could talk to. I just do what I do, I guess, basically just study, try to study."

Sage rarely left the house. She did not want to do anything that might lead her back to Shady Elms. From her perspective, they would take away her newly reacquired Adderall and force her to take medications with terrible side effects that would limit her future.

> *SAGE:* I mean, that's why I've been hesitant to go back.
>
> *INTERVIEWER:* If you felt like you were having a breakdown, would you be inclined to tell anyone?
>
> *SAGE:* No, not after that.

Sage knew the solution to her worries: don't ask for help even if you need it. You cannot end up back in the hospital again. Many refusers felt this way.

After Christmas, when my assistant and I visited her family again, Sage looked skeletal. Her pupils were so dilated that they were black as night—a look I strongly associate with psychosis. I wrote in my fieldnotes: "Sage doesn't look like herself."

Sage clearly wanted to air her grievances. Rhonda looked exhausted. Her eyelids drooped and her hair was pulled to the side in a hasty knot. She kept her head propped on her hand, squashing up her cheek like raw dough. The whole scene was fraught. I wanted to leave. I feared that Sage would snap and do something that would force me, under the regulations of my research, to reach out to a clinician for help or possibly emergency services, which I knew would be against her wishes.[2]

Sage was fixated on the idea that her psychotic break was caused by a psychological crash that occurred when Rhonda took away her Adderall after she disagreed with her about their religion.

> *SAGE:* The next morning, I woke up—my medicine was gone. I went and got it again [from another doctor]—my medicine was gone. You can't take people's medication and I had too much going on. And if I believe that [states religious beliefs that her parents do not support], and I choose to believe that, I am [her age as an adult].
>
> *NEELY:* Right.
>
> *SAGE:* That's my choice. I don't care. That doesn't mean you're psychotic. [. . .] That boundary is not understood by them.
>
> *NEELY:* Right.
>
> *SAGE:* It's not illegal.

As we were talking, Rhonda burst into tears. She could barely speak. She said schizophrenia ran in her family. She said her mother and sister and two cousins also had it. Rhonda was sobbing, raw in her unprocessed grief over what had happened in her own family due to mental illness. Feeling insulted, Sage became more agitated.

> *SAGE:* I'm not a child, that is—I'm not illiterate . . . I have a little bit of sense, you know? [. . .] All I need is to be left alone because I'm a person. I think pretty well, I say. I think of things both ways, and I think the best for me is to move on, so they don't worry about having to control me. Because I'm sure that's not healthy for them because I'm saying no and

they're saying yes. It's more one of those battles. So, if I demolish the battle instead of continuing it by not going home, I think that's all the mental health care me and my family need.

Sage wanted to move out so that she had more independence to experiment and make her own mistakes. This was part of developing moral agency—opportunities to try and fail—and she did not feel that she was getting this at home. As someone in her early 20s, she longed for a little room for experimentation and opportunity to be "bad" or make "bad" decisions.

> SAGE: So sometimes it's not all psychiatric, I don't think. Some things are decisions you just choose to make and it's not—
> NEELY: That other people think are bad decisions, but it doesn't mean you're crazy, it just means that you made a bad choice, right?
> SAGE: Yeah, so I think some things can be talked through versus just meds thrown at them to make them sleep.

. . .

Before our last interview, Sage did move out of her parents' house and in with a relative who lived nearby. She had less tension with this relative—someone she had always loved and trusted. She was also helping care for her grandparents, cooking, and cleaning for them in their home nearby. Sage felt that her grandparents were "the only people I really have that I can talk to."

She stopped trying to go to school or work and instead decided to apply for a disability income, though the government often denies disability cases for people like Sage who refuse treatment.[3] At her last interview with us, Sage showed no interest in a long conversation about what might be going on with her. She just wanted to move on.

By the time we parted ways, Sage's parents and extended family seemed to be helping her replenish her moral agency by giving her a chance to try out a new kind of story about herself with a new audience outside her immediate family. Sage had some peopled opportunities through this extended family. They did not seem as caught up in the nuts and bolts of her life choices or religious beliefs as her parents had been—or, if they were, it did not come up. They recognized her as a "good enough" person even if she had made some mistakes. They understood that she needed time and space and patience, which they offered.

All her family also seemed to understand that she did not want to take any more antipsychotic medications, and they supported her in that choice. They accepted that she needed Adderall to feel whole, and for better or worse, she continued to use it. They assisted her in finding a social role that helped her secure some of the social bases of self-respect by contributing to the family, which meant caring for them. They also gave her material support by offering her a safe place to live away from her parents. Offering Sage access to material and moral support did not cure her psychosis, but it did enrich her everyday life and redirected her toward feeling loved and valued as an adult, which moved her in the direction of restoring her sense of moral agency.

. . .

Many of the young people in our study experienced a lot of family tension; "family tension" was the most frequently applied code in our data set. This recurrence may in part reflect the fact that 75 percent of the youths my team interviewed lived with their family in the month prior to their psychotic break, so the family had at least witnessed and were often directly affected by the events surrounding the mental and moral breakdown.[4] After the young person was released from the hospital, they often had to return home—back to ground zero—the site, for many of them, of at least some of the events that had led to their hospitalizations.

Once they came home, most had to live with their family despite persisting tensions and misunderstandings over what had happened: Whose version of events was correct? Why did the family have the police take them away? Trust had eroded on both sides.

An emergency psychiatric hospitalization moves people in the opposite direction of breaking free, becoming independent, and having their own home, romantic partner, and career. After their hospitalization, the young people in our study initially relied on other people for material support such as transportation, food, housing, cell phone payments—really, for everything. Even if a young person tried to gain some financial independence by applying for disability income, the process can take years. Federal law requires young people to show evidence that they have been experiencing "serious and persistent" medically documented symptoms for at least the past two years.[5]

They must also be in treatment. Under federal social security laws, individuals are not entitled to benefits if they fail, "without good cause, to follow prescribed treatment that is thought to lead to the restoration of their ability to engage in substantial gainful activity."[6] There are of course loopholes in the law about who does the prescribing, whether or not it would help a person return to "substantial gainful activity," whether or not a person has a religious right to refuse, and whether or not they are incapacitated to the point that refusal is part of their inability to understand the consequences of not following the treatment. These determinations are made on a case-by-case basis and so are subject to the young person and their lawyer knowing the rules, the interpretation of a judge who hears the case, the skill of the lawyer presenting the case, and the young person knowing about any of this procedure and having access to a lawyer.

Amy (introduced in chapter 2) also had a family history of long-term hospitalization for schizophrenia and her own history of Adderall misuse. She had accused a family member of molesting their own children. Her family struggled to welcome her back home, but they were trying. Unlike Sage, Amy used treatment, including antipsychotic medications, which her family insisted on for her to receive material support, which she needed. However, the medications made her very tired, and she gained a lot of weight. Most days, she did not feel like going to work and even getting to an interview was a challenge without a car.

During that time, Amy depended on her brother Robert for material support. She had moved back in with him after she got out of the hospital. However, she felt disillusioned. "I hate being reliant on other people. When you need help you have to bite your tongue about things, you have to kind of just accommodate everyone around you because you are dependent on them. Then you get to a point where you just feel like a shell of yourself. You never stand up for yourself or be who you are. I'm just sick of that feeling." It was hard for Amy—and her family—to view her as a good person when she was not working, even if her medications were contributing to her lethargic behavior.

Like Sage, Amy felt embarrassed, wished her family did not know about her psychiatric hospitalization, and wanted to move on. And, also like Sage, Amy felt that her family was now questioning her intelligence:

> AMY: Basically, just there are some stigmas with my family of that happening. There's some sarcasm about it.
>
> INTERVIEWER: Like what kind?
>
> AMY: Like, "Oh, whatever, you're crazy," blah, blah, blah. I mean, it was an incident. I was taking a lot of Adderall. I wasn't sleeping properly. I was in a very negative circumstance with living with my sister. It was stressful. I wasn't eating healthy. I wasn't sleeping healthy and there's a ton of stress. I was in a town that I had never lived in before. I didn't know anyone. I didn't have a good base of friends to talk to, you know?
>
> INTERVIEWER: Right. You feel like your family doesn't understand that? They're just stigmatizing or . . . ?
>
> AMY: There's a lot of that going on. I mean, there's a lot of sarcasm. People don't talk to me as much about things, because, I don't know, I feel like they discredit my intelligence now, if that makes sense.
>
> INTERVIEWER: You feel like that's very starkly different from how it was earlier?
>
> AMY: Yeah.

Some people felt infantilized. Ariana talked about trying to convince her mom she was not a little kid anymore. Miranda talked about being babied by her family.

> MIRANDA: Like, my clothes, for example, I've asked them, "No, let me fold up my clothes. Let me do it. I can do it on my own." Or, "Let me make my cup of coffee." It's just small things. Like, "Don't try to baby me; I can do it by myself."
>
> INTERVIEWER: Do they baby you a lot?

MIRANDA: Yeah, they kind of do. But, you know, they're coming to realize that I'm not a baby even though I'm going to be *their* baby girl forever, you know?

INTERVIEWER: So, you're striving for more independence and . . . ?

MIRANDA: Definitely.

. . .

A young person's moral agency is not something they develop on their own; it is built in relationship with others, and the first group of people with whom they build it is usually their family. After a mental and moral breakdown, a lot of the young people we worked with turned to their families to help them repair their sense of moral agency, but this negotiation was really hard. A psychotic break at home blasted into that safe space. It called the young person's moral agency into question with their core people, the people who knew them best, and casting that into question was frightening and disorienting—not just to the young person but also to their family and key supporters. Letting go of a happy, healthy young adult, and allowing them to make their place in the world, is hard enough. But allowing someone who had, in a confusing, unexpected, radical, and highly visible way, failed to launch to now try making their own decisions again—as necessary as it is for replenishing moral agency—was daunting.

Overall, my research team was able to talk to 19 key supporters for 18 of the young people in our study. Some families—such as Pedro's—wanted nothing to do with my research team. Others had language barriers like Mohammed's mom, who only spoke Arabic. A few key supporters talked to us during our visits or phone calls but did not want to go on the record officially and so are not included in the count.

Research on carers for persons with early psychosis (a term similar to *key supporters*) shows that three-fourths of carers are women and three-fourths are a parent, indicating that many are the cared-for person's mother.[7] Similarly, most of the young people in our study described their mothers as their key supporters. These mothers walked the line between keeping their child safe and allowing them to try again. Many were stressed by the perceived need to monitor or surveil an independent adult child after their mental breakdown. Moreover, not all families had the material resources to manage the situation. For single parents who worked, providing this sort of care was a huge challenge. Everything was overwhelming— the situation, the troubling information that their child might have a disabling psychotic disorder, and the lack of solutions on hand.

Markus's mom, Hazel, a single Black parent (single because her husband lived in another state for work), explained:

I'm working, so that's why I said he needs to be monitored, and kind of walked back in life so that when he has an opportunity to live alone again, he will know how to control himself and manage himself. . . . Even though, you know, some things happen, but we as a person, the individual, have some responsibilities, too. I'm not totally saying that he is one hundred percent free of guilt or anything. So, there should be some element of control or responsibility he too has to pay. And mine, too. I'm doing mine now, trying to make sure that he knows what to do, and to be responsible for many things.

In Gideon's family, another first-generation Black African immigrant family, his younger brother, Jacob, went to community college instead of a four-year college so that he could watch over him. They took the same classes: Gideon had failed those classes the year he was ill so he took them again with Jacob. They slept in the same bed because Gideon could be difficult to manage at night. When I asked if Gideon was taking his medications, Jacob listed them off.

"We give it to him in the night. When he wakes up, sometimes he's calm, he's good. Sometimes he just like flips out, starts going crazy."

"Why?" I asked.

"I don't know. He becomes really agitated sometimes," Jacob said wistfully.

Biruk, another second-generation Black African immigrant, named his sister Ayana as his key supporter. When a person on the research team interviewed Ayana, she said:

> Currently, at this moment in time? I think he does need to be nurtured because I know that you can't be mean to people that are ill. You cannot be hateful or impatient with them. I understand that patience is needed, but specifically, with our family, I think they spoil him too much. I feel like, there is obviously a mental issue; it's not a joke anymore. At some point, they weren't sure if he was doing it on purpose maybe to gain attention or something, or to gain sympathy. I mean—no, there's definitely an issue.

While my assistant interviewed Ayana in the parlor, I was in the formal dining room with Biruk. He told me that his parents were about to fly him to another state to visit an aunt who was a "homeopathic" doctor. They had stopped giving him any medications in order to detox his system before the trip.

He looked and sounded much worse than only a few weeks prior. What he said in the interview was almost nonsensical. He had been kicked out of college for dancing erratically at inappropriate times and disrupting his classes, but he said he could not control it. He believed he could feel everyone's energy and had to dance it out when it overwhelmed him. It was hard to see him this way.

I trusted him so much that even when he unzipped his pants and put his hand through his fly, I just ignored him and maintained eye contact. Afterward, I asked myself, *Why? Why did I just ignore his behavior?* He wasn't trying to hurt me or show off. There were plenty of people in the house. We were not in an enclosed room. But still, I could have given him feedback that that was not OK.

It was difficult for me, someone who is thoroughly familiar with psychosis, to know what to do. It was hard to predict what was going to happen. It was hard to know what was right. Yet families, with little to no knowledge or support, need to navigate these boundaries as they watch a loved one struggle every day.

And many families were afraid to ask for help. They kept the situation a secret to avoid broader societal stigma or out of fear that people would judge their child, or their other children, or them. Reflecting on my interaction with Biruk, I realize I was also hiding his behavior. I just wanted it to go away—the part that was not like him—to focus on the part that was like him: the dynamic, funny, and smart young man I knew him to be. That was the young man I was looking forward to talking to when I walked into his house that day. I did not find him, but I did not tell Biruk. I did not want to make it worse.

Markus's mother, Hazel, belonged to a strong church community, but while she relied almost completely on her own faith, she also hid her struggles from her faithful friends.

INTERVIEWER: Do you have help from your community, helping him with prayer and in other stuff or . . . ?

HAZEL: I didn't make this public. I didn't make it public.

INTERVIEWER: Okay, but that is like a lot of weight on you, on your shoulders, then.

HAZEL: Yes. God doesn't give someone a load that he or she will not carry. Yes.

James's mother, Mala, also did not share her situation with her faith community:

MALA: Yeah. We're not really *in* the church, you know? We go to like a small bible group. People there know, so they just pray. Not all the details, but we just said James is facing some challenges and they pray, so—which is a good thing.

INTERVIEWER: Yeah.

MALA: But, you know, that's the thing with things like this: it's like this taboo we have. It's not like cancer, where you tell, "Oh, this and that was from cancer" and then you get all this sympathy, "Oh." And then you really try and do that with necessarily the brain? Yeah.

• • •

Many families tried to protect their children from stigma, to avoid making things worse, but in the process isolated themselves—and their children—and removed themselves from key sources of support, people who might also have helped the young person replenish their sense of moral agency, such as their church and their broader family and community. Mala's comparison between youths with cancer and youths in crisis is striking. Mental illness still implies bad parenting in our culture, no matter how much the brain disorder or chemical imbalance model has been pushed. People still judge the parents, especially the mother.

This cultural trend is clear when stories involving mental illness are covered by the news media. Where was the person's mother? How did she not know? What did she do or not do for her child that made them this way?

No wonder families remain silent.

Some parents did share their struggles with their extended families, though, which could be helpful. Sandra, Corrina's mother, had a large family, and with one sister's encouragement, she decided to tell others. But this happened only after she had been to a few family support meetings at Shady Elms' outpatient program with her daughter. Sandra explained:

> I started hearing some of what [patients and their family members] would share. [. . .] I found out that I was not alone, and they started sharing a lot of things, and what have you. And one of the things I found out was that you cannot, one [person] cannot carry the brunt of being the complete caretaker all the time. Sooner or later that person will snap, and so you need to increase your support group.

When Sandra did share what was going on with Corrina, "everybody became very supportive by texting Corrina, calling her, all these sorts of stuff, sending pictures and whatnot. So, yeah, that really was a big help for me, because it felt like a big weight had been lifted. So I'm an advocate of that."

Corrina also appreciated the extra family support and reconnection with her aunts and uncles—people whose relationships with her had diminished, as with so many American youths, as she was nudged toward independence in young adulthood. Families and other types of supportive community, when genuine and knowledgeable about psychosis and what it might entail, can make a big differ-ence in helping young people move toward restoration. This was also the case for Sage, whose grandparents and aunt had stepped up to help her reorient when her relationship with her parents became untenable. As mentioned in chapter 4, Jack seemed to recover the fastest, but he had a large and supportive family who did not accept that he had had psychosis but thought he had some rare form of undi-agnosable epilepsy. Ariana's family also stepped up, as chapter 5 explains, to help her replenish her sense of moral agency.

However, as important as we know families to be, and as much as our mental health system relies on them, my study showed that they often had very little exter-nal material, medical, or moral resources of their own. Family carer burden was a major unaddressed issue. Family therapy was expensive and time-consuming and often not covered by insurance. Mala talked about how lucky they were to find a doctor and some social workers who were willing to talk to her and her husband about James's situation despite his lack of insurance coverage and the fact that he was an adult. For while families are very much at the center of care, they have very little access to information and meager medical decision-making power once their adult child is involved in the mental health system. Mental health providers are also at times powerless: they must wait for something bad to happen before anything can be done if a young person does not want help voluntarily. No one can be proactive.

This lack of information and support was stressful for everyone involved. Fam-ily members facing early psychosis reported higher levels of stress than family members of a relative with a more "chronic" psychotic disorder.[8] In one study of 80 family carers for persons with early psychosis, anthropologist Anna Lavis and colleagues unpacked an ongoing level of distress that could last well beyond the initial crisis.

According to this study, daily life was quite unpredictable for someone caring for a person with early psychosis. Lavis's carers had to help young people with sometimes very basic things—things they had not needed help doing for a long time, since they had become adults, but now were needing help with again: remembering appointments, making sure they took their medications, and getting a good night's sleep. This resonated with my findings, as well. Hazel compared it to babysitting an adult child.

She was not alone. Carers often reported worrying about the young person regularly and wondering if they were OK even when they did not live together. Moreover, the at times aggressive and disruptive behaviors of the person with psychosis could be traumatizing for carers and cause symptoms of posttraumatic stress.[9] Gideon's brother spent all his time watching him—going to school with him and sleeping next to him at night even—to ease his parents' worry that he might hurt himself or someone else. This constant vigilance was exhausting.

"A palpable distress," anthropologist Lavis and colleagues wrote, "resonates through our transcripts" as "the well-being of the carers comes to depend on that of the service user."[10] Even after a young person was doing better, the distress could "solidify and settle, seeping into many areas of [carers'] daily life . . . even after [their loved one's] recovery, both because embodied vigilance can be hard to let go of and because carers may find that bit-by-bit their lives and selves have been cumulatively, but hugely, reshaped."[11] One of the most telling indicators of that distress, Lavis and colleagues found, was a family's sense that they had not been able to talk about their experiences in any other setting, such as with mental health services.[12] Caregivers were often on their own.

All the stress, stigma, and isolation that come with the diagnosis of psychosis make it likely that parents are going to be more critical of their children, as in the interactions between Sage and her parents. Substantial literature suggests that "high expressed emotion"—or high levels of critical comments, hostility, and emotional overinvolvement on the part of family members—is associated with poorer patient outcomes, including more frequent relapse and hospital admissions in longer-term patients diagnosed with schizophrenia.[13] Some argue that this research is harmful because it places the blame for a young person's relapse on the family, thereby adding to the family's sense of shame and guilt about the mental health concerns of their loved one. On the other hand, much research suggests that expressed emotion is counterproductive. Even so, are families accountable if they do not know how to talk to a person struggling with psychosis in the right way?

It seems that criticism from carers has negative effects on the person experiencing psychosis, including increasing their anxiety.[14] Moreover, high expressed emotion in families is even more likely among relatives who report a higher burden of care and fewer adaptive coping strategies.[15] And of course emotions are running

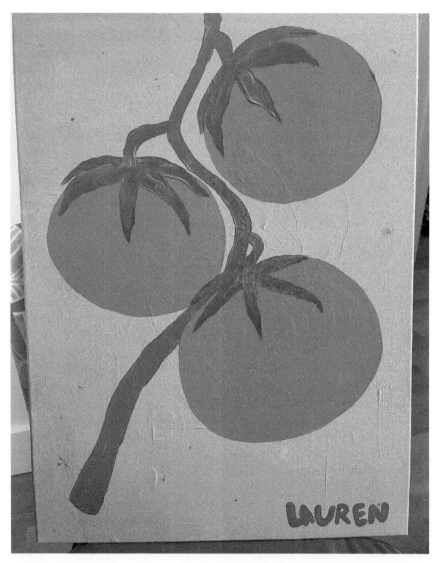

FIGURE 5. "Ripe Tomatoes" by Lauren Ann Villarreal. The artist wrote the author in an email: "This piece is an homage to my father. My dad works in the produce business, and we've had a distant relationship until recently, where we had a very open talk. This piece was about reconnecting with my father. I wanted to create something simple and fun. The majority of my art has been used to cope; this piece was about bringing fun back to my art." *Reproduced with permission of the artist.*

sky high in the household. Many families experience loss and are going through a grieving process.[16] Parents are often shocked by the onset of psychosis, and must now adapt their expectations about the future course of their children's lives, now made uncertain in the presence of this illness.[17] They also may feel that they have lost their child—at least the child they knew before the onset of the illness.[18] They may experience intense grief, guilt, and worry and may report largely ignoring their own needs to prioritize the care of their loved one.[19]

The foregoing review of the literature reminds me of Sage's mother, Rhonda, tearful if not openly weeping through most of our interviews. Clinical psychologist Anne William-Wengerd, who worked with parents around the time of their child's initial diagnosis of psychosis, described a process in which parents become "frozen" in their grief because of the uncertainty around the diagnosis and course of their child's illness.[20] Families then have few opportunities to grieve or to talk about their grief. They do not seek out or receive much support from their own communities. As Mala said, if her child had cancer, everyone—neighbors, friends, church members—would rush in with support. But, as I have demonstrated, psychosis is heavily stigmatized and implies that there is something terribly wrong at home or with the parents—or both. Many key supporters said they felt they could not even ask their extended family for help for fear of being judged.

Known serious mental illness like psychosis in the family thus also calls the family's moral agency into question. Can others still see them as a good family or parent? Can they see themselves in this way? Isn't it better to just not talk about it? This is what Pedro said his family had decided to do. My own family struggles all the time with whether we have made the right choices or not and how and when to share our struggles with others for fear of being judged.

And yet, unsupported and stressed as families are, going home is often the best choice for a young person leaving the hospital who has nowhere else to go. Without them, material support became very scarce. It certainly seemed better than the usual alternative—the streets and the homeless shelters. Some of the youths my team engaged initially in the hospital did not have a home to go to, or they did not report one. We quickly lost track of most of these young people, often because their cell phones were "disconnected or no longer in service," according to the messages we came to know all too well.

However, we did engage with a few young persons who avoided going home after their initial hospitalization at Shady Elms. James, who was furious with his parents, tried going to a homeless shelter after one of his hospitalizations. After a night or two, he called home. His dad picked him up at a local homeless shelter.

Biruk was also released out onto the streets in a euphoric daze after his hospitalization, imagining a utopia in which he could live on his own and avoid further parental control. His parents had no idea. A few days later, while wandering the railroad tracks early in the morning, another man sexually assaulted him at knifepoint. Biruk went to the hospital for treatment, and the staff called his parents. His dad picked him up—and took him home.

Then there was Daphne. Daphne was on summer break between high school and college when she experienced her first break. She grew up as a first-generation Latina immigrant living with her single mom, Monica, who had several children. Daphne graduated with straight As, had two good jobs lined up for the summer, and was going to be a first-generation college student on a full ride in the fall. Her life was full of promise. After high school graduation, she asked her mom if she could live with her father to try a change of pace.

"She was fine," Monica lamented, "but I guess [after she moved] she hung around with this wrong group or crowd and she started changing. I don't really know what happened, what she did or what, but that she started just doing things she wasn't supposed to, these weird things." The "things" included withdrawing socially from the rest of her mother's family and posting disturbing ideas on Facebook. Daphne was fired from her summer job after she broke her employer's trust. Monica and her father decided to defer college and keep her closer to home. She enrolled in some online college classes, but no one thought to seek out mental health support.

Then, one night, Daphne wandered away from her new friends after a concert where she had used some cannabis and become confused. Later, she said, she was picked up by a stranger in the middle of the night who claimed to be a police officer who could help her. He locked her inside his house, took her phone, and wouldn't let her out, she claimed, but she eventually escaped and found a way to call home.

Daphne had been gone for almost a month. Monica had reported her daughter as a missing person, but Daphne was an adult, so there was not much more she could do. Now, Monica was delighted to have her back.

It disturbed Monica, though, when Daphne spoke about being sexually victimized by the man, so she took Daphne to the hospital, where they gave her the morning-after pill (which was still legal in Texas at the time). The hospital also transferred her to Shady Elms because her behavior was unusual and the staff thought her stories did not quite make sense. Shady Elms sent her to the state hospital for 28 more days. She was on public insurance.

When Daphne was released, she went home to Monica's house. When I visited, Monica and Daphne lived in a pleasant cluster of small houses near a highway. The neighborhood had no trees, but it did have sidewalks and little green AstroTurf lawns and children's toys in the front yards. The house had a few bedrooms, a nice kitchen, some basic furniture.

When I visited, Daphne had been home for a week or two, but she had refused to take her prescribed medications. She felt great without them, she said during my visit—"like a sunny day at sunset."

Daphne did not identify as a person who took medications, as a sick person. She did not want to be put in the patient role. "I mean, me, as a person, I don't like being on drugs. I don't like taking pills, medicine. I never—growing up, in my childhood—I never had to go into the hospital. Never. So now, showing up and going to these appointments and stuff, I do not like it. That's just from a person that don't hardly go around clinics and stuff."

I asked her how she had been doing.

> *DAPHNE:* Good. I've been good. Life's been great out of the hospital. I mean, no matter what if I hear those voices, I'm still good. I understand that it's a life-living thing—you know, situation. But I'm fine. I know I'm healthy. And I'm good. I'm on my feet. And I'm looking for employment this week, just to get ahead. And that's it. Right now, I put a pause on going to school online because right now I just don't want to do school. I would just rather work and get back up to it because I have debts, so I have to pay my debts before I start doing the schooling and paying for school.
>
> *NEELY:* Can you tell me more about the voices you are hearing?
>
> *DAPHNE:* Oh, well, I used to hear voices all the time. And now, I don't know if I should say it's "a regular thing" or not, because maybe that's just that. It doesn't do any harm to me or anything like that. I don't know.

Daphne then started talking about black magic and witches (*brujas*) and how she thought her mother's family was practicing witchcraft against her, trying to kill her:

> Yeah, witchcraft. It was voodoo.[21] Voodoo through the whole thing, through the whole process of being there and being there at the hospital. I still heard my aunt's voice. [. . .] But I mean, it's crazy that you have to live life staying up awake at night just thinking that somebody's going to try and kill you. Which, it's unbelievable because I know where I stand. I've made it and my mind is right, and these medications and going to the hospital has—I'm ready to get over it, because—and get away from my mom and family because I don't want to be around them, because it's just witchcraft. And I don't believe in that. I'm always a happy person. And being here stuck inside my mom's house has really devastated me. It gives me depression. So, an anxiety."

Daphne also thought the social worker who visited their house was a bruja, which disturbed her. And so, like so many other parents, Monica worried about leaving Daphne alone, as she explained:

> I tried telling her I was going to help her look for somewhere I could go drop her off until I get off work and then I could go pick her up, but she refuses. She's like, "No." She's okay. She don't need help. So, what do I do? I ask myself, "What am I going to do then?" I mean, I can't have her in the street. So, what am I going to do? I don't know. What do I do?

I was struck by how young Monica seemed herself. She had clearly been a teen mom. I was also moved by her open and honest pleas. She was totally at a loss for how to help and was looking for support. She was an immigrant, a single mom, trying to pay for a single-family home, working two jobs, caring for four children. What could she do?

A week or two later, Daphne was back in the hospital: she had gouged a hole in her scalp trying to find the brain damage that she thought was caused by the medications they had given her at the hospital. The intake nurse at the county hospital emergency room assessed her as suicidal. Daphne did not agree. She wasn't trying to hurt herself; she just wanted to prove that she was right. They patched her head up and transferred her to Shady Elms involuntarily for self-harm.

Daphne would not sign a consent form for Monica to visit her. When I saw her there on one of my regular visits, her head was partially wrapped in gauze. She really had tried to cut a hole in her head. I felt dismayed. I asked about her mom. She said:

> I'm not upset with her. I told her I hope she sees a difference in me. I'm not gonna let her run me over and put me in these mental places. Cuz, you know, I don't belong here, and I don't need to take any medicine. If I have an anger issue or if I'm suddenly rough to fight against what I believe, then that's not my problem. That's something I'm fighting for because I'm not gonna allow someone to jump over me and make me have a lower voice. No.

Like Sage, Daphne was seriously frustrated with parental micromanagement. And even though Monica had nothing to do with her most recent admission, when she was released from the hospital, Daphne did not call her mother. I talked to her mom about this in another interview:

> MONICA: Ten days and then she got released and they wouldn't give me information [about] where she got released or whatnot. That's the third [time that it has been a] month and a half that I haven't heard from her, didn't know anything from her.
>
> NEELY: Okay.
>
> MONICA: They weren't able to help me out as far as letting me know what was going on.
>
> NEELY: Because of privacy?
>
> MONICA: Right. Right.
>
> NEELY: Okay.
>
> MONICA: They [the hospital staff] told me it was that HIPAA or something.

About six months later, Daphne called Monica. This time, Daphne was well into her pregnancy with the child of a man whom she said she knew and who wanted to get married, but no one could ever identify him. The house manager at her group home told Daphne's mom she was having a girl, but Daphne insisted it was twin boys. Monica had not seen Daphne in months, so she called us to ask if one of the team members could take her to the group home where Daphne was staying, which was not accessible by public transit. She needed a ride and some moral support. I agreed to take her (with my research assistant along), and on the way we had lunch and talked while we picked up Daphne's favorite fast food at Chick-fil-A.

I was astonished to find that the group home where Daphne had been staying sat in a tiny strip of little box houses tucked in between major highway overpasses. I could not imagine how that area had been zoned for houses. Its position cut it off from any kind of civilization. There was no access to any public transportation, nowhere to walk, no trees. The houses seemed to be made of concrete.

Inside, the house was wreathed in cigarette smoke. There was a tiny living room with an old television and a collapsing couch. The kitchen had a four-person table. One bedroom was reserved for the house manager—a person with no training or certifications who had agreed to take over the house after being a resident for a certain amount of time. The rest of the clients who lived there were staying in the other bedroom. There were seven beds shoved together, and everyone shared one bathroom. Daphne, late in her term, was the only female living in the room.

Daphne, who was quite young, looked disheveled and dirty and her ankles were badly swollen. I watched the house manager give her an antipsychotic medication that had not been approved as medically safe for pregnant women to take. When I pointed that out to the house manager, she blew cigarette smoke in my face and shrugged.

"Well, she signed the waiver," she rasped.

Monica begged Daphne to come home, but Daphne refused. She said her husband would be coming for her soon. She did not have his phone number, so if she left, he would not know how to find her. During our visit, Daphne said a lot of things that made no sense to me. It was heartbreaking.

Later, Monica called to share that Daphne had to leave the group home after the baby was born. They did not let mothers stay there. If they could not find her a bed in a place for mothers and babies, they would put the baby in foster care unless Monica stepped forward. Monica decided to bring them both back to her house after the birth, but that did not work out. Monica had to send Daphne out of the house again because Daphne was convinced the baby girl was an impostor. She thought someone had stolen her twin boys and replaced them with a demon baby girl. Monica was afraid Daphne would hurt the baby. She wanted to keep her granddaughter, but she was afraid what her own daughter might do. It was an impossible situation.

Could this situation, I wondered again and again, have been avoided? So many young people get lost in the system. Daphne and Monica helped me realize that this is partially related to privacy laws that separate young adults and families, especially when young people are moved in disjointed and unpredictable ways between institutions charged with their care, a phenomenon my team started to call *bouncing*. Of the 26 young persons for whom we had a clear map of their treatment trajectory during the first several months after their initial hospitalization,

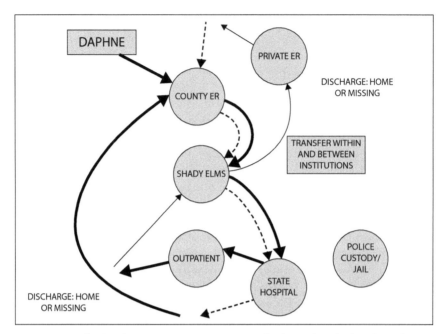

FIGURE 6. Daphne's pathways to care. Here, we can see the chaos of Daphne's pathway through care after initially seeking help at the county hospital (County ER). It illustrates the twelve "bounces" between institutions of care and periods of being discharged, missing, or living at home as she sought help in her first year after treatment was initiated. It helps us also imagine how difficult it might be for families to locate their loved ones in such a system when they do not have access to information. *Illustration by author.*

only 2 bounced once. Another 16 bounced up to four times, and 9 more bounced up to thirteen times.

When someone bounced, there was no way to keep track of them if they had not consented to their information being shared with an emergency contact. Otherwise, according to the families I worked with, it was up to their child to call them. Calling parents or listing them as emergency contacts is not something most young people want to do when they are in crisis, particularly if their parents were the ones who originally called the police for help or in some way talked them into going to the hospital.

Thus, at any given point, a young person could be released to the streets, transferred to a different facility such as the state hospital for weeks at a time, end up homeless, be abducted into sexual exploitation, or spend time in jail, and their loved ones would receive no notification. Their key supporters also could not call a facility to confirm that they were there—or at least that was their perception. There is, however, more flexibility in information sharing in psychiatric emergencies than most families—and likely most providers—realize. Ensuring that providers and families are aware of when and how, according to the law, they can ask for information during a psychiatric hospitalization is one of the reforms suggested in chapter 7.

Whether a young person objected to their parents being contacted, or parents were blocked from access due to a misunderstanding of the law, bouncing resulted all too often in a disconnect from family at a crucial time. While some parents may be toxic and young persons may not want contact with them, the parents we met seemed to have good intentions. They were frightened, not sure how to help, and sometimes unable to find their young person so they could advocate for them or make sure they were receiving quality support.

Daphne's mother had not been able to find her pregnant daughter, to protest her abhorrent living conditions in the group home, or to advocate for different medications that were not contraindicated for pregnancy. The deeper into her psychosis Daphne went, the less she trusted or wanted to connect with her mother. Maybe she was ashamed. Maybe she was out of touch with reality. She likely had a fraught relationship with her mother. Regardless, there was no way for her mother to find her when mental health providers would not help her make that connection.

Bouncing, paired with misinterpretations of privacy laws, may make relapses more likely by creating elevated stress, allowing for social isolation, and removing even the most basic source of moral and material support—the family—from a young person's life. It also may make it more likely that a young person will not have a safety net if or when they have another break or if their psychosis continues. It was not clear who to call for help or what the best course of action was.

The research says that the more breaks or relapses a person has, the more likely they are to develop chronic psychotic disorder. Is this because they have a diminishing level of moral and material resources available to them as medical treatment escalates? And is it then also a result of fewer resources that their moral agency is lower and they are losing hope that they can lead a good life on their own terms? Is the greater likelihood of psychosis due to the side effects of antipsychotic medications prescribed at high doses or as long-acting injectables that are too strong to help a person stay in school or at work? Or is it because the people around them, their key supporters, are becoming overwhelmed and cannot offer sufficient support as things become more challenging? It may well be all of these things, and they are very likely feeding into one another. As I point out earlier, the moral and material dimensions of care are as important as the medical aspects at this critical time. There needs to be a balance between the three.

· · ·

The family—or some equivalent—is the foundational place for developing moral agency and replenishing it when it is lost. Any young person hoping to recover from a mental health crisis needs the support of some close key supporters such as their family to move forward. This is challenging for families whose relationship with the young person has been seriously compromised by events around the crisis. It is difficult for the young person and their loved one to reorient to each other in the aftermath of a mental breakdown. Behaviors that occur during psychotic episodes, such as punching a grandmother, stealing a car, or gouging a hole in one's scalp, break the unspoken ethical "givens" of everyday life that once helped parents and their children orient to each other.[22] This loss is devastating for families, in part because, when they don't recognize the new person who has replaced their child, they feel as if they've lost their child.

I have given examples of these ethical breaches throughout this and previous chapters: Amy erroneously accusing family members of molesting children, Michael trying to harm his sister's child, Haniya considering harming her own children, James using illegal drugs, Sage challenging her parents' religious views, and so on. When these shared ethical orientations are no longer present, it can be difficult for families to embrace their children as "good enough" people, because their shared moral world has been called into question. *Are you who I thought you were, and can I trust you?* they seem to be asking.

In the meantime, the young person is also feeling that their shared ethical orientation with their families has been broken, because their parents have not protected them from harm and may have even perpetuated it. From the young person's perspective, their immediate family, by contacting the authorities to initiate emergency care, exacerbated a harmful situation. Sage thought her parents had disrupted her life plans—education, work, romantic relationships, having her own car—again and again when she did not appear to be an ethical person to them. This made her feel that they were being the unethical ones: they had her put in hospitals three times, they wasted time she should have been at school, they embarrassed her, and they were the reason she felt horrible for months afterward.

So, how can families hope to regain some form of equilibrium when there is a depletion of shared ethical space and clear moral understandings? How could Monica give Daphne moral agency, when the story that she wanted to tell was that her mother and her mother's sisters and the social workers trying to help them were witches, casting spells so that she would not feel well? How could Monica allow Daphne to keep her child when she thought that child was an impostor demon? How could Monica keep Daphne's infant safe without forcing Daphne out of her home?

Supportive families kept trying to remind the young person that there was a way back to the light and they would try to help them find it. Eventually, a young person might be able to connect with that promise, and that connection might help them reorient in the dark. But, to be able to provide unconditional love, which is what is needed when moral agency is so profoundly diminished, families need support.

Families are essential to reestablishing moral agency, providing some measure of continuity, and helping a young person get back to normal, but they need assistance in processing and understanding their loved one's mental health crisis and how best to support them. By investing in youths and family supports, we might help more young people avoid a chronic disease, keep them out of emergency care and hospitals, and avoid unnecessary expense for individuals, families, and our mental health system. We might also save lives. Ideas for doing so are the focus of the following, final chapter.

7

Turning Points

You don't know what to expect, and you don't know how to get to the next point. So, it is—it's very murky. After overcoming that, people need something good to look forward to and work towards. Otherwise, you could just get really depressed and go play in traffic. You know?

—AMY, AT STARBUCKS, WEEK 12

I mean, the future—I don't know—kind of scares me because you don't understand if you never had schizophrenia. Like it just—I know I'm probably going to have to do something, but it's just like—it's like what can you do? I don't think I can be productive, like, I don't know. I don't know.

—MICHAEL, AT HOME, WEEK 20

Advice for others? Hmm . . . Maybe if you guys wanted to explain to people this isn't something to be ashamed of and this isn't something that can be prevented even, so you have to work through this and realize that this is where you're at and there's nothing you can do about it except enjoy it and make the best out of it.

—CORRINA, AT HOME, WEEK 6

A young person in the United States learns how to be a "good enough" person based on shared moral understandings about what is good, beautiful, and true in their local moral worlds, which are shaped by their everyday mutual relationships with the people they care about and who care about them, such as family, close friends, and mentors. To become a respected adult, they must then go out into the world and prove they are moral agents capable of developing new shared moral understandings with a new community of their choice. As they seek to become a moral agent in social worlds beyond their families, they must learn how to belong in new ways.

Young Americans are expected to leave home and choose with whom they want to belong next—coworkers, classmates, people training for the same craft or military branch, people who share a hobby or religious affiliation, who are in the same fraternity or sorority, or who enjoy volunteering or playing an instrument or sport. Sometimes, their first attempt at fitting in leads them to join a community of people that may not be conducive to longer-term success. Sometimes, young people make choices that push back against religious or other cherished moral understandings held by their family or home communities, and their parents do not approve.

Regardless, young people typically are expected to develop their own "tribe," if you will, that recognizes them as a good person, is willing to give them a chance, and that respects them for who they are as they move into adulthood.[1] In this way, young people thrive in a culture that expects them to become independent, because regardless of how independent we are, everyone needs other people to get by. While there are exceptions, most are not supposed to get this kind of moral agency from their family: they are expected to break away from their families and prove their ability to achieve independence even if they come back home eventually. If they do so successfully, and with a group of other relatively successful people, they might be set up well to become a valued adult. This is one of the main functions of American college life: to connect young people trying to become independent with a new set of people for fun and to work toward success together as moral agents—people who together can move forward with positive stories and mutual self-respect through the opportunities and connections they can offer one another along the way.

For some young adults, as we have seen, this step can go disastrously wrong. A psychotic break is a serious setback for a young person's attempts to prove themselves as a good person with anyone. New friends, old friends, and family members will wonder if they still share or are able to share with the young person core moral understandings about what it means to be a responsible and trusted friend, family member, or adult—an understanding that binds people together.[2] The young person feels this doubt, too. As the previous chapters show, their mental breakdown is also a moral breakdown that at least initially compromises their relationship with others and even their own self. It depletes their moral agency.

When they start to feel better, the young person has trouble understanding why, when they were psychotic, they chose to harm relationships and jeopardize opportunities that mattered to them so deeply. They question their own self and motivations: Am I a good person? Who was I and who am I going to become? Can I trust myself?

As Michael tried to explain, "Imagine you just being normal one day, and then it's like somebody taking control of your mind, and it's like your mind is holding yourself hostage. Like anything could happen at that point. Your mind could tell you to go shoot up a building and you would think it's because you're doing it for a just cause." Of course, this did not apply to him: his delusions were even worse, he thought, because they led him to try to harm his own niece. Psychosis can be extraordinarily frightening. It can make a person dangerous to themselves or others if unchecked. And these experiences can lead to an existential crisis.[3]

I argue that, over time and on every level—within themselves and with family and friends, old and new—a young person's experiences with underaddressed mental health concerns diminishes their moral agency. Their moral agency needs to be replenished for them to move forward with their lives. Moral agency fuels self-confidence and helps others to have confidence in them. They need enough of it to become a valued adult who can be trusted to form and maintain relationships and make responsible decisions. It is crucial for well-being.

Nourishing others' sense that one is a moral agent, and thus nurturing one's own sense of moral agency, is hard for all young people. It is especially hard for young people with early psychosis. It's hard in part because of the lived experience of psychosis symptoms, which are disorienting in and of themselves, and in part because of our medical and societal ideas about and responses to psychosis. Not everyone experiencing psychosis ends up with a complete lack of moral agency at the end of the typical sequence of events. The initial breakdown, emergency intervention, psychiatric hospitalization, return home, and attempt to get back to "normal" all provide opportunities for both diminishing or replenishing moral agency. If we pay attention to these opportunities, we can offer more assistance during this difficult time to young people and their families and loved ones.

Ariana is one example of a person who found ways to start replenishing her moral agency right away. Ariana was trying—from the moment I met her—to protect her moral agency and establish her right to be seen as a good person capable of acting independently for the greater good of others. As chapter 4 relates, she immediately began exercising her autobiographical power by introducing herself to me as a person who volunteered helping children with learning differences in high school even as she was desperately distracted by voices telling her that the end of the world was at hand. When she returned home after a long-term stay at the county hospital and people started gossiping about her, she moved away—literally, quit her job and drove to another state—to take back control of the story others told about her life by starting over in a new setting.

Ariana's family was important in that process. Together, they used humor, trust, and love to help her move forward. Early on, they shared some laughs about her stint in the "crazy house" to help heal their relationship and reestablish the social bases of self-respect. Ariana used her relationship with her family to create a peopled opportunity for employment by helping her brother with his new infant while he and his wife went to work—a key source of material support for them both.

It was not completely clear that this would be enough to help Ariana restore her sense of moral agency outside her family and thereby transition to independent adulthood. Toward the end of our interviews, though, Ariana had this restoration in mind. She was considering the possibility of becoming a trained peer support specialist and having a career in helping others manage their own mental health concerns based on her own lived experience of psychosis—which excited her. She wanted to get the certification needed for this position. Working as a peer support specialist seemed safe to her because it involved people who understood what she had been through and so offered her social bases of self-respect. Plus, she felt that it built on her skills working with children and youths with learning differences in high school. This could be just the peopled opportunity she needed to build bridges into communities of like-minded others beyond her immediate family.

If Ariana had continued to use psychiatric hospitalizations and medications to get better, her family may not have given her so many opportunities. However, by refusing antipsychotic medication and a psychiatric diagnosis of psychosis, both of which for her family were associated with being "crazy" or "addicted," Ariana secured her ability to be seen as a good person. Ariana had a replenished sense of moral agency at the end of our study and demonstrated that upholding her status as a moral agent, at least for her, was more important than being medically compliant. A return to moral status that enabled her to belong was what she needed most at that time. It's possible that if the medicines had not initially rendered her stable, she would have had another breakdown later—it's hard to say. But while Ariana's is a high-risk approach, especially in the absence of medical supervision, it made the most sense in her local moral world, and it would have been ideal if the care on offer—mutual support or a medical professional—could have partnered with her to help her recognize warning signs in case another psychotic break approached. In that case, if the onset of symptoms had been recognized early on, a low dose of medicine for the shortest possible amount of time could likely have kept her out of the hospital and firmly connected to her everyday life with work and family. That option was not offered to her, however, and we can only hope that she managed any future concerns with the help of her family and not another emergency hospitalization.

In contrast, Michael had very little sense that he could replenish his moral agency with anyone but his family throughout the study period. He felt stuck. His family begged him to leave the house, to sign up for an art class, anything. Michael refused. His mind, he was sure, did not work the same as other people's minds. His thoughts felt more confused. Chapter 5 notes how he struggled with erectile dysfunction as a side effect of his antipsychotic medications (a common one).[4] His ideas about success and masculinity and his potential as a health care worker or husband and father after a schizophrenia diagnosis seemed severely limited, which led him to doubt that he could ever have a career and family and belong in the adult world.

Michael did not recognize himself, as he explained: "I just don't feel like myself. [. . .] I was going through my Facebook posts [from 3 years ago] and it just seems like I don't even know who that is. Like, it seems like the real me, but I just don't know who that person—it just doesn't feel like it was me that did it."

His family reassured him that they were still willing to see him as a moral agent even though he had tried to harm his niece when he was overwhelmed by psychosis. They were confident that while he was not quite himself and had not been for a couple of years, he was fundamentally a good person whom they loved. He had scared them, but he used their memory of him as a moral agent to move on with living together peacefully at home while refusing mental health care.

Michael's family did not want him to use psychiatric labels. They did not believe he had schizophrenia, and they thought that medication made him not like himself. When they initially sent him to the state hospital and followed medical advice, their friends were horrified and told them to get him out as soon as possible. Although Michael followed his family's directions, he struggled with the loss of his former social status, his virility (which did not come back right away when he stopped his medications), and his sense that he was a stranger to himself.

His family encouraged him to hang on to hope, but toward the end of our study Michael was still at home, had not been visiting with friends for a couple of years, and was not working or in school. He felt deeply disheartened. He was losing his sense that he could ever be a moral agent in this world. He thought maybe he could thrive in a place where there were only people like himself.

He explained:

> I feel like I would be better off just with the schizophrenia if the government just had like an island, like—I don't know. Just took people with mental illness or schizophrenia, I don't know about bipolar disorder, but just put them on an island, and just let us live out the rest of our lives like that. If they'd have done that, I wouldn't even know the difference. I don't know. I think once your mind goes off reality, I don't think it goes back. I don't think the medicine that we have takes you—fixes everything—and takes you back to how you were before. I think it just like stops the symptoms, but like the other stuff you lose, I don't think you gain it back.

Clearly, for Michael, his local moral world was more important than medical advice. He did not trust the treatment on offer and his family did not, either. Most important, he needed to feel that he could belong somewhere in a way that was seen as at least good enough by those around him, and he did not see how a person with schizophrenia could live with anyone besides other people with psychosis—on an island where they could all be themselves.

Corrina used mental health treatment because her family required her to do so to be accepted back into their home. Taking medications did not fix everything. For months—and through five different medications with frightening side effects, including convulsions—they did not work. She had aggressive episodes and disappeared for hours at a time. Once the medications did start working, she still had trouble establishing herself as a moral agent in her family and in the world beyond her house and her boyfriend. The constraints on her moral agency were evident during our home visits: her well-intentioned mom was supervising her narrative, controlling some of her autobiographical power. Her family remembered how she had been reckless and frightening and had not fully convinced themselves that Corrina was trustworthy, which limited her peopled opportunities and social bases of self-respect at home. It was hard to forget "Karina," who thought they were demons sent from another galaxy and destroyed their property.

Corrina's mother wanted her to finish her college degree. About half of the young persons we interviewed had at least some college education when they had their psychotic break. During the time she engaged with my team, Corrina tried to go back to college, but she did not have the confidence—and likely did not have the right accommodations and support—to return to school. Instead, she had a nervous breakdown in her college classroom, which further diminished her self-confidence and her willingness to practice being a moral agent in the outside world again. With few opportunities to replenish her moral agency at home, Corrina had trouble doing so in the outside world as well. Instead, she continued to live with her parents and hang out with her boyfriend and his friends watching Netflix and smoking cannabis. For her boyfriend and his friends, that was good enough, but that was not going to launch Corrina into valued adulthood.

Corrina was insightful and smart, and she had the potential to do more—she knew it and her mother knew it—but she was not sure what to do. One time she asked me shyly if she could sit in on my classes—maybe having the right professor who understood what she was going through would help, she thought. *Sure*, I said, though I had no idea whether SMU would allow it. But she never reached out to ask me again.

I have also shared the example of Markus, whose mother (or her God, from her perspective) was very much in charge of his narrative, leaving him little opportunity to work on his autobiographical power. For Markus's mom, Hazel, having faith that God would heal him was more important than any medical involvement. She shared that medical involvement for mental illness was not acceptable for what they understood to be a "spiritual attack" (see chapter 5). Hazel was trying to preserve his social bases of self-respect by having him refuse medical care. She used the hospital only as a holding tank so that she could continue to focus on fasting and praying for his spiritual healing. Hazel said: He doesn't need medical intervention but periodic advice, yes [. . .] to give him examples of, 'Look at this person—he went to school, did this, and this is where he is so you too can do it.'" Hazel and Markus would likely have benefited from a peer support specialist who could have offered encouragement and advice on how to thrive after experiencing psychosis—the very kind of person that Ariana hoped to become.[5]

Ariana, Michael, Corrina, Markus, their families, and, really, most Americans have the same need: to experience life as a moral agent in community with loved ones who matter to them. Some people think of this as recovery. "Recovery" has been a popular movement in American mental health care, a movement that insists that people can get better—perhaps even better than they were originally—even after they experience a serious mental illness.[6] However, for young people, I am unconvinced that *recovery* is the right word. *Recovery* implies a cure or a return to something—a righting of a wrong. But a psychotic break is not a wrong turn at the crossroads, as James suggests in chapter 1. Rather, it is a moment of vulnerability and potential—an opportunity for a person to become diminished or replenished in terms of the moral agency they need to move forward with their lives—and that depends on the medical, moral, and material resources available to them, as well as their ability to procure them through intimate relationships based on mutual moral recognition that one can at least become a "good enough" person again.

· · ·

There is no cure for psychosis, and it is not wrong to have psychosis symptoms. Some see it as a gift. For most of the young people I met, the psychotic break started off as an intense spiritual experience, which was not a negative experience. Some have called psychosis a spiritual emergency.[7] There are many ways to describe the experience, and they do seem to matter, so what if, instead of a breaking point, a psychotic episode was considered a turning point on the pathway to adulthood? A point where loved ones and other adults capable of offering support realize that someone needs extra moral, material, and medical support and that we can and must offer such support to prevent negative outcomes and help them move toward a meaningful life? Such rethinking could also serve as a turning point for society: an invitation to families and the broader culture to help protect, promote, and replenish moral agency for all young people who are struggling to become valued adults and belong.

We can begin by doing more of what this book has been trying to do all along: holding space open for individuals experiencing psychosis and listening more compassionately to them. As anthropologist Luke Kernan writes, "To view these experiences as endpoints, as brief silences, or as something discrete and outside of their larger context, is dangerous both ethically and academically. They have sonic reverberations, consequence. And, as the night can fall fast, we should be astute and boundless in mobilizing agency and becoming—of injecting compassion into that lifeblood to assuage the burden of self. Of taking responsibility. Of listening."[8]

This book is a product of my team's best attempts to listen during the challenging critical period in the first several months after a person's initial emergency hospitalization for psychosis. What follows are some ideas for social change and reform based on what we heard and what we know from the literature works. Here, I have done my best to draw together the evidence base for what works in order to provide steps we can follow to promote moral agency during a young person's pathways to and through care and so reduce the negative consequences of experiencing psychosis in a society that, in general, offers few affordances for nonconsensus realities. If we take these steps to turn what I identify as breaking points into turning points that signal the need for us to work together to protect and replenish a young person's moral agency, we will see many more youths returning to their pathway to valued adulthood.

STEP 1. PREVENTING BREAKDOWNS

Ideally, we would prevent a full mental and moral breakdown from happening in the first place. We need to offer material, moral, and medical support to young people, as appropriate, before they have gone too far down the road toward those "catalytic events" that call their moral agency into question: being dismissed from school; losing roommates; losing a job; threatening or harming oneself, a family member, or romantic partner; engaging in egregious substance misuse; wrecking a car—all examples shared in the young people's stories in this book. We have to offer people help *before* they get to that point. Many people delay seeking help for a mental health crisis. There are many reasons for this decision and many solutions.

We can start by recognizing that even when they may seem delusional, young people are trying to find a frame of reference via a locally available cultural mythos that can help others perceive them as good people worthy of relationships. Rather than telling them they are crazy or rejecting them, we might be curious about the identities they have chosen, such as a superhero, Jesus, or an angel. "I see you; I hear you; and how can I be supportive?" is always a helpful approach. If we do this more often, from within the morally meaningful cultural spaces that people naturally seem to seek out during a psychotic episode, such as religious spaces, we might help people find meaning in their psychosis experience in ways that are gentle, do not induce fear and isolation, and gently nudge them toward connecting with further medical and material support. This approach would require us to think carefully about what cultural toolkits, such as those mentioned in chapter 2, can help people make sense of their psychosis in a more life-affirming way. While I understand that some people may end up thinking they are Satan or a demon, I suspect that this happens when others reject or ridicule them and they become confused and self-deprecating. Social media both exacerbated ideas that persons were communicating with them when they were not, as with Pedro's Liquor Ladies, Miranda's Romeo, and James's celebrities. It also opened the young person up to criticism, as Sage and many others explained, leading many of them to later regret posting anything online when they were experiencing symptoms. Some, including Michael, withdrew from social media, which could be isolating. Others kept posting things they later regretted, leading them to leave online life, as with Corrina.

What I noticed in my research was that if a young person's psychosis experiences were interpreted negatively by others, the person became afraid, began to isolate themselves more, increased their substance use (typically cannabis, which many thought helped with anxiety), and lost too much sleep. Each of these results seem like something we can prevent.

Mobilize Faith-Based and Community Supports to Address Help-Seeking Delays

In my research, religion and spirituality constituted a widely used source of cultural mythos for young people trying to make sense of psychosis. I am confident that with good training and care we can work with pastors, priests, imams, chaplains, rabbis, and other faith-based leaders to craft cultural toolkits that support young people and can potentially prevent a crisis.[9] Training faith-based leaders in mental health care has been done in other parts of the globe where there is a shortage of mental health professionals,[10] but there is no reason not to try this in the United States, especially in areas with limited mental health care and in communities that identify as more religious.

In my own small research study in partnership with Valerie Odeng, a public health master's student and Black African immigrant, Valerie interviewed 17 Black African immigrant pastors in north Texas after sharing a vignette with them about a person with early psychosis.[11] We found that the pastors were very eager to receive further training to help. All the pastors we talked to thought relationships were key, whether they involved partnering with young people, families, or health professionals. Faith-based leaders can foster a communal form of alliance that includes the families of the person experiencing distress and takes place in nonclinical, likely less stigmatizing settings such as in the privacy of the young person's own home or at their church. This may be especially helpful for a young person's sense of moral agency—protecting and replenishing them as they go along—before they fall into a crisis.

Faith-based leaders also have a pre-established level of trust with congregants that may make it easier for them to advocate for certain kinds of care (such as psychiatric attention) and engage families and persons with mental health concerns more effectively than others. This trust could be a good supplement for other kinds of social services, especially in rural or impoverished areas with fewer resources or for cultural groups that might respond better to a trusted community member than to a less familiar mental health professional.[12]

The pastors my team engaged with also expressed a strong desire for further collaborations with other mental health professionals. At least one pastor mentioned sending chaplains to offer support to the local mental health system. Licensed chaplains are found in hospitals and schools (most often higher education), as well as military settings.[13] They have helped the Department of Veterans' Affairs support people experiencing moral injury in the context of posttraumatic stress and may also be an important care resource for people with psychosis, who often have trauma histories.[14] Working with churches, synagogues, mosques, and interfaith chaplains to provide spiritual support to persons with psychosis and their families could also help nourish moral agency. Since many people have experiences they identify as spiritual or religious, and since those people often approach religious or spiritual leaders first, it makes sense to offer these spiritual leaders training in how to support, screen, and refer young people who may be in the early stages of a crisis. In partnerships with Black faith communities, mostly in the urban United States, this approach has met with some success in reducing mental health stigma and addressing mental health concerns such as depression, though the studies we have thus far have been limited.[15]

It is important for young people to access mental health support as soon as possible after symptoms first appear. One way to encourage young people to seek out help more quickly is to reduce the stigma around asking for help. For example, Ariana waited a long time to go to the "crazy house" because, in her Hispanic culture, a person is either fine or "crazy." There is no in-between. I have heard people from rural America express similar ideas. There are things we can do to help people think of mental health care as a positive solution, not a signal that someone is "crazy" and therefore outside the range of acceptable human experience.

It seems to me that the families in the study provided a lot of guidance on how stigma-free early intervention might make sense for them. They wanted control over the labels, especially given their impact on the young person's moral agency. Families and young people tended to use more culturally acceptable, common-sense terms, such as *nervios* (literally, "nerves"), PTSD, or depression, which may be more acceptable and easily recognized. These terms may not convey the seriousness that *psychosis* or *schizophrenia* signal, but it left families and young people freer to speak openly about what was going on at a vulnerable time. Using more flexible sets of information and diagnostic terms may also help ease medical mistrust in communities that have experienced mental health measures as forms of social control, such as the African American community, where the diagnosis of "schizophrenia" has historically been used to lock up Black civil rights activists.[16]

In addition, young persons and families who did seek help prior to an emergency tended to approach trusted community members first. Following their lead, we can listen to and build partnerships with key supporters that young persons and their families do trust. For both Latino and Black participants, as I have mentioned, faith-based leaders were often trusted advisers. Other potential community partners include school counselors, teachers, coaches, and librarians. Alternative healers such as *botanicas* or *curanderas*—visited by some of our Latinx participants—may also be trained to help families recognize when a young person may need more support. Every possible community partner needs to be trained to informally support young people and families as mental health concerns develop, and then to guide families who need help to connect with more formal forms of support as early as possible.

Reducing help-seeking delays demands that we work with families, especially in public school settings, to make sure they understand that mental health is as important as physical health, and that we help families, teachers, counselors, and coaches recognize warning signs that a young person may be struggling. I think of this as a young person's *care network*—the people who might be linked together to support a young person when things start to go wrong. It would be crucial for multiple people in a young person's care network to have the knowledge and ability necessary to quickly recognize when things start to go poorly. This preparation is always complicated: how do we provide education and training that avoids increasing stigma around certain children and youths, just as we do with those who are struggling in other ways? However, if done well, having well-developed community-based supports for youth mental health can help families avoid catalytic events, police involvement, and emergency interventions, which in our study were always damaging to the young person's moral agency.

Educate Frontline Prescribers about Psychosis

That a young person has accessed mental health care does not mean that care they're given is the best for early psychosis. It is ideal for the psychiatrist on the care team to be someone the young person likes. However, there are not enough psychiatrists available—about half of Americans, 150 million people, live in federally designated mental health professional shortage areas.[17] Thus, there are many different prescribers of psychiatric medications, including general practitioners, nurse practitioners, and physician's assistants, and not all prescribers have the training needed to help with psychosis. For example, negative symptoms of psychosis such as attention deficits and working memory loss may be misrecognized as symptoms of ADHD. One recent survey of 140 college campuses found that 1 in 6 students reported a psychotic experience over the previous year. In those cases of psychosis symptoms, use and misuse of amphetamine-based drugs like Adderall prescribed for ADHD (and several other prescription drugs) were associated with mostly mild (but noticed) psychotic experiences after adjustment for alcohol, tobacco, and cannabis use.[18] More research is needed to understand the relationships between prescription amphetamine use or misuse and psychosis. Meanwhile, any prescriber who is not intimately familiar with current information on psychosis may not know the risk.

In addition, not all prescribers know the best practices, which include prescribing a person experiencing a psychotic break the lowest possible dose of antipsychotic medications for the least possible time so as to avoid, as one psychiatrist told me, "using a fire hose to put out a candle."[19] Overprescribing can turn young people like Sage off to using medication completely. Antipsychotics are also sedatives and so, at higher doses, make work, school, and social activities more challenging. In addition, they do not work for everyone. Prescribers need to be trained specifically to understand which drugs can trigger psychosis: who is at risk; how to recognize and help when a person is developing psychosis, including from a drug they have been prescribed; and when to refer a person who is struggling to a psychiatrist—preferably before they go into the hospital for emergency treatment.

Ideally, there would be a national network of psychosis-specific psychiatrists able to treat patients via Telehealth across county and state lines so that young people with psychosis everywhere have access to the best prescribers for their concerns and the same prescriber over time, regardless of whether they are at home in a rural area, attending school in another state, studying abroad, traveling with the military, or doing a summer internship (or, say, during a global pandemic). However, developing this network would require addressing barriers to receiving mental health treatment across state lines and issues with computer and internet access in impoverished or rural areas.[20]

Substance Misuse

While we are at it, we need to address one of the main issues for young people with early psychosis, which is that substance use—so popular in American culture for young people—can complicate their symptoms and lead to more aggressive behaviors. Many young persons could benefit by not "playing" quite so hard. There are other ways for young people to connect besides partying together, and we need to build up both those points of connection and opportunities to help young people decide to stay sober or engage in healthier activities together. I loved Pedro's idea of offering more gym memberships to young people who otherwise lack the resources and who would find wellness and community in that kind of space.

Another possibility would be to increase the availability of youth-focused events—open to the wider community—at explicitly "sober" spaces where young people already naturally enjoy hanging out, such as coffeehouses. Activities could include poetry slams, open mic nights, film screenings, book clubs, "knit ins" for people who like to knit or crochet, video game competitions, and so forth. Such activities could be fun, provide for a creative outlet, and build community. These activities could also be offered in churches, public libraries, or other community spaces like the local YMCA. Evidently the app "Phoenix" helps people connect in just such a way in communities across the United States.

Creativity was also an important resource for the young people in our study. Even though the interview protocol did not prompt young people to talk about it specifically, one-third of the young persons we interviewed mentioned making music or pursuing visual or performing arts. Research indicates that interventions that reflect the culture of a target population are more effective than standard treatments.[21] Using rap or hip hop as a base for developing new interventions, for example, could offer fresh ways to engage youths who enjoy those kinds of

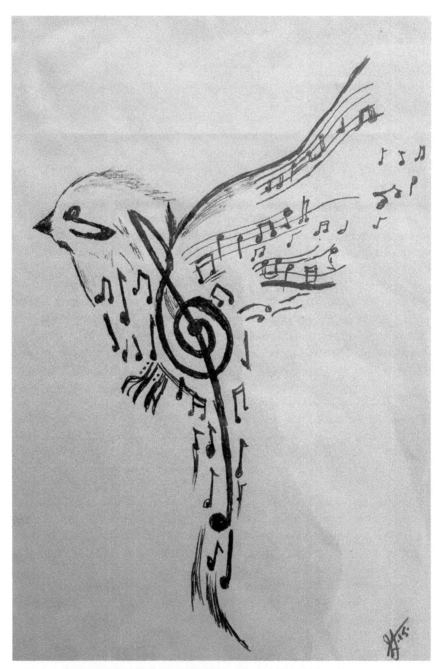

FIGURE 7. "Songbird" by Joseph Steven Laurenzo. This image was a gift from my younger brother to celebrate my husband's love of music. Joseph texted my mother a note to accompany the image in this book: "People with mental illness have the gift of seeing and imagining things differently. This is expressed in their art." My brother has been making art for more than thirty years. *Reproduced with permission of the artist.*

music. Fun activities—and the friends that can result from having something in common—are also helpful for replenishing moral agency.

STEP 2. IMPROVING CRISIS MANAGEMENT

The current pathways to care that most young people have available to them—typically after a crisis, through an emergency setting, and often with police involvement—set young people up to fail. Such a pathway invites social stigma by making an early mental health crisis seem criminal. It exposes young persons to confrontation with and possible physical harm by the police. It sets them up to have a police record, incur court costs, and face other challenging criminal justice outcomes that can tax their material resources and meaningful relationships. As a result, the young person and their families seriously question their moral agency in the days that follow. As a society, we must decide, Are they "mad" or "bad"? What do we mean by those terms? What are the consequences of the approaches we use? With this information, we can work toward reform. In the meantime, here are a few places to start.

Even within a supportive community, and even when there is some mental health care in place, families still may need emergency services. Unfortunately, the way most families know to contact emergency support is to call 911. As soon as that happens, the police are also notified. In twenty-eight states, police are legally required to be involved in an emergency call. But police involvement is often highly visible to neighbors, families, and friends and perpetuates the impression among all involved that they have done something wrong or even bad. The optics and consequences of police involvement, including the reputational and physical danger to people in crisis, need further attention. Simply put, if a person is experiencing an emergency, we could provide gentler entry points to care.

One initiative includes the number 988, which connects people to a mental health crisis hotline with access to trauma-informed counselors, mobile crisis units, co-responder services, and longer-term mental health programs. Since the line replaced the National Suicide Hotline in July 2022, the numbers of calls, texts, and chats have risen by 45 percent, with 80 percent of calls answered by someone in the same state, 93 percent of calls and 98 percent of texts and chats being answered overall, and reduced wait time to talk to a counselor.[22] Currently, however, there is concern about insufficient mental health resources like a counselor on call, a safe or respite space available where people can go, or even knowledge of local resources when they do exist among persons staffing the lines, as well as questions about the training and qualifications of 988 staff in general.[23] In addition, not all calls are answered, it is not clear or uniform how 988 works from region to region (some states have significantly lower answer rates, such as Arkansas and South Carolina at 55–69%), and the waitlist for many mental health services to which a person could be referred is far too long. It took a while to work the kinks out of the 911 emergency system, and even that still has issues, and proponents of 988 argue that it will take sustained effort. We need to make sure people keep trying to make this emergency number work more efficiently at the local and the state level.

For the time being, police will likely continue to be the primary first responders to psychiatric emergencies in most states. Interventions to improve police inter- actions include the use of mobile crisis clinicians, unarmed response units, and mental health–trained intervention teams.[24] Even police officers who receive only a special 40-hour training about mental health as mental health first responders (crisis intervention team [CIT] model) are more likely to offer a person mental health services (instead of jail) and less likely to use force and arrest during police encounters with individuals with a mental disorder.[25] To date, more than 3,000 jurisdictions worldwide have implemented this CIT model.[26]

Other models use co-responders and embed a person with lived experience, a social worker, or a behavioral health specialist in the unit that responds to mental health emergencies. People in crisis prefer this model.[27] Dallas County, for exam- ple, has piloted such a program, the RIGHT Care program, since 2018. The team includes a community paramedic, a licensed mental health clinician, and a spe- cially trained police officer. According to its website, the team responded to 4,000 calls in the first eighteen months of its existence, with only 2 percent resulting in arrest, 900 people being diverted from the emergency room directly to mental health support, and 500 diverted from jail. Whether it has been deemed to have worked well in the long run or will be expanded remains to be seen.[28]

There are alternatives available, but as a society, Americans need more invest- ment in pilot programs, developed in partnership with the communities expected to use them, to understand what works well, for whom, and under what circum- stances. Interestingly, the least-restrictive options, such as a crisis line or mobile crisis team, are also the least costly but need to be more widely available and able to connect people to mental health supports and services quickly.[29]

STEP 3. REDESIGNING EMERGENCY HOSPITALIZATIONS

Ideally, young persons experiencing early psychosis would never reach a crisis point where they are being brought into the hospital by police. Expensive emer- gency hospitalizations offer little material, moral, or therapeutic support and are a far cry from psychologist Carol Gilligan's notion of ideal care as "an activity of rela- tionship, of seeing and responding to need, taking care of the world by sustaining the web of connection so that no one is left alone."[30] In fact, being left alone is often what happens to young people with early psychosis, as friends, family, educational structures, social networks, and vocational opportunities evaporate after they have been picked up by police, hospitalized, and deemed "psychotic."

We desperately need to redesign our approach.

Educate Providers and Families about Privacy Laws

First, it might greatly help if young persons and their families could be better connected with each other during their hospitalizations and subsequent experiences with bouncing, especially when everyone is new to the system. To better ensure connection, we need a widespread understanding about what HIPAA laws mean and what mental health professionals can and cannot tell families when their loved one is in the hospital, in jail, or the like.[31] Often institutions of care assume they cannot share *any* information, but this is not true. In a whole set of circumstances, family members are permitted to know about the care of their loved one in psychiatric emergency situations, as recently outlined in a document from the Office of Civil Rights of the US Department of Health and Human Services.[32] For example, a family can be notified if the patient has not objected, if the family has been involved in care previously, and if the hospital staff can infer from surrounding circumstances that it is in the best interest of the patient (for example, the patient did not describe abuse at the hands of a parent). If a patient is unable to agree or object, because of some incapacity or emergency—which arguably applies to some of the young people in this study—then a psychiatric hospital is free to notify a "member of the household, such as a parent, roommate, sibling, partner or spouse, and inform them about the patient's location and general condition." A hospital can also "disclose the necessary protected health information to anyone who is in a position to prevent or lessen [any] threatened harm" if such disclosure can reduce a serious and imminent threat to the health or safety of the patient or others, even without the patient's agreement.

This last clause is the key that might have helped Daphne and others, though it leaves a lot of room for interpretation. In fact, the law even states that no one can "second guess a health care professional's judgement," and so they are free to share when, in their judgment, sharing may protect the patient from harm. Therapists can even contact parents to let them know that a patient has not been attending appointments and may be in danger. These circumstances need to be made clearer to the public and to institutions of care so that young people aren't getting lost in the system while they are bouncing between facilities or after discharge. In many of the examples I share in this book, key supporters needed access to more information about the youths' whereabouts and well-being but were unable to get it, possibly because health care professionals did not understand the spirit of the law or feared receiving hefty fines or being sued.

Some argue that the law is often interpreted incorrectly by health care facilities or by employees without adequate training (who are often on the frontline interacting with families), which prevents patients' families from getting information that is not actually restricted under the law. Some doctors are calling for the laws to be revisited to address unnecessary bottlenecks in patient care. In cases of early psychosis, better connecting parents to the hospital and to other mental health providers may go a long way toward helping keep a young person safe (assuming that the family is a "safe space" for a young person in the first place, which was true for most of the young people in our study).

Focus on Trauma-Informed Care

Given ample evidence that people seeking inpatient psychiatric services have often already experienced trauma, it seems clear that traumatic histories affect a person's willingness to seek help and engage in care.[33] As Sascha DuBrul advised, "We desperately need to create sanctuaries for people who are having the kind of spiritual and emotional crises I was having when I was a teenager."[34]

One approach is to implement principles of trauma-informed care in emergency settings and among first responders for people in crisis. Maxine Harris and Roger D. Fallot, former codirectors of Community Connections, an addiction and mental health rehabilitation program in Washington, DC, identified five principles to guide trauma-informed care practice: physical and emotional safety, trustworthiness, choice, collaboration, and empowerment.[35] Physical and emotional safety includes separating patients by their self-identified gender at all stages of care,[36] making safe "time-out" spaces available, respecting patient privacy and modesty (when they are bathing, sleeping, and using the bathroom), training staff in de-escalation strategies, and helping patients identify triggers and calming strategies to help them feel in control. Establishing trustworthiness includes helping clients feel safe, respecting their emotional limits, explaining procedures and tests, respectfully and consistently practicing informed consent, and maintaining respectful professional boundaries. Collaboration means treating the client as an expert on their own life and allowing the client to plan and evaluate the care they receive. Finally, empowerment refers to helping clients identify and employ coping strategies. For services specific to early intervention for psychosis, research suggests that trauma-informed care involves seeking agreement and consent from the service user before beginning any intervention; building a trusting relationship with the service user; maintaining a safe environment for service users; fostering a calm, compassionate, and supportive ethos; and being empathetic and nonjudgmental.[37] While these principles may sound like basic human kindness, some of the stories I have shared throughout the book suggest that this is exactly what needs to be upheld as important in emergency psychiatry settings. Many of these elements were missing from the care the young people described receiving, and following any of them may have made a difference for preserving and promoting moral agency. Research suggests that conditions are not better elsewhere in the United States.[38] Changing these conditions will require time, training, and commitment.

Safe Spaces for Mothers and Children

My research also revealed that one group in dire need of better solutions is young mothers with early psychosis and their children. Nursing mothers faced the added physical and psychological challenges of stopping breastfeeding.[39] In the United Kingdom and other countries of Western Europe, there are mother-baby units that keep mothers with postpartum psychosis and their babies together with a focus on safety, psychosocial support, and psycho-education. However, this accommodation was nowhere evident in my study, and one advocacy group, the Maternal Mental Health Leadership Alliance, wrote in 2023 that only four such units exist in the United States.[40] My team did not witness anyone even offering a breast pump to a nursing mother.

One group that may have an experience comparable to that of mothers dealing with psychosis is incarcerated mothers. Research on this group suggests that forced separation of mothers from their children is an experience similar to still-birth or miscarriage and increases the risk of self-harm as the woman struggles with the loss of their identity as a mother.[41]

Separation is hard on the children, too, and can have lasting consequences. First, breastfeeding, when possible, is essential to infant development. Second, the cycle of institutionalization seems to perpetuate itself. Women with a psychotic disorder who had their children taken away from them while in a joint mother-baby unit in France and Belgium for women with postpartum psychosis were 4.4 times more likely to have been separated from their own mothers and institutionalized as a child.[42] Children who are separated from their own mothers and institutionalized thus may be more likely to have their children taken away later. The research recommends that, if separation is necessary, the child be placed with a family member or a foster family rather than in an institution to help limit the consequences of maternal separation for the child.[43] This is an area in need of careful consideration and reform to stop the devastating cycle.

Value and Offer Mutual Supports

Many, many times throughout this research (and in my global health work as well), young people and their families expressed an interest in working more with someone who had been through psychosis as a young person and was now doing fine. Such people are known as peers or peer support specialists. A peer is someone who understands, someone who has been there before, someone who is doing well. For youths and families, they also wanted this living example that things could get better. Employing more peer support specialists in emergency and crisis services can help improve the system and promote moral agency, because peers can serve as real-world examples of the fact that, though a person may be having a hard time—including homelessness, substance use disorders, and incarceration, along with serious mental health symptoms—they can still pass through it and find meaning and purpose, gainful employment, and community in a group of people who have survived similar experiences. Peers can also offer advice to young people about how to manage symptoms and medications, relationships with therapists, psychiatrists, friends and family, resources for wellness, and much more. Several young people I talked to said they would happily volunteer to visit other young persons in the hospital to help them know they were not alone. This would probably be possible via Telehealth, as well, which may help reduce concerns about safety, anonymity, and the possibility of accidentally triggering someone by sending them into the hospital as a volunteer. Some, like Ariana, already had plans to become a professional peer support specialist. A support group composed of a mix of people who are struggling and people who are doing well and can understand and encourage one another could be ideal.

These kinds of options do exist, just not in formal mental health care settings, typically. One is the Hearing Voices Network, run by people who share the experience of voices, visions and other extreme states.[44] Another is the Fireweed Collective, for persons who identify as mad or neurodivergent. The Inner Compass Initiative seeks to empower people to make a friend with someone who is having similar experiences and claims to offer unbiased, straightforward information about psychiatric drugs and diagnoses. Some of these groups hold gatherings in numerous local communities around the United States (and other countries) and online to help people, in mutually supportive ways, manage experiences such as hearing voices and taking or tapering off of antipsychotic medications. The Wildflower Alliance, with support from the state of Massachusetts, has four community centers, operates the peer-run respite Afiya House (mentioned earlier), and also offers training workshops for people seeking to deepen their peer support skills. DuBrul, who started the Icarus Project, which turned into the Fireweed Collective, explains that mutual support networks make friends into everyday heroes who are accessible on a local level: "We send off ripples" of support, he observes, "through the fabric of our friends."[45] This network building provides more community, he explains, so that people do not spend their whole lives feeling out of place.[46]

Corrina similarly said:

> If these [other young people in my study] don't have a lot of friends, which, it can be hard . . . That makes it ten times worse, so much worse, and then that also puts more strain on the people that are in their family, 'cause they become more needy, 'cause you need friends. I realize now, without my friends, I feel so depressed and so much more anxious. If y'all needed to get me in touch with any of these people, I would be willing to talk to anybody, because I understand if they need a friend, I can be a friend.

While confidentiality issues prevented us from connecting the young people in the study, Corrina would have been a valuable friend for a lot of the young people my team met. She herself made a few friends in group therapy whom she stayed in touch with for support. Young people are making such friends organically, but more of us could, and should, help them along.

Alternatives to Inpatient Hospitalizations

Another possible approach is to divert "first-timer" young people away from emergency hospitalization altogether to smaller, safer spaces. *Peer respites* represent one such alternative, so called because they are staffed by peers. Peer respites are typically run out of houses in residential neighborhoods and serve as places where people experiencing a mental health crisis can go any time of day or night for a short-term stay (an average of five days in 2018[47]) as an alternative to psychiatric hospitalization.

Peer respites provide services such as support groups, one-on-one time with peer specialists, recovery-oriented self-help training, and recreational activities. Many respites allow people to stay who are actively suicidal or experiencing psychosis, or both, but admission is determined on an individual level.[48] They also permit people to choose whether they want to take medications, and they offer a safe space for those who do not. Currently, there are thirty-three peer respites in thirteen US states.[49]

One randomized clinical trial comparing the use of peer respites to locked inpatient psychiatric facilities among a sample of uninsured, civilly committed adults found that those using the peer respite self-reported improvements in mental health and treatment satisfaction.[50] A study of the effectiveness of another peer respite program in New York found a reduction of 2.9 psychiatric hospitalizations per respite client as compared to clients who went to the emergency room in the first year, and Medicaid expenditures were an average of $2,138 lower.[51] In a qualitative study from the Southwest, peer respite users described the first two days of their five-day stay as a time to slow down and rest and the last two days as preparing to reenter their daily lives. Users thought the peer respite created a "much more relaxed atmosphere" than a typical psychiatric hospitalization,[52] though a minority did not like the unstructured environment.[53] In a matched-pairs analysis between patients who used peer respites and those who didn't, people who went to peer respites instead of the emergency room were 70 percent less likely to end up in inpatient psychiatric hospitals.[54] I wonder if this has something to do with the Medicaid reimbursement rules for emergency rooms that seem to encourage long-term holds in inpatient facilities to protect reimbursement for uninsured patients, a practice I detail in chapter 4.

In another qualitative study of people who have used peer respites, most concluded that being around peers who have been through similar experiences was

comforting and helpful to their recovery. Afiya, a peer respite center in Massachusetts, conducted poststay surveys suggesting that it was greatly beneficial. Ninety
percent of participants said they would choose Afiya again over a hospital or other
support option.[55]

Many details are still to be worked out, such as the ideal length of peer respite
stays. Many participants in one peer respite said that even a 30-day stay (this
setting offered 3 to 29 days) would not be long enough.[56] Some who like peer
respites don't want to leave, or may come back frequently, for example to avoid
homelessness. Shorter stays likely helped people get back to their lives more
quickly, but it's complicated. Some people need more sanctuary. Thoughtful
training and supervision of staff and clients are also necessary, especially to prevent staff burnout.

The truth is that we know how to create the sanctuaries that DuBrul said he
needed as a teenager. We know how to provide better emergency care for people
with psychosis that is trauma informed and safe and offers mutual support that can
protect moral agency. For a young person to want to continue engaging in further
mental health care, the initial landings in "care" for them need to be soft, welcom-
ing, and safe. American society needs to invest in more trauma-informed care and
peer support in emergency settings, as well as alternatives to those settings, such
as peer respites. We also need to build better support systems for mental health
care workers. This includes training for the hospital workers who are trying to
make meaningful changes in the face of arcane and difficult medical billing practices and a lack of structural or trauma-informed supports. Change for the better
also means giving peers more opportunities and funding and space or bandwidth
to provide support, both in the hospital and in the community.

STEP 4. OPTIMIZING EARLY INTERVENTION

Coordinated specialty care (CSC), as mentioned in this book's introduction, has
been rolled out as the premier model of care for early psychosis intervention in the
United States. Efforts to implement this model had barely begun in Texas when I
first started my research, and no one in my study qualified under the initial eligi-
bility criteria, which have since changed.

As these services have become more available nationwide thanks to federal
and state investments in early intervention for mental health, much research and
hard work has been done to decide what early intervention means (do we screen
at-risk youths and pretreat?), what to offer, and how to best roll these services
out to Americans across the country who come from a wide range of social contexts, levels of resources and need, and cultural backgrounds. At this writing, I
am participating in one CSC research project called EPINET-Texas, funded by
the National Institutes of Mental Health, which uses a "learning healthcare system" to create feedback loops with providers, youths, and families that can help us

optimize services. EPINET-TX is also in conversation with several other, similar programs around the country to harmonize data and learn more about what works and does not work for all Americans.[57]

While much is shifting and being learned, in general, the model aims to offer some specific components in every location, including medication management, individual or group therapy, family psychoeducation, and vocational or educational support.[58] Of course, not all states fund these programs adequately, and not all young persons can access all of them, but since the model is currently considered to be an ideal form of care, I offer recommendations relevant to each of these components.

Medication Management

Once a person is diagnosed with psychosis, the way forward with medication must be thought through very carefully and in partnership with the youth and their family. As this book argues, medication management is a medical, material, *and* moral issue. Of course, young people need to be able to afford and access prescribers who know how to handle psychosis symptoms well with the right medication, as mentioned in step 1. But we also need to understand that the young person or their loved ones may not view using medications as a tool to help them replenish their moral agency and so they might reject those medications. Ariana's family and coworkers thought using medications signaled she was "crazy" or an "addict" or both—labels that she could not embrace—and so she refused longer-term medication use. Michael's sense that the side effects might limit his ability to be a father was too much to bear because, in his local moral world, becoming a father was key to meaningful adulthood. In contrast, for Pedro, using medications indicated that he might obtain disability income that could help the family, so he embraced medications—but on his own terms, making it clear that he was taking the medication to treat his PTSD, another signal to his community that his diagnosis did not mean he was a bad person. Amy—whose grandmother had died in a state hospital after being held there for schizophrenia—eventually embraced her medications because her family saw it as a way for her to avoid the same fate. Sage's grandmother had also been hospitalized for schizophrenia, but her parents and grandparents supported her refusing medications (though she did not refuse Adderall). At this point, the decisions the young people made about treatment depended on whether they thought using them to access a better life would not jeopardize the respect they needed to thrive from the people they loved.

Most research to date has focused only on whether people should have antipsychotic medications at all. While these findings are hotly debated, people who take antipsychotic medications their whole lives appear to live on average twenty-five years less than they might have, even when controlling for lifestyle factors like smoking and obesity.[59] The side effects of the drugs may contribute to cardiometabolic problems that can lead to heart disease and diabetes, for example.[60]

On the other hand, a systematic review of studies exploring use of antipsychotic medication by people diagnosed with schizophrenia (which is not the inevitable outcome of early psychosis but is a possibility) claimed that mortality rates were higher in patients with no antipsychotic use than in those who did not use the drugs.[61]

Specific to early psychosis, a Finnish twenty-year follow-up study on discontinuation of antipsychotics following a first episode found that people who never used antipsychotics past their initial hospitalization had a 214 percent higher risk of death than those who did.[62] Based on this evidence, the authors argue that long-term antipsychotic treatment is associated with increased survival. In Norway, some psychiatrists are encouraging medication-free options for early psychosis. One study that included interviews with patients who discontinued antipsychotics at different time points showed that a robust relationship with the treatment team, as well as patient personal responsibility and agency within that relationship, was imperative for positive outcomes after discontinuing medications.[63] Those who discontinued medication also described an improved relationship with their therapists compared to previous experiences. Yet discontinuing or not using antipsychotic medications is controversial, even among Norwegian psychiatrists.[64]

There are many studies and arguments on both sides, and we do not have all the answers yet. Coordinated specialty care, the popular model in the United States right now, advocates for using the lowest possible doses of medication for the shortest possible time.[65] In a recent review, this CSC approach to medication prescription was associated with more work and school involvement among the young persons and lower symptom severity.[66] With my own results in mind, it seems clear that prescribers should, at a minimum, be taught how to interact flexibly and ethically with young people and their families concerning medications. Clear information about psychiatric medications, the side effects, interactions with other drugs, and whether they need to take a drug for life is surprisingly hard to find, and many people are receiving prescriptions without a clear sense of what the medications do. There needs to be more transparency around potential risks and side effects—a stronger good-faith effort to provide "informed consent."

Decision making about prescriptions and changes works best when it is shared between patient and physician, which also ensures that the patient takes their medications as prescribed. Sofia was not interested in taking medications until she worked with someone who understood that she was experiencing "nervios" and needed homeopathic approaches alongside psychiatric medications. Furthermore, those who have unwanted side effects but no information on how to mitigate them often reject the medications. If antipsychotics are not helping them restore their moral agency by helping them look good, feel good, and be productive—all culturally valued states of mind for young people—then they are an unappealing choice. These suggestions line up with literature that advocates for "shared decision making" between doctors and patients as a key to ethical psychiatrist-patient relationships, but the connection should hold true for the young person and any prescriber, as well.[67] Providers also need to be open to the possibility that psycho-social interventions may be more acceptable to a young person and their family.

Vocational and Educational Support

Vocational and educational support is another key part of the CSC model, but may not always be implemented, at least in public insurance settings where there are limited resources and staff. However, this piece is important in attracting young people to using early-intervention services. All of the youth in our study were highly focused initially on getting their lives "back to normal," or at least back on track, and the best way to do this is to help them stay as connected to school and work as possible.[68]

While nearly everyone in our study reported having employment during their lifetime, it is not clear that they all had a job they wanted or that paid well, and several lost their jobs during their crisis. In the state-of-the-art (but not yet widely available) CSC model, members of a team that supports a young person with early psychosis include "supported employment specialists" who are dedicated to helping young persons find a competitive job. In turn, young persons must choose to participate, use mental health treatment, and have a goal of competitive employment.[69] Supported employment programs then offer personalized disability benefits counseling and aid in a job search that meets the young person's preferences. Participation in early psychosis services has also been found to increase work participation.[70]

Educational support is another important goal for many young people as more Americans enroll in college after high school (70 percent in 2009) as an important part of their transition to young adulthood in a country where "college for all" is a widely held cultural ideal, though some media outlets argue that this ideal is changing.[71] Supported employment programs can also offer education components. In one program that made quarterly assessments, OnTrack New York, having educational support in the first quarter in which young people were enrolled in services was significantly associated with school enrollment in the second quarter and continuing throughout the first year of services.[72]

Overall, developing educational environments that better support people with mental health concerns stands to benefit many young people. One study found that over four-fifths of college-enrolled students experiencing a first episode of psychosis also face a disruption in their college education. While many return to college afterward, it takes them about a year and a half on average to do so.[73] This is a long time for a young person to be out of school. Smoothing the transition from the hospital back into school or preventing a full disruption in the first place needs to be a high priority. Back-to-school toolkits for higher education, developed for students and families as well as administrators, suggest that effective accommodations create more inclusive environments and offer more flexibility around helpful forms of testing, attendance policies, and classroom resources (e.g., recording lectures).[74]

Stigma is also a huge concern in higher education. Administrators, professors, and teaching assistants are not sure what to do with a student who is having a mental health crisis in class—or afterward. I have seen this personally as an educator. It can be difficult for students to access mental health care while on campus or back at home during a break. Students like Pedro, James, Sofia, and Markus shared their problems with school expulsion and student loans related to their mental health crisis. James was expelled from school. Corrina had to drop out due to the anxiety it caused her to attend classes. All of them lost scholarships and financial aid and had loans they could not cancel because they had passed an administrative deadline at the school for withdrawing. Young people were then carrying debts even though they had no course credits or progress toward a degree to show for them. We need to develop more compassionate policies and evidence-based guidelines to support young people in staying in school, not penalize them when they cannot, and to help them get their student fellowships and scholarships back when they are able to return.

Counseling centers also need to be prepared to help young people with psychosis or make referrals to people who can, and student insurance needs to cover that care. We could create technological options for young people who need to attend school virtually for periods of time to manage serious symptoms. My favorite option comes from Norway, which has pioneered using "telepresence robots" that can attend class, record lectures, and take notes for disabled or sick children when they are not well. The program has met with some success—but, of course, not without some controversy.[75] Why not pilot such a program here for young people who require long inpatient stays? Or at least have someone—perhaps a teaching assistant, a school employee, or a student volunteer—record lectures and take notes for them? These are not expensive or complicated asks. Someone just needs to care enough to make it happen.

Supporting Families

Throughout this book, I show families that were often a key part of protecting, replenishing, and nourishing a young person's moral agency. They also provided critical support of a young person materially (providing housing, cell phone payments, food) and medically—for example, by given them a safe place to stay, reminding them of appointments, providing transportation, and monitoring medication use. Most people working in early psychosis services seem to believe that involved families are the best possible asset for a young person in their recovery. But to be able to provide material, medical, and moral support effectively, families themselves need sufficient support.

Most CSC programs offer "family psychoeducation," if anything, but much more is needed.[76] Family psychoeducation is important; it is meant to help families understand what is going on with the young person and how to support them by increasing their "mental health literacy"—a construct I critique in chapter 3.

However, none of the families I met accepted the psychoeducation on offer. In general, I think there must be longer, more in-depth, and more sustained family support for families to heal.

Some innovative programs are using "family navigators" or "family support specialists," people who have a loved one who has experienced a serious mental health concern and so are able to offer a lived-experience perspective as a family member to those newer to the experience.[77] One study from Australia found that family peer support workers who provided families with comfort, guidance, and advice were helpful.[78] In my own research on the "Opening Doors to Recovery" program in Savannah, Georgia, my team found that family community navigation specialists—as they were called in that context—were a positive addition to a team of supporters for persons with long-term psychiatric disability.[79] They helped provide emotional support and served as a strong communication liaison between the family and providers.

In addition, my research has shown that all families and young persons would benefit—separately and together—from more therapeutic support, ideally offered at home, in the evening, and possibly online. Therapy can help families rebuild trust and shared moral understandings—so important for moral agency—in the aftermath of a psychiatric crisis. Formal, clinic-based "interventions" provide information about ways to address practical issues, help families feel more supported, and increase the family's confidence that they can support their relative.[80] Therapeutic "talking" interventions for families that also have been shown to help reduce relapse and hospital admission rates for people with psychosis and help improve social functioning.[81] In addition, family interventions are thought to reduce the burden of care for families and better prepare them to provide care.[82] Engaging family members may be especially important, as well, in working with persons from minoritized groups. In one review of mental health disparities among ethnoracially minoritized individuals with severe mental illness, identifying a family support person to include in doctor's visits and providing family psychoeducation were both critical for lowering attrition.[83] However, I think most of the families I worked with would have loved having any of this work with families conducted in their home during a time when they were all present.

Probably the most comprehensive and best-researched family intervention is the Open Dialogue approach, which does typically occur in the home and often includes a psychiatrist, a psychologist, and a nurse.[84] This team follows the patient through inpatient and outpatient settings, from the first 24 hours after their possible initial first psychotic episode *for as long as treatment is necessary*. Having a secure team in place helps the young person and their family navigate the system. Team meetings are held at the patient's home or another safe space and include at least two trained therapists, family members or another key supporter, and the young person. Hospitalization and medication are not the focus of treatment, are often delayed, and are used sparingly. Hospitalizations are not forced. Instead, the foundation of the treatment is the Open Dialogue—an "equal" dialogue between the patient, the patient's key supporters, and the therapists with a goal of increasing a sense of agency, motivating change, and creating a shared understanding of the situation. All participants discuss all issues openly and in the presence of all the other members of the team and family.

Research suggests that overall recovery rates using the Open Dialogue approach are often better than for people receiving treatment-as-usual, including a reduced need for psychiatric treatment and fewer psychotic symptoms.[85] A 19-year follow-up study in Finland that compared first-episode psychosis patients using the Open Dialogue approach to those using treatment-as-usual found that Open Dialogue users had significantly less overall need for hospitalization, antipsychotic medication, or disability allowances. For patients with more threatening behavior, however, the dialogical approach was less successful.[86] In addition, suicide rates were high in both Open Dialogue and control groups, indicating that psychotic experiences were still highly distressing, even with this more therapeutic and egalitarian, family-based approach.[87] Yet this treatment has helped many young persons and their families deal effectively with acute stressors and life crises.

In addition, encouraging everyone involved—the young person, their clinicians, and their key supporters—to voice their ideas and concerns in equal ways offered opportunities for new kinds of understanding while promoting shared decision making.[88] Much of what frustrated many of the young persons my team engaged with over time, which often led them to reject future mental health care, involved not feeling listened to by family and treatment staff throughout inpatient stays and beyond. This sense of dismissal may be softened by using an Open Dialogue approach that promotes mutual trust—an important part of the psychotherapeutic process.[89] In general, Open Dialogue users felt better listened to and understood than they did in other kinds of care experiences, though some patients with psychosis did find the meetings to be overwhelming and strange.[90]

Unfortunately, it is not yet clear how well Open Dialogue translates to locations outside Finland. It has been offered in the United States in mental health agencies in Massachusetts, Georgia, New York, and Vermont. In Vermont, where it is called the Collaborative Network approach, one qualitative study found that it was well received, appreciated, and perceived as an empowering form of mental health care.[91] A study in Massachusetts suggested that families liked having a space where they could process their experiences together, the involvement of the team in their lives, and the transparency of the Open Dialogue treatment process.[92] Interviews with youths and family members in Vermont revealed that young people felt less singled-out when their families were included in the treatment process and that they felt they had learned as much from having their family present as their family and clinicians had learned from them.[93] An Atlanta-based team found that the approach was feasible and acceptable and had some positive effects even with less frequent meetings and without home visits.[94]

However, more research is needed. In the meantime, some Open Dialogue principles might be adapted to offer families more therapeutic support at home or in a safe space after a psychiatric crisis.

STEP 5. MATERIAL SUPPORT

Research on state-of-the-art care for early psychosis suggests that it may work best for people with a high socioeconomic status.[95] It makes sense that low socioeconomic status would make it harder to find the material resources needed to access care. Thus, we must consider ways to offer more material support to young people in crisis and their families. It is not just the responsibility of individuals or clinicians or community supporters to promote youth mental health; it is the responsibility of us all, and some of that promotion is going to require ongoing investment in mental health care for those at higher risk who cannot afford to prioritize mental health care when they face so many other challenges.

One way we all can help is to agree to make mental health care cost-free for people who have experienced psychosis without requiring them to have a "disability" that renders them unable to work. Nearly everyone in my study reported having worked at some point prior to their first hospitalization. Evidence suggests that people who have psychotic symptoms want to work, but many ultimately seek out social security disability income or supplemental security income (depending on how long they have worked). Such assistance offers a living stipend to offset the financial burden of not being able to work and helps them secure mental health insurance through Medicare (after 24 months in the case of SSDI) or Medicaid (automatic for SSI) to help cover the high costs of medications and potential future hospitalizations.

Disability is expensive for the government to offer, though the details are hard to parse. Federal expenditures for SSI alone in calendar year 2022 totaled $57.1 billion for 1.23 million individuals, of which about $14.65 billion was allocated to persons with serious psychiatric disabilities such as schizophrenia and bipolar disorder.[96] Many people do need the monthly stipend to live on and many also need the Medicaid and Medicare to access and pay for mental health care.

Of course, this means that insurance is another area in need of reform. Mental health care is expensive, and accessing services early is difficult for families unless they have the right insurance. If they don't, accessing mental health care requires them to use emergency services, which is expensive, prevents early intervention, and can be a traumatic experience. At the hospital where I worked, the young persons who lacked insurance—presumably mental health insurance— seemed to be sent consistently for a long stay at the state hospital to meet Medicaid requirements, which was costly for youths and their families. The fiscal year 2024 "maximum daily rate of charge to individuals" for an inpatient stay in a Texas state psychiatric hospital was $579 per day for "adults" and $928 for "children and adolescents," which would add up quickly: 28 days for an adult would cost a person $16,212.[97] This price is likely cheaper than a long stay at Shady Elms but is still staggering for most people I worked with to cover. No wonder Sage compared it to the costs of a year of college.

In 2014, when my fieldwork started, the Affordable Care Act had just made it possible for some of the young people to apply to stay on or reapply for their parent's insurance until age 26. Insurers could no longer declare a history of psychosis as a preexisting condition and thus a barrier to insurance.[98] Some of these reforms have been helpful. Even so, among those who are in the early stages of psychosis and qualify for Medicaid based on income, the lack of a documented disability can preclude their access to Medicaid benefits that would cover early psychosis services, because the funding is limited to those with multiepisode schizophrenia and there must be at least one year of documented illness to apply. These requirements limit services that could help prevent people from becoming disabled in the first place.[99]

Commercial health insurance and Medicaid programs also do not typically cover comprehensive early-psychosis services—and even when they do, what they cover is highly variable.[100] In one study, Medicaid covered around half of the costs of CSC, which excluded community outreach activities, team meetings, ongoing training, and supervision—all of which are needed to build effective programs.[101] Both state and federal entities are actively investigating additional financing strategies and increasingly liaising with private as well as public insurers, but we need to continue to push these agencies to make changes that foster preventive and intensive early psychosis support for young persons before and after a crisis.[102] One recent change (September 2023) for public insurance was to adopt a single code for billing for the package of CSC services at the federal level so that any CSC component, tailored to a person's specific needs, could (in theory) be covered by a single code.[103] While the effects of the change remain to be seen, many consider this a step in the right direction for improving access to the full package of CSC interventions.

In one international review of primarily Western countries (one from China), 14 of 15 studies of early-psychosis intervention programs found that the availability of such intervention "resulted in reductions in total costs or were cost effective because they decreased high cost adverse outcomes," such as by reducing the number of emergency room visits and high-cost inpatient hospitalizations, while improving a young person's quality of life.[104] Despite the evidence, even if everyone had insurance, there are not enough early-psychosis programs available currently to meet demand. For example, in Texas each year about 3,000 young adults ages 12–25 are estimated to need early-psychosis services.[105] In 2014, when this study took place, there were only two CSC teams in Texas, and they were capable of serving 60 total young persons, representing 2 percent of state-level needs.[106] By 2016, when my study ended, there were only ten, with the capacity for 300 (10 percent of those in need). In 2022, around 1,366 clients were served in Texas by CSC teams,[107] which the Meadows Mental Health Policy Institute estimates as representing about 17.5 percent of persons needing those services in any given year. Nationally, it is estimated that more than 75,000 young persons go without access to CSC programs every year.[108]

We can do better. This is not a money grab; it is a potentially self-sustaining investment in young persons' futures that may reduce costs drastically in the long run. CSC models cover two years and cost about $15,000 per person per year—less than the 28-day inpatient state hospital bill many of the young persons we worked with likely received after their initial hospitalization. If we work instead to get people on track and avoid generating the need for crisis intervention, rehospitalization, and disability services, the savings for individuals, their families, taxpayers, and the government will be inestimable.

· · ·

Opportunities to help young people prevent, approach gently, pass through, reorient to, and find treatment and support for experiences of psychosis through moral agency–enhancing practices are described throughout this book. This final chapter attempts to distill these into five steps we could take to radically transform care by strengthening its medical, material, and moral dimensions to help a young person protect their moral agency at a vulnerable time, which is key for moving forward into valued adulthood.

Moral agency is the catalyst for individual, familial, and societal belonging for any young person in the United States, including a person with early psychosis. Social belonging heals us all. We all need to be loved. The origin of the word *believe* is beloved.[109] We need others to see us as at least "good enough" for love—good enough to be beloved and believed—for our lives to have meaning.

If we pay attention to moral agency and offer young persons better support, many more can pass through their crisis and move forward with a life that is perhaps even more enriched and meaningful than it would have been otherwise. Not everyone who has experienced psychosis and moved on wants to share that story with others, so we do not hear about many of their stories, but I have talked to many people over the years who passed through this kind of experience, and more and more people are coming forward. Some of them have published research, first-person narratives, films, and artworks that have been crucial for me to understand psychosis myself, and I have no doubt there is much more to come as society embraces neurodiversity and understands that everyone has something to offer the collective whole. People with lived experience are doing their part to help, but all of us, as humans, can also become allies and do as much as we are able to help young persons experiencing symptoms of psychosis. Helping young people stay connected to people they care about and engaged in activities that are meaningful to them and reminding them that they are a "good enough," beloved person is crucial for them to envision a pathway to and through care. This care may be medical, it may be moral, and for many it will need to be material at times, as well, but if we commit to making sure that support is on offer and sometimes offer it ourselves, we can make a difference.

In this way, we can make psychosis a turning point—a moment when we realize a young person may need more accommodations to move forward, a moment when we commit to providing that support. This will require a societal turning point in the United States: the political will to make reforms, the social will to be allies for those of us with anomalous experiences, and the compassion to offer real financial support to improve youth mental health care and access to that care. When we exercise this will, we can turn some of these breaking points into turning points. And, in so doing, we can help a precious young person—full of incredible potential—to know that they are beloved and will find a life worth living.

ACKNOWLEDGMENTS

I experienced firsthand how hard it was for the young people and their families to live through the events in this book, and I want to thank them first, for sharing their stories, lives, and time with my team and me. I tried to change details enough to conceal their identities while preserving key experiences that could help us re-envision care. I hope I honored their struggle and courage well with this text.

Second, I am so grateful to my family. This work spanned a decade, and a good chunk of my children's childhoods. Now they are coming of age themselves—a daunting and exciting time—and a challenge I hope this book will help them meet with courage and joy. They waited for me patiently to come home when I needed to travel for research or work or to recharge. When I was home, they helped me engage in play—making me laugh and play board games or put puzzles together or play music or go outside or adopt a puppy or go shopping for clothes or host elaborate Harry Potter birthday parties—the list goes on. They helped me feel uplifted and less alone.

Allen, my spouse for twenty years, is my rock. He always makes me feel safe, loved, and encouraged. While I wrote this book, he provided so much emotional and material support—covering for things with the children, listening to me process difficult material, allowing me to sojourn as needed, and pushing me to think pragmatically (but what can we *do* about it?)—and he did so gracefully and with kindness and compassion. We even survived a global pandemic. I could never do what I do without him.

Of course, other family and friends have been supportive (and some of those friends are listed as colleagues below, so they aren't listed here) and they include: my mom and dad, Patricia and Steven Laurenzo; my older brother, Eric, and his wife, Shelly; my hilarious nephews, Asher and Elijah; my younger brother, Joseph, ever-inspiring; and my wonderful in-laws, including Nancy, Dan, and Lisa Myers; Mike Allen-Myers; Tim and Terry Andrews; JP and Cat Goodyear, and all their offspring. My gratitude, as well, to my smart, loving, and supportive aunts and uncles, especially Bobby and Leann Laurenzo, Mark and Linda Harris, and Cindy and Tom McCulloch. I am also sending good vibes to my Uncle Greg, who passed away while I wrote this book.

I also lost three grandparents while I wrote this book—may they rest in peace: Eleanor Fahey Harris, O. Elizabeth Niswonger, and Frederick Laurenzo. Eleanor "Meme" was especially supportive to me my entire life, and I miss her sharp wit and loving presence.

Friends offering direct encouragement and family support included Toni Arrant and Scott Smeltz, Jon and Jenn Blaeuer, Chris Bolding, Amy and Andy Davis, Marsha and Kurt Gadsden, Kaitlin and Andrew Guthrow, Sarah Hagen, Jennifer and Tate Hemingson, Laurel and Kerry Johnson, Sally Kittles, Sarah Klitzke, Audry Lee, Kristen McClain, Barb McCluer, Besrat Redda, Erin and Hank Stafford, Leah and Keith Sumner, Joslyn and Bryan Taylor, Arianne and Mike Theiss, Nancy Wiens and Sam Yates, Kristie Zenick, and Corey Zimmerman and Shobu Odate. It takes a village, and I have a good one.

I love my colleagues at SMU, and among those who did not help directly with the project, I appreciated the support and encouragement of Caroline Brettel, Sunday Eiselt, Simon Craddock Lee, Karen Lupo, David Meltzer, Carolyn Smith-Morris, and Paige Ware. At the University of Texas Southwestern Medical Center, John Burruss, Carol North, and John Sadler helped orient me to the world of mental health care in Dallas. Meredith Baughman, Sherry Cusumano (may she rest in peace), and Marsha Rodgers helped me understand the world of mental health policy in North Texas. More recently, colleagues at the University of Texas at Austin helped me think through substance use issues, among other things, including Deborah Cohen, Vanessa Klodnick, Molly Lopez, and Samantha Reznick. I also want to thank early readers of book proposal drafts and draft opening chapters, which included Ippolytos Kalofonos, Rebecca Lester, Tanya Luhrmann, Allen Myers, and my mom. Sharon Broll joined my team as a developmental editor after a few chapters had been written, and she was crucial in helping me lay out my message clearly across each chapter. Anonymous reviewers from the University of California Press were also incredibly helpful and influential in the production of this final draft, as was the lovely acquisitions editor Kate Marshall, who connected me with them. Kate has supported this project from early stages with incisive comments and enthusiasm, which bolstered my spirits. Steven Baker, a wordsmith extraordinaire, also did an excellent job offering insightful and remarkably thorough copyedits.

Colleagues who have helped me think through many aspects of my work over the years include, among many others, Eileen Anderson, Suze Berkhout, Elizabeth Bromley, Julia Brown, Elizabeth Carpenter-Song, Tom Csordas, Lauren Cubellis, Michael D'Arcy, Byron and Mary Jo Del Vecchio–Good, Whitney Duncan, Sue Estroff, Elizabeth Fein, Linda Garro, Joseph Gone, Doug Hollan, Kim Hopper, Janis Jenkins, Laurence Kirmayer, Daniel Lende, Sara Lewis, Michael Nathan, Christine Nutter, Matthew Wolf-Meyer, and Kristin Yarris.

As you can see in Appendix 1, I have a host of SMU students, researchers, and faculty to thank for their help designing this project, collecting the data, interpreting the data, and producing what is now a final draft of this book. Research designers included Michael Compton, Lisa Dixon, Nev Jones, and (for the Hispanic- or Latinx-focused pieces) Maggie Caballero. Data collection, coding, and interpretation helpers included for a substantial time the wonderful Anubha Sood, Katherine Fox, Nia Parson, and Gillian Wright—all of whom dedicated a lot of compassionate energy to this effort. Additional helpers at various times, often supported by a student scholarship from the Hamilton family through SMU, included Shalimar Diaz De Leon, Jordan Goldstein, Miguel Gutierrez, Candace Johnson, Caroline Jones, Darci Martin, Ekiomoado Olumese, Lauren Philpott, Brenna Raney, River Ribas, and Diego Salinas. Literature reviews, which were sometimes very complicated and in-depth, were immensely aided by the support of especially Matthew Hutnyan and Emily Stein, and also at times Imani Holmes, Claire Janssen, Taylor Shimizu, and Justin Wilkey. In addition, Justin pretty much singlehandedly and with great dedication helped me prepare and finalize the notes and bibliography to help distract him from his medical school applications. He is going to be a wonderful doctor.

Another SMU undergraduate student, Lauren Ann Villarreal, provided some of the art featured in this book, including "Identity," "Spiraling," "The Hospital: the hallway bathroom," and "Ripe Tomatoes." My brother, Joseph Steven Laurenzo, also provided the art piece "Songbird," which I have always loved.

This book also benefited from presentations of project material at the National Institute of Mental Health in Bethesda, Maryland, the biennial Society for Psychological Anthropology conference, and the annual American Anthropological Association conference, as well as invited lectures at University of California San Diego, University College London, McGill University, University of California Los Angeles (UCLA) School of Medicine, Stanford University, University of Texas-Southwestern Medical School, and with community partners such as the board members of Metrocare Services in Dallas, the Los Angeles County Department of Mental Health, the UCLA Behavioral Health Center for students, and the Early Intervention for Psychosis Team at the Ohio State University.

Team Ethnographic Methods

Over the nearly ten years it took to collect, analyze, and write up the data that constitute this book, my research team was indispensable. Of course, given the time frame, the team expanded and changed over time. My initial research award (R03 MH102568) from the National Institute of Mental Health (NIMH) included three consultants: Michael T. Compton, Sue Estroff, and Lisa Dixon. Compton was a psychiatrist specializing in social determinants of mental health and focused on the experiences and needs of Black youths experiencing early psychosis and their families. Dixon, also a psychiatrist, was the architect of what was then—and still is—the most influential study of early intervention for psychosis in the United States, the NIMH-funded Recovery after an Initial Schizophrenia Episode (RAISE) trial. Estroff was a medical anthropologist with long-recognized expertise in mental health services research and was also engaged in research with young persons with early psychosis and their families. With NIMH funding for this project, I also hired the gifted medical anthropologist Anubha Sood, who was my insightful, thoughtful, and meticulous partner for much of the ethnographic heavy lifting in this project. In the first year, we also added an undergraduate Health and Society student, Gillian Wright, to help with data collection and analysis, and she stayed on with the project for three years.

Over time, and with further funding from the Hogg Foundation for Mental Health Research to expand the study, we also added Dr. Nia Parson, my colleague in anthropology who is a bilingual Spanish speaker with expertise on resilience, and a PhD student in medical anthropology, Katherine (Katie) Fox. We also added two consultants—Nev Jones, a community psychology PhD and mental health services researcher who herself had benefited from an early intervention program, as well as Maggie Caballero, a local peer services specialist who ran her own, peer-run drop-in program for primarily Latino-identifying clients in Fort Worth, Texas, called the HOPE Center. Nev and Maggie met with the team quarterly over the course of two years to help us think about how to ask questions and improve our methods and understand some of the data from a lived-experience perspective. Maggie also consulted on relevant aspects of local Hispanic culture.

From 2014 to 2017, at varying intervals, Anubha, Katie, Nia, and I worked together on hospital-based fieldwork and recruitment. We rotated to cover most days of the week to see if there were any new young persons in the emergency room to recruit for the study. This was the most labor-intensive part of the project because many times young persons in crisis were hard to connect with (for example, they were released as soon as they were stable) or because they refused to participate. We had to wait until they were feeling well enough to consent, but sometimes missed them when they were transferred or released before we obtained permission to follow up with them if they had not yet signed the consent. We kept fieldnotes about significant events in a shared document and also tracked all kinds of data on various spreadsheets and even a Trello board at one point.

The study required signed consent from all participants. We lost many potential participants at this stage (regrettably, our IRB did not include tracking refusals or people who we lost prior to consent). Once a person had consented, we asked them to fill out a demographics form with our help (we filled it in while talking to them) and engaged them in an initial interview, often in the hospital. We were able to engage 47 young people in that initial interview. Over time, we also interviewed 19 key supporters.

Interview participants were offered $20 gift cards (e.g., CVS, Walmart) for each interview, a bonus for self-initiating scheduling the first interview with us ($30), and a $30 bonus for completing all four interviews, for a total of $140 per person. Key supporters also received $20 gift cards per interview.

Several of us also went on follow-on state hospital visits (during visiting hours with the young person's permission) and home visits, which we always did in pairs for safety. During these visits, we engaged young persons and their families in audio-recorded interviews and made field notes afterward that were shared with the team. Per the study design, we were not allowed to visit any young person more than four times, and were able to talk to the family only twice, during the first four months so as not to affect anyone's decision-making process. Anyone we talked to after the initial six months had to contact us first.

During the years of active data collection, we met almost weekly in team meetings—except during the summer—to discuss all visits and interviews, to troubleshoot any challenges, and to plan for future visits and interviews. A larger team of people also took part in the meetings, including numerous research assistants who helped to think about the data, transcribe it, and code it, because we engaged in ongoing coding per grounded-theory methods.

As part of the continual coding process for the project, Anubha, Katie, Gillian, and I developed a codebook during the weekly lab meetings to tag the data set using Dedoose, a cloud-based, collaborative, mixed-methods software. We also entered all the demographics collected for the young persons and key supporters, so we could sort by demographics, though our sample was not large enough to create statistically significant comparison groups. Once the data set was fully coded, Lauren Philpott, Matthew Hutnyan, Emily Stein, and Claire Janssen, all SMU undergraduates, helped me to download and organize the data into various files in response to my requests about various topics, which helped to inform the stories chosen to feature in this book as representative of the stories of many people who were coded similarly.

Resources for Youth and Families

This is a nonexhaustive list of resources I trust to offer information and support.

UNDERSTANDING PSYCHOSIS

Cooke, Anne, ed. *Understanding Psychosis and Schizophrenia (Revised)*. British Psychological Society, Division of Clinical Psychology, 2017. Accessed January 29,2024. https://doi.org/10.53841/bpsrep.2017.rep03.
National Institute of Mental Health. *Understanding Psychosis*. 2019. NIH Publication No. 20-MH-8110. https://www.nimh.nih.gov/sites/default/files/documents/health/publications/understanding-psychosis/understandingpsychosis.pdf.

EMERGENCY ALTERNATIVES

National Empowerment Center, Directory of Peer Respites in the United States. https://power2u.org/directory-of-peer-respites/.

EARLY PSYCHOSIS INTERVENTION PROGRAMS

Stanford Early Psychosis Program Directory (United States only). https://med.stanford.edu/peppnet/interactivedirectory.html.
Early Assessment and Support Alliance Directory. https://www.easacommunity.org/national-directory.php.

MUTUAL SUPPORT RESOURCES

For Youth

Intervoice and Hearing Voices Network (Global). https://www.intervoiceonline.org/#content.
Hearing Voices Group Directory (US). https://www.hearingvoicesusa.org/find-a-group.

For Families

National Alliance on Mental Illness. https://www.nami.org/findsupport.

INTRODUCTION: UNDER PRESSURE

1. Shady Elms was the main recruitment site for this study. The name of this emergency facility has been changed to protect the anonymity of staff and service users with an additional layer of confidentiality.

2. This study was approved by the hospital's internal and regional review boards and the Southern Methodist University (SMU) Human Subjects Review Board and met the federal requirements for human subjects research. All participants gave written informed consent to participate in the study. All researchers were CITI (Collaborative Institutional Training Initiative) certified in research compliance and the ethical conduct of research. Hospital-based research team members also underwent background checks and drug screenings before receiving clearance to enter the hospital.

3. US Department of Health and Human Services, *Protecting Youth Mental Health*.

4. Centers for Disease Control and Prevention (CDC), "Youth Risk Behavior."

5. CDC, "Youth Risk Behavior."

6. CDC, "New CDC Data."

7. See, for example, Overhage et al., "Trends in Acute Care Use"; Khan et al., "Comparative Mortality Risk."

8. Weiner, "Growing Psychiatrist Shortage."

9. See Hartmann et al., "At-Risk Studies." However, the onset of schizophrenia—only one of multiple potential outcomes that can result from psychosis symptoms—seems to differ in age by gender and come later for women (ages 25–35). Ochoa et al., "Gender Differences."

10. Compton and Broussard, *First Episode of Psychosis*.

11. National Institute of Mental Health, "Understanding Psychosis."

12. McGorry, "Transition to Adulthood."

13. Substance Abuse and Mental Health Services Administration (SAMHSA), *Coordinated Specialty Care.*

14. Doyle et al., "First-Episode Psychosis."

15. Classic ethnographic works on schizophrenia in anthropology include Barrett, *Psychiatric Team*; Rhodes, *Emptying Beds*; and Estroff, *Making It Crazy*. More recent work includes Brodwin, *Everyday Ethics*; the collection edited by Jenkins and Barrett, *Schizophrenia, Culture, and Subjectivity*; Davis, *Bad Souls*; Nakamura, *Disability of the Soul*; and the collection edited by Luhrmann and Marrow, *Our Most Troubling Madness*. On bipolar disorder, see Martin, *Bipolar Expeditions*. For discussion of autism, see, for example, Fein, *Living on the Spectrum*. On depression, see, for example, Kleinman and Good, *Culture and Depression*; O'Nell, *Disciplined Hearts*; Kitanaka, *Depression in Japan*. On addiction, see, for example, Meyers, *Clinic and Elsewhere*; Garcia, *Pastoral Clinic*; Knight, *Addicted, Pregnant, Poor*; Raikhel, *Governing Habits*.

16. See, for example, Hejtmanek, *Friendship, Love, and Hip Hop*; Béhague, "Psychiatry, Bio-epistemes, and the Making of Adolescence"; and Jenkins and Csordas, *Troubled*.

17. See, for example, Giordano, *Migrants in Translation*; Duncan, *Transforming Therapy*; Reyes-Foster, *Psychiatric Encounters*; Pinto, *Daughters of Parvati*; Lakoff, *Pharmaceutical Reason*; and Pandolfo, *Knot of the Soul*.

18. See, for example, the edited volumes Biehl, Good, and Kleinman, *Subjectivity*; Good, *Postcolonial Disorders*; Good et al., *Reader in Medical Anthropology*; and Jenkins, *Pharmaceutical Self*.

19. Walker, *Moral Understandings*.

20. The anthropological tradition of examining morality and health was brought to the fore by Arthur Kleinman in his seminal work "Experience and Its Moral Modes," which introduced the concept of "local moral worlds" and their importance for health. Drawing on this work, Angela Garcia, in *Pastoral Clinic*, illustrated the importance of local moral worlds in the context of heroin addiction, and Tanya Luhrmann, in *Of Two Minds*, discussed the importance of morality in psychiatric care and the social response to psychiatric conditions. In *Extraordinary Conditions*, Janis Jenkins also highlighted the role of morality in shaping ideas about mental health and mental illness. Jenkins and Csordas discussed the moral qualities of emotion, a topic with its own intellectual genealogy, which they unpack in *Troubled* (see, especially, pp. 154–61).

21. For an in-depth discussion of American cultural ideas that shape notions of valued adulthood for those deemed mentally healthy, please see my first book, Myers, *Recovery's Edge*. The discussion there draws on the work of feminist philosopher Martha Nussbaum, as well as historian Alexis de Tocqueville (*Democracy in America*), sociologist Max Weber (*Protestant Ethic*), and American "founding fathers" Frederick Douglass (*Narrative of the Life*) and Benjamin Franklin (see Pangle, *Benjamin Franklin*).

22. Walker, *Moral Understandings*; Blacksher, "On Being Poor"; Mattingly, *Moral Laboratories*.

23. Myers, *Recovery's Edge*.

24. One reviewer of this manuscript asked what the difference might be between social capital and moral agency. Social capital has an inherently collective and transactional quality: you get something collective (group membership, social networks, the capacity for collective social action) out of what you put into the collective group (community participation, civic engagement). For more about social capital, see Putnam, *Bowling Alone*.

While social capital and its components are important to social belonging and mental health (see, for example, Flores et al., "Mental Health Impact"; and Hirota et al., "Associations of Social Capital"), moral agency is more nuanced and less transactional. It is based on the ways one seeks to craft others' perceptions of one as a "good enough" person, someone they will wish to connect with intimately. It is a process of self-making and identity development that is at once intimate and shared with others and leads to agency in the world or the loss of that agency (for further discussion, see Holland, *Identity and Agency*). When it comes to moral agency, a person does not have to give in order to get; for example, if people see you as a "good enough" person, they might give you much more than you give them. People who care about you will make a lot of space for you to try and fail, to have ups and downs, to edit and regroup and try again. If you feel recognized as a person who can be loved, then you are better able to try. This is more about a way of knowing oneself and a way of being known than about social transactions or collective social action.

25. Many thanks to Kim Hopper for countless conversations and access to his unpublished writings on moral agency that helped me think through and develop this concept further. I also initially drew on an article led by Sara Lewis, "Partners in Recovery," that mentions moral agency as a concept related to peer support, but does not expand on it.

26. Myers, *Recovery's Edge*.

27. Myers and Ziv, "'No One Ever Even Asked Me That Before.'"

28. To make this argument, I built on works I used to explore the concept in my first book, such as Arthur Kleinman's work on local moral worlds (Kleinman, "Experience and Its Moral Modes"), Angela Garcia's work on what it means to be a "good" person in heroin-using families (Garcia, *Pastoral Clinic*), and Erica Blacksher's use of the term *moral agency* in the context of her childhood of chronic socioeconomic deprivation to describe the freedom to aspire to a good life (Blacksher, "On Being Poor"). I also built on Cheryl Mattingly's then recently published work, *Moral Laboratories*, offering the concept of everyday life as a "moral laboratory" that offered intersubjective opportunities for moral experimentation, or spaces of possibility and critique where, "with action, humans are able to create something new—to begin something unexpected" (Mattingly, paraphrasing Hannah Arendt, in *Moral Laboratories*, 16).

29. Here, I am speaking of life narratives much as anthropologists Eleanor Ochs and Lisa Capps do, as "ordinary social exchanges in which interlocutors build accounts of life events, rather than on polished narrative performances," so that narratives are worked out between people as they share the making of a coherent story (Ochs and Capps, *Living Narrative*, 2). Sociologist Michael Bury, in "Chronic Illness as Biographical Disruption," argued that the continuing presence of any chronic illness disrupts the life narrative and requires a revisiting of one's self-concept. Sociologist Arthur Frank also wrote about the importance of storytelling for healing—arguing, especially, that even if a person is not able to be the author of their own lives, they at least need to be the editor (see Frank, *The Wounded Storyteller*). Social scientist Andrew Sayer has argued that these editorial skills are essential to confronting the injustice and inequity experienced by marginalized groups(see Sayer, *Why Things Matter*, 209). In my article in *Transcultural Psychiatry* ("Recovery Stories"), I explored notions of the life narrative in the context of psychiatric disability. For more on how self-narratives can be "disrupted" or "colonized" in the context of chronic illness and so must be reclaimed, see Weingarten, "The 'Cruel Radiance of What Is'"; Brodwin, *Everyday Ethics*; Luhrmann, *Of Two Minds*; Jenkins, "Psychopharmaceutical Self"; Kirmayer

and Gold, "Re-socializing Psychiatry"; and Lewis, "Narrative Turn in Psychiatry." In addition, Padgett, in "There's No Place Like (a) Home," and Lewis and Whitley, in "A Critical Examination of 'Morality,'" have argued that power over the self-narrative may be key for mental health recovery. In the context of early psychosis, specifically, other social scientists have argued that autobiographical renderings are important. See, for example, Judge et al., "Recognizing and Responding to Early Psychosis"; Larsen, "Finding Meaning"; Tranulis et al., "Early Intervention."

30. For an initial discussion of John Rawls's concept of "the social bases of self-respect" (Rawls, *A Theory of Justice*), see Myers, "Recovery Stories."

31. Ideas about dignity, accountability and self-respect initially stemmed from reading the work of Kim Hopper (including *Reckoning with Homelessness* and "Rethinking Social Recovery"). Also influential were Jacobson, "Dignity and Health"; and Ware et al., "Connectedness and Citizenship"—both recommended to me by Kim Hopper. Peopled opportunities are not social support, but rather "a holistic vetting and recognition of a person or people offering the opportunity to make further connections" (Myers, "Recovery Stories," 248). Sayer, in *Why Things Matter to People*, notes that without the opportunity to even practice being the kind of person one desires to be, it is impossible to move forward in life. "Mundane" moralities, he indicates, must be learned between people, and so are learned, developed, and nourished in social contexts and practiced, which requires opportunities to practice for a person to get it right. Lewis, Hopper, and Healion, in "Partners in Recovery," observed that this kind of opportunity may be most available in the context of peer support, where a mutual understanding of experiences of psychotic symptoms are grounds for empathy and kindness.

32. When I say "research team," I mean it, and I feel very grateful for all the wonderful people who have helped bring this book to fruition. See Appendix 1 for more details.

33. The word *minoritized* is meant to denote how systemic inequalities, oppression, and marginalization place individuals in a socially constructed "minority" status, thereby rendering them "minoritized" individuals. For more, see Shim, "Dismantling Structural Racism"; and Sotto-Santiago, "Minority in Academic Medicine."

34. McGorry, "Transition to Adulthood."

35. Hartmann et al., "At-Risk Studies."

36. Aceituno et al., "Cost-Effectiveness of Early Intervention"; Correll et al., "Comparison of Early Intervention Services"; Malla and McGorry, "Early Intervention in Psychosis."

37. Bennett and Rosenheck, in "Socioeconomic Status," found that one important moderator of the outcomes reported in a major early intervention clinical trial, the RAISE Early Treatment Program study (see Kane et al., "RAISE Early Treatment Program"), may have been patient socioeconomic status (SES). Their secondary analysis suggested that the main trial outcomes were significant for the top 25 percent of the SES distribution of persons enrolled in the trial, but statistically insignificant for the bottom three quartiles of SES distribution. More research is needed on why early intervention services may be less effective for those with lower SES and on the advantages people with higher SES may bring to the program that make it more likely for them to have a positive outcome. These findings, I would argue, also highlight the potential relationship between moral agency and SES, something that Blacksher highlights in her seminal paper on the topic, "On Being Poor," in which she argues that moral agency is difficult for persons living in poverty to access. The

findings also indicate how important social determinants of health like SES may be for the effective treatment of psychosis: we must address the material conditions along with the moral and the medical.

38. Jones et al., "Recovering the Vocational Self?"

39. Doyle et al., "First-Episode Psychosis."

40. Anglin et al., "From Womb to Neighborhood"; Anglin, Link, and Phelan, "Racial Differences in Stigmatizing Attitudes"; Gee and Ford, "Structural Racism"; Metzl, *Protest Psychosis*; Oluwoye et al., "Systematic Review of Pathways to Care."

41. At the time of this research, none of our participants were using the label *Latinx* to identify themselves. Thus, for this book I have chosen to preserve the ways they self-identified for this study. However, if researchers specifically use *Latinx* in their publications, I try to use the term when reporting that research so as to honor the way their participants identified.

42. While the metrics for the study set by the National Institutes of Mental Health classified everyone as African Americans, the Black African participants in the study did not identify with that term, but did identify with the term *Black*, and so I used that term in place of *African American* unless someone explicitly identified as African American during the study.

43. The word *immigrant* implies the desire to permanently move to a country, whereas the word *migrant* indicates a person who typically comes and goes seasonally for work. I have decided to use *immigrant* here, because none of our participants indicated seasonal or temporary residence.

44. Myers et al., "Pathways through Early Psychosis Care."

45. Myers, "Schizophrenia across Cultures."

46. Mindlis and Boffetta, "Mood Disorders"; Selten, Van Der Ven, and Termorshuizen, "Migration and Psychosis."

47. Myers, "Schizophrenia across Cultures"; Selten et al., "Migration and Psychosis."

48. For further discussion, see Selten et al., "Migration and Psychosis." There was not a higher prevalence of schizophrenia in sending countries, suggesting poverty or stress alone caused the higher risk. Moreover, receiving countries outside Europe like Canada and the United States have more restrictions on who can enter their countries, which may affect how many migrants are admitted with mental health concerns.

49. Anglin et al., "From Womb to Neighborhood"; Lawson et al., "Race as a Factor in Inpatient and Outpatient Admissions"; Barnes, "Race, Schizophrenia, and Admission"; Snowden and Cheung, "Inpatient Mental Health"; Gillon et al., "Ethnicity and Diagnostic Patterns"; Strakowski, Shelton, and Kolbrener, "Effects of Race and Comorbidity."

50. On misdiagnosis, see Lawson et al., "Race as a Factor in Inpatient and Outpatient Admissions"; Barnes, "Race, Schizophrenia, and Admission"; Snowden and Cheung, "Inpatient Mental Health"; Gillon et al. "Ethnicity and Diagnostic Patterns"; Strakowski, Shelton, and Kolbrener, "Effects of Race and Comorbidity." On socioeconomic disadvantage, see Anglin et al., "From Womb to Neighborhood."

51. Anglin et al, "From Womb to Neighborhood."

52. Anglin et al.

53. Selten et al., "Biological Mechanisms."

54. Myers and Ziv, "'No One Ever Even Asked Me That Before.'"

55. Shakespeare, *As You Like It*.

56. Bellah et al., *Habits of the Heart*.

57. Walker, *Moral Understandings*; Kendi, *Stamped from the Beginning*; DiAngelo, *White Fragility*.

58. Persons who are working on replenishing moral agency after its loss are featured in a recent special section of a journal issue of *Medicine Anthropology Theory* (Brown et al., "Experimental Engagements with Ethnography, Moral Agency, and Care"), which includes pieces about moral agency related to men with histories of military sexual trauma in the United States (Yahalom, Frankfurt, and Hamilton, "Between Moral Injury and Moral Agency"); persons with dual diagnoses of serious mental illness and substance use disorder in Ireland (D'Arcy, "'Swallow Them All, and It's Just like Smack'"); drug users and ethnographers in the United States (Ziv, "'I'm Trapped Here'"); structural racism and ethnographic work (Brown, "The Stories We Tell or Omit"); Ukrainian War refugees and Khmer Rouge survivors (Lesley, "The Anthropologist as Audience"); and asylum seekers in Madrid (Wagner, "Deserving Asylum").

59. Walker, *Moral Understandings*.

60. Oluwoye et al., "Systematic Review of Pathways to Care"; Bergner et al., "Period of Untreated Psychosis."

61. McLeod et al., "Police Interactions"; Nichols, LeBrón, and Pedraza, "Policing Us Sick."

62. Texas Health and Safety Code, Title 7: Mental Health and Intellectual Disability, Subtitle C: Texas Mental Health Code, Chapter 573: Emergency Detention.

63. Rosenberg, "Mental Health Issues on the Rise"; US Department of Health and Human Services, *Protecting Youth Mental Health*.

64. Myers et al., "Decision Making about Pathways through Care."

1. WORK HARD, PLAY HARD

1. In all quotations, an ellipsis without brackets indicates that the speaker paused. Ellipses with brackets indicate that the text has been elided in some way and that the gap is not a natural pause but an omission of some text that seemed irrelevant to me, such as the person saying something repetitive or the response of the interviewer to the person speaking.

2. Kavanaugh and Anderson, "Solidarity and Drug Use."

3. Many thanks to an anonymous reviewer for this helpful statement.

4. For more on adolescence across cultures, see the special issue of *Ethos* "Psychological Anthropology and Adolescent Well-Being," edited by Jill E. Korbin and Eileen P. Anderson-Fye.

5. Erikson, *Identity*, 16, 89.

6. Erikson, 130.

7. The military is one path that is highly ritualized, often in secret ways, but there were no veterans in my study, so it is not covered here.

8. Van Gennep, *Rite of Passage*, 13. See also Turner, *Ritual Process*.

9. Morinis, "Ritual Experience," 152.

10. See Hodgson, *Once Intrepid Warriors*; and Spear and Waller, *Being Maasai*.

11. Turner, "Betwixt and Between."

12. See, for example, Turner, "Betwixt and Between," 96; Morinis, "Ritual Experience," 13; van der Zeijst et al., "Ancestral Calling."

13. For a nonacademic but entertaining description of this phenomenon in American culture, see Ethan Watters's *Urban Tribes*.

14. Arnett, *Emerging Adulthood*.

15. Waters, *Coming of Age in America*, 3.

16. Adams, *Epic of America*.

17. Obama, "2013 State of the Union Address."

18. Rose, "Donald Trump on the American Dream."

19. Moore and Myerhoff, "Introduction," 3; McNamee and Miller, *Meritocracy Myth*; Mead, *Coming of Age in Samoa*.

20. Borgen and Rumbaut, "Coming of Age in 'America's Finest City.'"

21. Douglass, *Narrative of the Life*; Weber, *Protestant Ethic*; Bellah et al., *Habits of the Heart*; Pangle, *Benjamin Franklin*.

22. Bellah et al., *Habits of the Heart*; Nussbaum, *Frontiers of Justice*.

23. Khalifa, "Work Hard, Play Hard."

24. Chamary, "'Work Hard, Play Hard.'"

25. Imtiaz, "Way We View Free Time."

26. "Best Television Series of 2022."

27. LeClair et al., "Motivations for Prescription Drug Misuse."

28. In my more recent study with rural and urban youths using early-psychosis clinics in Texas, 89 percent of the youth mentioned using cannabis—more than the two-thirds of whom mentioned using alcohol. One-third also mentioned using cocaine and LSD. Myers et al., "Perspectives of Young Adults Diagnosed with Early Psychosis."

29. Young people and many research articles have used the term *marijuana*, as well as *ganja, skunk, pot*, and others, to refer to products from the plant *Cannabis sativa*. When not specified by participants, I also use the more neutral, scientific term *cannabis*.

30. The National Survey on Drug Use and Health collects data face-to-face, using computer-assisted audio self-interviewing, which means respondents interact with federal employees but answer questions using a computer in a private setting on their own. Substance Abuse and Mental Health Services Administration (SAMHSA), *Key Substance Use and Mental Health Indicators*.

31. Arnett, *Emerging Adulthood*.

32. Kavanaugh and Anderson, "Solidarity and Drug Use."

33. The classic "diathesis-stress model" of schizophrenia (see Walker and Diforio, "Schizophrenia") claims that people with a psychotic disorder like schizophrenia have a "constitutional vulnerability" to everyday stress that causes a "stress cascade" even when environmental stressors are minimal. Corcoran et al., "Stress Cascade and Schizophrenia"; Jones and Fernyhough, "New Look at the Neural Diathesis-Stress Model;" Phillips et al., "Stress, the Hippocampus, and the Hypothalamic-Pituitary-Adrenal Axis"; Walker, Mittal, and Tessner, "Stress and the Hypothalamic Pituitary Adrenal Axis."

34. See this book's introduction for further discussion. See also Selten, Van Der Ven, and Termorshuizen, "Migration and Psychosis."

35. Worthman, "Inside-Out and Outside-In?," 437.

36. Schulenberg and Maggs, "A Developmental Perspective on Alcohol Use."

37. Oluwoye et al., "Systematic Review of Pathways to Care"; Goulding, Chien, and Compton, "Prevalence and Correlates of School Drop-Out"; Amaro et al., "Social Vulnerabilities"; Anglin et al. "From Womb to Neighborhood"; Oluwoye et al., "Systematic Review of Pathways to Care."

38. Amar, "Cannabinoids in Medicine"; Fleming et al., "Examination of the Divergence in Trends for Adolescent Marijuana Use."

39. Mostaghim and Hathaway, "Identity Formation, Marijuana, and 'the Self.'"

40. The strongest predictor for transition from substance-induced psychosis to a subsequent psychotic disorder is type of substance. Generally, estimates of transition are highest for cannabis, intermediate for amphetamines and hallucinogens, and low for other substances (e.g., alcohol). See Murrie et al., "Transition of Substance-Induced, Brief, and Atypical Psychoses to Schizophrenia."

41. Myles, Myles, and Large, "Cannabis Use."

42. Compton et al., "Subtyping First-Episode Non-affective Psychosis."

43. Sanchez et al., "Racial and Gender Inequities."

44. Compton, Furman, and Kaslow, "Preliminary Evidence of an Association between Childhood Abuse and Cannabis Dependence."

45. Goulding et al., "Prevalence and Correlates of School Drop-Out"; Ramsay et al., "Prevalence and Psychosocial Correlates of Prior Incarcerations"; Compton et al., "Abnormal Movements in First-Episode, Nonaffective Psychosis."

46. Schensul et al., "The High, the Money, and the Fame," 407.

47. Schoeler et al., "Effects of Continuation, Frequency, and Type of Cannabis Use," 952.

48. Marconi et al., "Meta-analysis of the Association between the Level of Cannabis Use and Risk of Psychosis," 1265; Mustonen et al., "Adolescent Cannabis Use," 230; Hasan et al., "Cannabis Use and Psychosis," 406.

49. Kraan et al., "Cannabis Use and Transition to Psychosis."

50. Sah et al., "Cannabis Induced Psychosis."

51. Schoeler et al., "Effects of Continuation, Frequency, and Type of Cannabis Use," 221–22; Hasan et al., "Cannabis Use and Psychosis," 408.

52. Among those who displayed violent behavior, 61 percent met criteria for cannabis use disorder (compared to 23 percent of patients who met criteria for cannabis use disorder among those who did not display violent behavior). However, in another study, aggressive behavior in first-episode psychosis was significantly associated with higher rates of alcohol use, and there was only a nonsignificant trend for an association with cannabis use disorder. See Lopez-Garcia et al., "Clinical and Neurodevelopmental Correlates." Thus, this association cannabis use and violent behavior is still a matter of debate.

53. American culture offers some alternative pathways to adulthood. The straight-edge punk scene, for example, openly avoids substance use and offers a supportive community that shares an interest in a specific kind of music, which has at times been compared to religion and can have effects beyond young adulthood. See, for example, Stewart, *Punk Rock Is My Religion*; and, for a longer discussion of the effects of membership, Haenfler, "The Entrepreneurial (Straight) Edge." Other young Americans may have more religious guidance in their lives; for example, those who are guided into missionary work as a rite of passage, perhaps especially in the Mormon church (see Pepper, "You Are Hereby Called"). There are also efforts at cultural revitalization in some Native American communities, such as among the Navajo, that incorporate elders, ceremony, and healing ritual (see, e.g., Dole

and Csordas, "Trials of Navajo Youth."). However, none of the young people in my study mentioned these as part of their own transition.

2. INTO THE MYTHOS

1. Walker, *Moral Understandings*, 117.
2. Estroff, *Making It Crazy*, 217.
3. Myers, "Beyond the 'Crazy House'"; Zigon, *"HIV Is God's Blessing."*
4. Nabbali, "A 'Mad' Critique," 7.
5. Radua et al., "What Causes Psychosis?"
6. Kirkbride and Jones, "Prevention of Schizophrenia."
7. Luhrmann, "Diversity within the Psychotic Continuum."
8. Van Os et al., "Systematic Review and Meta-analysis of the Psychosis Continuum."
9. Hornstein, "Bibliography of First-Person Narratives."
10. Rose, "Service User/Survivor–Led Research."
11. See, for example, Rose, *Mad Knowledges*; May, "Bringing an Inside Perspective to Mental Health Services"; and Jones (Jones et al., "Back to School"; Jones et al., "'Did I Push Myself over the Edge?'"; Jones et al., "Recovering the Vocational Self?"; and Jones, Kelly, and Shattell, "God in the Brain").
12. This book, as one reviewer noted, employs the user-survivor literature as scholarship and as data. It is important to learn from the rich perspectives added by those with lived experiences of psychosis. I have attempted to incorporate some of the wisdom I have found in that literature here, especially the perspectives on being young and experiencing psychosis. Undoubtedly, I have missed a great deal, and more will come to light as other user-survivors publish their own work and as they are more frequently invited to the table to generate the best research and innovate real and lasting change. For a more thorough discussion of the potential of the lived experience perspective, see Rose, *Mad Knowledges*.
13. Deegan, "Common Ground Program Outcomes."
14. Cooper, "Anderson Cooper Tries a Schizophrenia Simulator."
15. Longden, "Voices in My Head."
16. Jones et al., "'Did I Push Myself over the Edge?'"
17. Jones et al.
18. Jones et al., 7.
19. Kernan, "Psychotic Bodies/Embodiment" (italics original).
20. Jones et al., "'Did I Push Myself Over the Edge?'" 330; Kernan, "Psychotic Bodies/Embodiment."
21. Jones et al.
22. Sass, "'Negative Symptoms,' Common Sense, and Cultural Disembedding," 304.
23. Quoted in Rose, "Service User/Survivor–Led Research."
24. Saks, *The Center Cannot Hold*, 55.
25. Corin and Lauzon, "Positive Withdrawal."
26. Indigo Girls, *1200 Curfews*.
27. Quoted in Rose, "Service User/Survivor–Led Research."
28. Mohr et al., "Toward an Integration of Spirituality and Religiousness"; Huguelet et al., "Spirituality and Religious Practices."
29. Kusters, *Philosophy of* Madness, xii.

30. Kusters, 4.
31. DuBrul, *Maps to the Other Side*, 63.
32. Jones, Kelly, and Shattell, "God in the Brain."
33. Jones, Kelly, and Shattell, 498.

34. The term *double bookkeeping* was coined by Eugen Bleuler in 1911 (see Bleuler, *Dementia Praecox*) to describe a feature of schizophrenia in which a patient can hold two mutually exclusive realities side by side at once—sometimes labeled as delusions. Psychologist Louis Sass argued that explanatory models of psychosis used by young people can serve as a kind of double bookkeeping in that a young person such as Corinna or Levi has enough insight to know that while others will likely not agree that their original perceptions were true, they nevertheless regard them as having been true because they can hold on to two, at times contradictory realities, consensus and nonconsensus, at once. Sass, "Double Book-Keeping." Corrina offered the "double vision" of drunkenness as an example. The fact that others cannot see or feel the doubling of vision does not make it any less real for the person experiencing it. They have to believe two things are true. (1) Reality is not "doubled"—my brain only perceives it that way—but I cannot deny that it is, for me, doubled. Therefore, (2) I can hold multiple perceptual realities—my own (I am seeing double) and that of the reality I share with others (no one else is seeing double). Jones and colleagues argued that double bookkeeping is an important way of socially renegotiating psychotic symptoms that were previously outside consensus reality, and found that these double-booking explanatory models often leaned toward the spiritual, magical, religious, or science-fictional. Jones, Kelly, and Shattell, "God in the Brain." Helene Stephenson and colleagues have argued that this quality emerges, as it did for Corrina and James, before a psychotic break, adding "an alarming openness to another presence within one's most intimate subjective life." Stephenson, Urfer-Parnas, and Parnas, "Double Bookkeeping," 2. Thus, what is helpful may at times also be disturbing.

35. Luhrmann, "Thinking about Thinking."
36. "Religious Landscape Study."
37. Rhodes, *Outsider Art*, 232.
38. "Religious Landscape Study."
39. Bruner, "Narrative Construction," 20.
40. Kernan, "Psychotic Bodies/Embodiment."
41. Rhodes, *Outsider Art*, 61. This book describes several such artists and provides images, as does Prinzhorn's own book, *Artistry of the Mentally Ill.*
42. DuBrul, *Maps to the Other Side*, 151.
43. Hopper, "Interrogating the Meanings of Culture."
44. Corin, Thara, and Padmavati, "Living through a Staggering World," 124.
45. Corin, Thara, and Padmavati, 128–29.
46. Corin, Thara, and Padmavati, 126.
47. Corin, Thara, and Padmavati, 130.
48. Van der Zeijst et al., "Ancestral Calling."
49. Bidois, "A Cultural and Personal Perspective."
50. Bidois, 41.
51. Fletcher, "Uncivilizing 'Mental Illness.'"
52. DuBrul, "The Icarus Project."
53. The Icarus Project, *Friends Make the Best Medicine.*

54. Powers, Kelley, and Corlett, "Varieties of Voice-Hearing."
55. Walker, *Moral Repair*, 97.
56. Rohr, *On the Threshold*, 1.
57. May, "Bringing an Inside Perspective."
58. Grof, *Psychology of the Future*, 137.
59. Laing, *Politics of Experience*, 86.
60. Vine, *Fighting for Recovery*.

3. DANGEROUS

1. Addington et al., "Duration of Untreated Psychosis."
2. Bergner et al., "Period of Untreated Psychosis;" Franz et al., "Stigma and Treatment Delay."
3. Corrigan, "How Stigma Interferes with Mental Health Care."
4. Misra et al., "Systematic Review of Cultural Aspects of Stigma."
5. Misra et al.
6. See, for example, Lewis, *Spacious Minds*.
7. Gibbs, Kriegsman, and Brown, "Dismantling Racial Inequities."
8. Luhrmann, "'The Street Will Drive You Crazy.'"
9. For a discussion of masculinity and psychosis in contemporary Mexico, see Yarris and Ponting, "Moral Matters."
10. These are community providers sharing their thoughts with my team, it is worth noting, not anthropologists like Matthew Gutmann or Emily Wentzell who have critically engaged with the construct of machismo and argued that it is an overgeneralized stereotype and that there are multiple kinds of masculinities in Latino culture. See Gutmann, *Meanings of Macho*; Wentzell, "Aging Respectably." Scholars have also theorized that perhaps of greater importance than machismo for Mexican men, with some variation according to class, is one's ability to uphold cultural expectations of economic productivity or face shame and stigma. Yarris and Ponting, "Moral Matters"; Falkenberg and Tracy, "Sex and Schizophrenia"; Jenkins and Carpenter-Song, "Awareness of Stigma." For further consideration of social class and gender, see Seale and Charteris-Black, "Interaction of Class and Gender."
11. Alvidrez, Snowden, and Kaiser, "Experience of Stigma"; Silton et al., "Stigma in America"; Gangi, "On the Gravity of Mental Illness Stigma."
12. Definitions of mental health literacy and measurement vary to the point that some have questioned the validity and usefulness of the construct (see, e.g., Spiker and Hammer, "Mental Health Literacy"), but one definition asserts that it has six components: "1) knowledge and ability to identify symptoms of poor mental health; 2) knowledge and beliefs of causes of poor mental health; 3) knowledge and beliefs of self-compassion and self-care practices to maintain good mental health; 4) knowledge and beliefs of mental health services; 6) intentions to access mental health services when needed." Gorczynski and Sims-Schouten, "Evaluating Mental Health Literacy."
13. Tambling, D'Aniello, and Russell, "Mental Health Literacy."
14. Rikard et al., "Health Literacy and Cultural Competence."
15. Lillie-Blanton et al., "Race, Ethnicity, and the Healthcare System"; Haynes et al., "Addressing Mental Health Needs"; Hammond, "Medical Mistrust."
16. Bazargan et al., "Psychosocial Correlates of Medical Mistrust."

17. Anglin et al., "From Womb to Neighborhood"; Oluwoye et al., "Systematic Review of Pathways to Care"; Metzl, *Protest Psychosis*.

18. For further discussion of redlining in Dallas, see Krupala, "Evolution of Uneven Development in Dallas"; and the Urban Institute's report on transportation disparities, Stacy et al., "Disrupting Structural Racism"; as well as parts of Flournoy's work on banking and housing redlining, "Racism and Redlining." Both of the latter two works are based on research in South Dallas. For a fascinating discussion, by a Dallas-based journalist, at the history of redlining and segregation in Dallas, see Schutze, *The Accommodation*. On the practice of redlining elsewhere, see Schechter et al., "'They Underestimate What We Can Do"; Taplin-Kaguru, *Grasping for the American Dream*.

19. Alang and McAlpine, "Pathways to Mental Health Services."

20. Oluwoye et al., "Systematic Review of Pathways to Care."

21. For a thorough ethnographic examination of the effects of immigration enforcement on health care, see Kline, *Pathogenic Policing*. For two examples of the negative mental health effects of US immigration policies on undocumented persons, see Lopez et al., "Health Implications of an Immigration Raid"; and Delva et al., "Mental Health Problems of Children of Undocumented Parents." For more on the effects of perceived discrimination related to immigration enforcement on the mental health of Latinx high school students, see Cardoso et al., "Immigration Enforcement Fear."

22. Esterberg and Compton, "Family History of Psychosis"; Compton, Whicker, and Hochman, "Alcohol and Cannabis Use"; Compton et al., "Preliminary Evidence of an Association between Childhood Abuse and Cannabis Dependence"; Langlois et al., "Adversity in Childhood/Adolescence"; Goulding, Chien, and Compton, "Prevalence and Correlates of School Drop-Out"; Ku et al., "Neighborhood Predictors of Age"; Ramsay et al., "Prior Incarcerations"; Ramsay et al., "Clinical Correlates of Maltreatment and Traumatic Experiences"; Compton et al., "Abnormal Movements in First-Episode, Nonaffective Psychosis."

23. Crouch et al., "Income, Race/Ethnicity, and Exposure to Violence."

24. Oluwoye et al., "Systematic Review of Pathways to Care"; Compton et al., "Preliminary Evidence of an Association between Childhood Abuse and Cannabis Dependence"; Langlois et al., "Adversity in Childhood/Adolescence."

25. For more on early psychosis and substance use disorder, see Abdel-Baki et al., "Symptomatic and Functional Outcomes of Substance Use Disorder Persistence"; Addington and Addington, "Patterns, Predictors, and Impact of Substance Use"; Archie et al., "Substance Use and Abuse"; Colizzi et al., "Substance Use, Medication Adherence, and Outcome" Mazzoncini et al., "Illicit Substance Use"; and Ouellet-Plamondon et al., "Specific Impact of Stimulant, Alcohol, and Cannabis Use Disorders."

26. While "duration of untreated psychosis" (DUP) is a widely used construct in the research literature and has been widely employed to show how delayed treatment can lead to more severe symptoms, measuring DUP is challenging. It is, by design, always retroactive (because to enroll in a study on DUP a person must have accessed a clinic). Establishing the DUP is done in many ways across research studies and often relies on the recall of a young person with early psychosis and their family about when a person started to have a variety of experiences that could be attributed to symptoms of psychosis. Whether or not these are actually signs of psychosis, when psychosis begins, and how well people remember all of what happened often months if not years later are all reasons for critique.

27. Howes et al., "Clinical Significance of Duration of Untreated Psychosis."

28. Compton et al., "Family-Level Predictors and Correlates of the Duration of Untreated Psychosis."

29. Nagendra et al., "Demographic, Psychosocial, Clinical, and Neurocognitive Baseline Characteristics"; Oluwoye et al., "Systematic Review of Pathways to Care"; Franz et al., "Stigma and Treatment Delay"; Bergner et al., "Period of Untreated Psychosis."

30. Franz et al., "Stigma and Treatment Delay"; Bergner et al., "Period of Untreated Psychosis."

31. Addington et al., "Pathways to Care," 358.

32. Lewis-Fernández and Kirmayer, "Cultural Concepts of Distress."

33. Jenkins, "Ethnopsychiatric Interpretations."

34. In the public health literature, the term *violence* implies that there is an *intention* to hurt, damage, or kill someone or something, but in the case of the actions of persons experiencing psychosis symptoms, it can be very difficult to establish intentionality—a major topic in mental health law cases. Rutherford et al., "Violence." In contrast, *dangerous* means "able or likely to cause harm or injury." While it is difficult to acknowledge, given that we do not want to perpetuate further stigma against people with psychosis, young persons experiencing an untreated first episode of psychosis and those who have been treated involuntarily *are* more likely to be dangerous as the rest of the paragraph in the main text and accompanying annotations demonstrate. Something we do not talk about is something that goes unaddressed. Persons with psychosis who perpetuate harm on themselves or their loved ones often experience amnesia about events, as well as deep shame and confusion when they do remember them, and deserve our support. Juliana Onmuwere and colleagues spoke eloquently about this at an important panel about violence and mental health at the International Early Mental Health conference in July 2023, which she organized, though their research is currently under review.

35. Spidel et al., "Early Psychosis and Aggression"; Large and Nielssen, "Violence in First-Episode Psychosis."

36. Whiting et al., "Association of Schizophrenia Spectrum Disorders and Violence Perpetration."

37. Maniglio, "Severe Mental Illness and Criminal Victimization."

38. Schoenbaum et al., "Twelve-Month Health Care Use and Mortality."

39. WFAA Staff, "Former A&M Football Player Gets Life."

40. According to Hedman et al., "The core criterion justifying an involuntary hold is mental illness that results in danger to self or others, but many states have added further specifications. Only 22 states require some form of judicial review of the emergency hold process, and only nine require a judge to certify the commitment before a person is hospitalized. Five states do not guarantee assessment by a qualified mental health professional during the emergency hold." Hedman et al., "State Laws on Emergency Holds," 529.

41. Texas Young Lawyers Association, "Involuntary Commitment in Texas"; Hedman et al., "State Laws on Emergency Holds"; Saya et al., "Involuntary Treatment in Psychiatry."

42. Texas Health and Safety Code, Title 7: Mental Health and Intellectual Disability, Subtitle C: Texas Mental Health Code, Chapter 572: Voluntary Mental Health Services.

43. Anderson et al., "Meta-analysis of Ethnic Differences in Pathways to Care."

44. Oluwoye et al., "Systematic Review of Pathways to Care."

45. Merritt-Davis and Keshavan, "Pathways to Care."
46. Allen, "Short-Term Emergency Commitment Laws."
47. Since we were interested in pathways to care from the beginning, this information was collected on the demographics form from all participants.
48. Shedd and Hagan, "Toward a Developmental and Comparative Conflict Theory."
49. Mesic et al., "Relationship between Structural Racism and Black-White Disparities"; Boyd, "Police Violence."
50. Jindal et al., "Police Exposures."
51. Jindal et al.
52. McLeod et al., "Police Interactions."
53. Kindy et al., "Fatal Police Shootings."
54. Saleh et al., "Deaths of People with Mental Illness."
55. Kindy et al., "Fatal Police Shootings."
56. Merritt-Davis et al., "Pathways to Care."

4. DISORIENTATIONS

1. I have written elsewhere about narrative disruptions and life narratives. For more, please see Myers and Ziv, "'No One Ever Even Asked Me That Before'"; and note 29 in the introduction.
2. *Girl, Interrupted*, dir. James Mangold (Columbia Pictures, 1999).
3. Ariana's story and other aspects of this chapter, including some details about the emergency room, appear in Myers, "Beyond the 'Crazy House.'"
4. At this time, NorthStar and Value Options served a seven-county area of North Texas and used Medicaid and other federal and state funding to cover regional mental health needs for the uninsured.
5. Hart, "Terrell State Hospital."
6. Martin, "Texas' Crumbling State Mental Hospitals."
7. US Department of Health and Human Services, "Readmission Measures."
8. In 2019 in the United States, the birth rates among Hispanic teens and non-Hispanic Black teens were more than two times higher than the rate for non-Hispanic white teens, so this fact was not surprising. Centers for Disease Control and Prevention, "Teen Pregnancy."
9. Chambers, "Impact of Forced Separation."
10. Molloy et al., "Trauma-Informed Care."
11. O'Connor, Neff, and Pitman, "Burnout."
12. Volpe, "Risk of Burnout."
13. Yang and Hayes, "Causes and Consequences of Burnout."
14. Butler, Critelli, and Rinfrette, "Trauma-Informed Care."
15. Herman, *Trauma and Recovery*; Shonkoff and Phillips, *From Neurons to Neighborhoods*; van der Kolk et al., "Disorders of Extreme Stress."
16. Bryson et al., "What Are Effective Strategies for Implementing Trauma-Informed Care."
17. Gatov et al., "Interpersonal Trauma."
18. Lipschitz et al., "Epidemiology of Hospitalized Adolescents."
19. Briggs et al., "Trauma Exposure."
20. Trotta et al., "Impact of Childhood Adversity."

21. Duhig et al., "Prevalence and Correlates of Childhood Trauma."

22. Garcia et al., "Sex Differences in the Effect of Childhood Trauma."

23. Hailes et al., "Long-Term Outcomes of Childhood Sexual Abuse."

24. Yates et al., "Sexual Assault and Psychosis."

25. Savage, "Lady Gaga."

26. Sondhi et al., "Patient Perspectives of Being Detained"; Digel Vandyk et al., "Exploring the Experiences of Persons Who Frequently Visit the Emergency Department."

27. Harris et al., "Patients' Experiences of Psychiatric Care."

28. Guzmán et al., "Examining the Impact of Emergency Care Settings."

29. Harris et al., "Patients' Experiences of Psychiatric Care"; Digel Vandyk et al., "Exploring the Experiences of Persons Who Frequently Visit the Emergency Department;" Guzmán et al., "Examining the Impact of Emergency Care Settings."

30. Bradbury et al., "Lived Experience of Involuntary Transport"; Wise-Harris et al., "'Hospital Was the Only Option.'"

31. Elisseou, Puranam, and Nandi, "Novel, Trauma-Informed Physical Examination Curriculum."

32. Digel Vandyk et al., "Exploring the Experiences of Persons Who Frequently Visit the Emergency Department."

33. Guzmán et al., "Examining the Impact of Emergency Care Settings."

34. Harris et al., "Patients' Experiences of Patients' Experiences"; Guzmán et al., "Examining the Impact of Emergency Care Settings."

35. Frueh et al., "Special Section on Seclusion and Restraint."

5. USERS AND REFUSERS

1. *Cocaine Cowboys: The Kings of Miami*, dir. Billy Corben (2006).

2. Nixon, "Remarks about an Intensified Program for Drug Abuse Prevention."

3. Kendi, "Reagan's Drugs," ch. 33 in *Stamped from the Beginning.*

4. "The Wars Don't Work."

5. "Lost Cause."

6. "How Drug Trafficking Is (And Isn't) to Blame."

7. Roberts et al., "Race/Ethnic Differences in Exposure to Traumatic Events"; Cerdeña, Rivera, and Spak, "Intergenerational Trauma in Latinxs."

8. The provider spent time with Pedro and seemed to be of the same ethnicity, either of which (or both) made Pedro feel affinity for the doctor. There is growing evidence that racial and ethnic concordance between patient and provider in behavioral health settings and a longer length of treatment between the two correlates with a stronger working alliance than discordantly paired patients and providers. Cheng et al., "Association between Patient-Provider Racial/Ethnic Concordance, Working Alliance, and Length of Treatment." Overall, a more diverse mental health care workforce in the United States would better serve the needs of everyone in our diverse population.

9. In 2016, when Pedro was interviewed, receiving SSI meant that an eligible individual received a $733 monthly living allowance, which was well below the national poverty level of $990 per month for one person. US Department of Health and Human Services, "2016 Poverty Guidelines."

10. Social Security Administration, "Disability Benefits."

11. See Hansen, Bourgois, and Drucker, "Pathologizing Poverty." In this seminal article, Hansen and colleagues argue that the 1996 welfare reforms led to an increase in the number of requests for medicalized forms of support as a new "survival strategy" for families living in poverty. The authors find that the increased use of permanent-disability incomes as a survival strategy for poor families empowered individuals. Securing such income by proving they had a serious psychiatric disability helped them overcome some of the stigma about being "crazy" as they became a sustaining source of financial support for their families. At the same time, impoverished persons wanting to access such incomes had to prove they were disabled enough to deserve care and agree to use therapy and psychotropics, thereby deepening societal prejudices against the "unworthy poor." Pedro's family and others in my study were using this disability strategy to survive, as Hansen et al. predicted.

12. In some ways, Pedro's approach is a manifestation of what anthropologist Emily Martin hoped might be possible in her ethnography *Bipolar Expeditions* (148–49). In a chapter about support groups, she wonders what it would be like if people could "use DSM terms in their own ways or to speak in terms other than the DSMs." And while she hopes this opportunity will emerge in new social movements with new possibilities for personhood for people having experiences labeled as bipolar disorder, such has not been the case for Pedro. He has not started a social movement in the broader world to shift the world's perspective of his personhood, but he has made a new space in his own local moral world in which he can thrive with his family.

13. Good, "Biotechnical Embrace."

14. Luhrmann, *Of Two Minds.*

15. In another study of VA providers, primary care physicians, primary care nurses, and psychiatrists held more negative beliefs about persons with schizophrenia than they did about those without schizophrenia. Smith et al., "Comparison of Provider Attitudes."

16. Corrigan and Watson, "Paradox of Self-Stigma and Mental Illness."

17. Colizzi, Ruggeri, and Lasalvia, "Should We Be Concerned about Stigma."

18. Pescosolido, Manago, and Monahan, "Evolving Public Views on the Likelihood of Violence."

19. Guarnaccia, "*Ataques de Nervios*"; Nogueira et al., "Culture-Bound Syndromes."

20. Jenkins and Csordas note a similar pattern in their work with adolescents in New Mexico, *Troubled in the Land of Enchantment* (84–129). Families and young people had ongoing conversations over time about their diagnoses and demonstrated similar patterns: parents often tried to normalize their children's symptoms as "typical" teenager behavior, and over time people tended to endorse diagnostic categories or express ambivalence about them, depending on how they were trying to make use of those categories to adapt to the situation at hand. For example, a young person might understand their diagnosis and agree with it and find it useful, but still not want to talk about it.

21. Sousa, "Diagnostic Neutrality."

22. Sato, "Renaming Schizophrenia."

23. "Schizophrenia Given New Japanese Name."

24. Yamaguchi et al., "Associations between Renaming Schizophrenia and Stigma-Related Outcomes."

25. Koike et al., "Long-Term Effect of a Name Change."

26. Aoki et al., "Change in Newspaper Coverage."

27. Muench and Hamer, "Adverse Effects."

28. Carbon et al., "Tardive Dyskinesia Risk."

29. A list of excellent resources to get started can be found here: "Transforming Grief," IDHA: Institute for the Development of Human Arts, accessed March 30, 2024, https://www.idha-nyc.org/grief.

30. Francey et al., "Psychosocial Intervention with or without Antipsychotic Medication."

31. Myers et al., "Decision Making about Pathways through Care"; Myers et al., "Pathways through Early Psychosis Care."

6. HOMECOMING

1. Some clinicians argue that long-acting injectables (LAIs) are a good solution for early psychosis to keep young persons who may otherwise be treatment nonadherent on their medication across the "critical period" until their psychosis can resolve. However, one long-term study suggests that there were no improvements compared to regular antipsychotics at three-year follow-up for young persons with early psychosis. Abdel-Baki et al., "Long-Acting Injectable Antipsychotics." In addition, my data suggest the side effects were very uncomfortable for young people and made them not want to seek out medication again. It would be interesting to see longitudinally if LAIs as a frontline treatment for early psychosis reduce later engagement with mental health care or antipsychotic treatment adherence and how that affects outcomes.

2. Notably, after this interview, we put a safety protocol in place, decided to always do interviews in pairs, and never felt quite so vulnerable again. We did have a clinician on call during all the interviews but never had to call one for help.

3. Social Security Administration (SSA), "Disability Evaluation."

4. In the cases of 3 persons, family referred to a spouse or romantic partner, but the rest listed "family" without specifying which person. The other 25 percent included 2 who were unhoused, 4 who lived alone, and 5 listed as "other."

5. SSA, "Disability Evaluation."

6. SSA, "SSR 18-3p: Titles II and XVI."

7. Jansen, Gleeson, and Cotton, "Towards a Better Understanding of Caregiver Distress."

8. Jansen, Gleeson, and Cotton; Martens and Addington, "Psychological Well-Being of Family Members."

9. Jansen, Gleeson, and Cotton, "Towards a Better Understanding of Caregiver Distress."

10. Lavis et al., "Layers of Listening," 137–38.

11. Lavis et al., 138.

12. Lavis et al., 138.

13. Bebbington and Kuipers, "Clinical Utility of Expressed Emotion"; Butzlaff and Hooley, "Expressed Emotion and Psychiatric Relapse"; Cechnicki et al., "Predictive Validity of Expressed Emotions."

14. Kuipers and Bebbington, "Cognitive Behaviour Therapy for Psychosis"; Docherty et al., "Emotion Criticism."

15. Raune et al., "Anxiety Interacts with Expressed Emotion"; Kuipers and Bebbington, "Cognitive Behaviour Therapy for Psychosis."

16. Williams-Wengerd, "Grief in Parents."

17. Darmi et al., "Intimate Stranger"; Wiens and Daniluk, "Love, Loss, and Learning"; Richardson et al., "Parents' Grief."

18. Godress et al., "Grief Experiences of Parents"; Stein et al., "Social Networks and Personal Loss."

19. Cairns et al., "Family Members' Experience"; Dillinger and Kersun, "Caring for Caregivers."

20. Williams-Wengerd, "Grief in Parents."

21. While I did not interrupt her to clarify at the time, I am pretty sure that Daphne meant this as a slang term for "black magic" rather than the formal African diasporic religion, which would be spelled *Vodou*. For more on this religion and the misunderstandings of it in the west, see Viddal, "Vodou and Voodoo."

22. For a richer discussion of ethical breaches and moral breakdowns in the context of this study, see Myers, "Beyond the 'Crazy House.'" For a further discussion of the "ordinary ethics" that are developed between people in the mundane context of everyday life, see Michael Lambek's introduction in *Ordinary Ethics*, 1–38; and Andrew Sayer's work on "mundane ethics," *Why Things Matter to People*. The idea that ethics are shared or developed in the space between people, that some of these are presumed in intimate relationships, and that it is highly disruptive when they are compromised emerged from Cheryl Mattingly's beautiful book *Moral Laboratories*, on morality and ethics for African American families facing seemingly insurmountable health crises; and from Steve Parish's writing, especially "Between Persons." In addition, Jarrett Zigon's concept of the moral breakdown (see "Moral Breakdown"), as well as Zigon and Throop's introduction to their special issue of *Ethos* ("Moral Experience"), were seminal to my perspectives on the relationship between moralities and ethics.

7. TURNING POINTS

1. For one description of "finding one's tribe" and its importance for American teenage girls, see Damour, *Untangled*.

2. Walker, *Moral Understandings*.

3. Many have written about the phenomenology of the existential crisis in psychosis. See, for example, Jenkins, *Pharmaceutical Self*; Jenkins, *Extraordinary Conditions*; DuBrul, *Maps to the Other Side*; and Kusters, *Philosophy of Madness*.

4. Muench and Hamer, "Adverse Effects."

5. We offered all the youths we interviewed a flier about peer-led online support groups for persons with lived experience of psychosis. The flier was developed as part of Darci Martin's Engage Learning Project at SMU.

6. Myers, *Recovery's Edge*; Vine, *Fighting for Recovery*.

7. Grof and Grof, *Spiritual Emergency*.

8. Kernan, "Psychotic Bodies / Embodiment," 20.

9. Griffith et al., "How Can Community Religious Groups Aid Recovery."

10. Global mental health initiatives in sub-Saharan Africa, for example, often explore potential collaborations between faith healers and biomedical practitioners. See, for example, work by Oye Gureje from Nigeria and Ursula Read from Ghana, including Ojagbemi and Gureje, "The Importance of Faith-Based Mental Health Care"; and Read, "Rights as Relationships."

11. Myers, Meeker, and Odeng, "Pastors as Partners in Care."

12. Chaumba, "Health Status"; Ezeobele et al., "Depression and Nigerian-Born Immigrant Women"; Nadeem, Lange, and Miranda, "Mental Health Care Preferences"; Thomas, *West African Immigrants' Attitudes*.

13. Licensing chaplains to provide care is essential to avoid harming young persons with religious moralization or guilt that may be toxic for them. The Texas legislature recently authorized unlicensed chaplains—who may advocate for their own religious views to young people, however extreme—to work in schools to support youth mental health. Downen, "Unlicensed Religious Chaplains." Given the precarity of this situation, I cannot support employing unlicensed chaplains. Licensed chaplains are interfaith and know how to value and respect the religious positions of all their clients, even if they diverge from their own.

14. Ames et al., "Treatment of Moral Injury"; Nieuwsma et al., "Chaplaincy and Mental Health"; Yahalom, Frankfurt, and Hamilton, "Between Moral Injury and Moral Agency."

15. Codjoe et al., "Evidence for Interventions to Promote Mental Health and Reduce Stigma in Black Faith Communities."

16. For a beautifully rendered unpacking of this phenomenon at Iona State Hospital in Michigan, see Metzl, *Protest Psychosis*.

17. Weiner, "Growing Psychiatrist Shortage."

18. Oh et al. "Illicit and Prescription Drug Use."

19. For an overview of prescribing recommendations, see Dixon and Stroup, "Medications for First-Episode Psychosis."

20. Lack of access often comes up in rural areas. For a discussion of barriers to implementation of early psychosis care via Telehealth in Texas during the COVID-19 pandemic, see McCormick et al., "Virtual Technology's Critical Role."

21. Robinson et al., "Review of Hip Hop–Based Interventions."

22. Saunders, "Taking a Look at 988 Suicide and Crisis Lifeline Implementation."

23. American Psychiatric Association, "New Report Calls for Research on 988."

24. Wasser et al., "Criminal Justice System."

25. Balfour et al., "Cops, Clinicians, or Both?"; Compton et al., "Police-Based Crisis Intervention Team (CIT) Model."

26. Usher et al., *Crisis Intervention Team (CIT) Programs*.

27. New York Council of State Governments Justice Center, "Law Enforcement Mental Health Learning Sites."

28. Meadows Mental Health Policy Institute, "Transforming Police Responses."

29. Boscarato et al., "Consumer Experience."

30. Gilligan, *In a Different Voice*, 62.

31. Many think the Health Insurance Portability and Accountability Act (HIPAA), passed in 1996, protects the privacy of people using health care. However, HIPAA was not intended to be a privacy law: it was supposed to help people carry health insurance coverage across jobs in an economy in which health care is tied to employment. It wasn't until 2013 that new regulations were added, including that "clinicians and health care organizations may not disclose Public Health Information (PHI) without patient permission unless that information is being used for treatment, payment, or health care operations." US Department of Health and Human Services (USDHHS), *Modifications to the HIPAA Privacy, Security, Enforcement, and Breach Notification Rules*; Berwick and Gaines, "How HIPAA Harms Care."

206   NOTES TO PAGES 163 TO 170

32. USDHHS, *HIPAA Privacy Rule and Sharing Information*, 9–12.

33. Petersen, Joseph, and Feit, *New Directions in Child Abuse and Neglect Research*; Gatov et al., "Epidemiology of Interpersonal Trauma."

34. DuBrul, *Maps to the Other Side*, 184.

35. Harris and Fallot, *Using Trauma Theory*.

36. This recommendation warrants further consideration, especially given issues that may be of concern to persons who identify as transgender, bisexual, gender nonconforming, gender nonbinary, and so forth.

37. Mitchell et al., "Reaching Consensus on the Principles of Trauma-Informed Care."

38. For earlier work, see Cohen, "Psychiatric Hospitalization"; and Jennings and Ralph, "In Their Own Words." For more recent work, see Frueh et al., "Trauma within the Psychiatric Setting"; Frueh et al., "Improving Public Mental Health Services for Trauma Victims"; Cusack et al., "Trauma within the Psychiatric Setting;" and Robins et al., "Special Section on Seclusion and Restraint." For a wide-ranging survey, see Bloom and Farragher, *Destroying Sanctuary*.

39. UvnäsMoberg et al., "Maternal Plasma Levels of Oxytocin"; Carter, "Oxytocin Pathways."

40. See Griffen, Twomey, and Dulaney, "Survivors of Pregnancy and Postpartum Psychosis Speak Out."

41. Abbott et al., "Compulsory Separation of Women Prisoners from Their Babies"; Lovell, "Some Questions of Identity."

42. Cès et al., "Pregnancy in Women with Psychotic Disorders."

43. Cès.

44. Deegan, "Common Ground Program Outcomes."

45. DuBrul, *Maps to the Other Side*, 71.

46. DuBrul, 109.

47. *2018 Peer Respite Essential Features Survey*.

48. Ostrow and Fisher, *Peer-Run Crisis Respites*.

49. National Empowerment Center, "Peer Respites."

50. Greenfield et al., "Randomized Trial of a Mental Health Consumer-Managed Alternative."

51. Bouchery et al., "Effectiveness of a Peer-Staffed Crisis Respite Program."

52. Fletcher and Barroso, "'It's a Much More Relaxed Atmosphere.'"

53. Croft, Weaver, and Ostrow, "Self-Reliance and Belonging."

54. Croft and İsvan. "Impact of the 2nd Story Peer Respite Program."

55. Afiya, *Afiya Peer Respite*.

56. Siantz et al., "Peer Respites."

57. For more information about the Texas sites and the overall network, see Molly Lopez (principal investigator), "Advancing an Early Psychosis Intervention Network in Texas (EPINET-TX)," EPINET: Early Psychosis Intervention Network, accessed April 1, 2024, https://nationalepinet.org/regional-networks/epinet-tx/.

58. Azrin, Goldstein, and Heinssen, "Early Intervention for Psychosis."

59. Newcomer, "Antipsychotic Medications"; Newcomer and Hennekens, "Severe Mental Illness and Risk of Cardiovascular Disease."

60. De Mooij et al., "Dying Too Soon."

61. Vermeulen et al., "Antipsychotic Medication and Long-Term Mortality Risk."

62. Tiihonen, Tanskanen, and Taipale, "20-Year Nationwide Follow-Up Study."

63. Oedegaard et al., "'It Means So Much for Me to Have a Choice.'"

64. Yeisen et al., "Psychiatrists' Reflections on a Medication-Free Program." This medication-free program had to close in fall 2023 when the Norwegian government decided to stop providing public funding to private enterprises. Medication-free and psychiatric drug–tapering consultations are now offered on an outpatient basis in the area, but advocates—some say—do not believe that it is comparable. See Whitaker, "Medication-free Ward in Tromsø."

65. Heinssen et al., "Evidence-Based Treatments for First Episode Psychosis."

66. Read and Kohrt, "History of Coordinated Specialty Care."

67. Adams et al., "Shared Decision-Making Preferences."

68. Myers et al., "Decision Making about Pathways through Care."

69. Substance Abuse and Mental Health Services Administration (SAMHSA), *Supported Employment.*

70. Correll et al., "Comparison of Early Intervention Services."

71. For more about the college-for-all ideal, see Rosenbaum et al., "New Forgotten Half." For more on the rising numbers of young persons enrolling in college see Kendig et al., "Childhood Poverty and the Transition to Adulthood."

72. Humensky et al., "Supported Education and Employment Services."

73. Shinn et al., "Return to College."

74. Jones et al., "Back to School"; Bower, Furuzawa, and Tyler, "Campus Staff and Administrator Version."

75. Johannessen, Rasmussen, and Haldar, "Educational Purity and Technological Danger."

76. There are many variations in format, but they all partner family members with the person experiencing psychosis to improve outcomes such as preventing rehospitalization. See, for example, Lucksted et al. "Recent Developments in Family Psychoeducation." Sessions might include informational, cognitive, behavioral, problem-solving, emotional, coping, and consultation therapeutic elements, and are led by mental health professionals or "family peers"—people whose children have experienced psychosis. These classes typically include content about the diagnosis; advice on medication, treatment management, and services coordination; attention to all parties' expectations, emotional reactions, and distress; assistance with improving family communication; and help with crisis planning. Cultural sensitivity is also needed, especially in planning sessions with families from minoritized groups. For more, see Oluwoye et al., "Developing and Implementing a Culturally Informed Family Motivational Engagement Strategy (FAMES)."

77. Chien and Norman, "Effectiveness and Active Ingredients of Mutual Support Groups"; Chien and Chan, "Effectiveness of Mutual Support Group Intervention for Chinese Families."

78. Leggatt and Woodhead, "Family Peer Support Work."

79. Myers et al., "Potential Role for Family Members."

80. Claxton, Onwumere, and Fornells-Ambrojo, "Do Family Interventions Improve Outcomes."

81. Hamann, Pitschel-Walz, and Kissling, "Medication Adherence Studies"; Pharoah et al., "Family Intervention."

82. Berglund and Edman, "Family Intervention"; Lobban et al., "Systematic Review of Randomised Controlled Trials of Interventions."

83. Maura and Weisman de Mamani, "Mental Health Disparities."

84. Open Dialogue began in Finland in the early 1990s as an experiment called the Open Dialogue in Acute Psychosis project. See Bergström et al., "Family-Oriented Open Dialogue Approach."

85. Seikkula, Alakare, and Aaltonen, "Comprehensive Open-Dialogue Approach."

86. Bergström et al., "Long-Term Use of Psychiatric Services."

87. Bergström et al., "Family-Oriented Open Dialogue Approach."

88. Seikkula et al., "Five-Year Experience."

89. Aaltonen, Seikkula, and Lehtinen, "Comprehensive Open-Dialogue Approach."

90. Florence et al., "'It Makes Us Realize That We Have Been Heard'"; Gidugu et al., "Client, Family, and Clinician Experiences"; Hendy and Pearson, "Peer Supported Open Dialogue"; Tribe et al., "Open Dialogue in the UK"; Twamley, Dempsey, and Keane, "Open Dialogue–Informed Approach."

91. Florence et al., "'It Makes Us Realize That We Have Been Heard.'"

92. Gidugu et al., "Client, Family, and Clinician Experiences."

93. Florence et al., "'It Makes Us Realize That We Have Been Heard.'"

94. Cotes et al., "Open Dialogue–Inspired Approach."

95. Bennett and Rosenheck, "Socioeconomic Status."

96. Social Security Administration, "2023 Annual Report of SSI Program."

97. Texas Department of Health and Human Services, "State Hospitals."

98. George et al., "Cycles of Reform."

99. Dixon, "What It Will Take to Make Coordinated Specialty Care Available."

100. SAMHSA, *Coordinated Specialty Care*, 16–17.

101. Bao et al., "Financing Early Psychosis Intervention"; Smith et al., "Estimated Staff Time Effort, Costs, and Medicaid Revenues," cited in George et al., "Cycles of Reform."

102. Bao et al., "Financing Early Psychosis Intervention Programs."

103. Meadows Mental Health Policy Institute, "Coordinated Specialty Care for Texans."

104. SAMHSA, *Coordinated Specialty Care*, 10.

105. Meadows Mental Health Policy Institute, "Coordinated Specialty Care for Texans."

106. SAMHSA, *Coordinated Specialty Care*, 27.

107. SAMHSA, *Coordinated Specialty Care*, 31.

108. SAMHSA, *Coordinated Specialty Care*, 11.

109. Good, *Medicine, Rationality, and Experience.*

BIBLIOGRAPHY

2018 Peer Respite Essential Features Survey. Accessed on page "Peer Respites: Action + Evaluation." Live & Learn, Inc. 2019. https://livelearninc.net/peer-respites.

Aaltonen, Jukka, Jaakko Seikkula, and Klaus Lehtinen. "The Comprehensive Open-Dialogue Approach in Western Lapland: I. The Incidence of Non-affective Psychosis and Prodromal States." *Psychosis* 3, no. 3 (2011): 179–91.

Abbott, Laura, Tricia Scott, and Hilary Thomas. "Compulsory Separation of Women Prisoners from Their Babies following Childbirth: Uncertainty, Loss, and Disenfranchised Grief." *Sociology of Health and Illness* 45, no. 5 (2023): 1–18.

Abdel-Baki, Amal, Clairélaine Ouellet-Plamondon, Émilie Salvat, Kawthar Grar, and Stéphane Potvin. "Symptomatic and Functional Outcomes of Substance Use Disorder Persistence 2 Years after Admission to a First-Episode Psychosis Program." *Psychiatry Research* 247 (2017): 113–19.

Abdel-Baki, Amal, Émile Poulin, Sofia Medrano, Paula Pires de Oliveira Padilha, Emmanuel Stip, and Stéphane Potvin. "Impact of Early Use of Long-Acting Injectable Antipsychotics on Functional Outcome in First Episode Psychosis: A 3-Year Longitudinal Study." *International Journal of Psychiatry in Clinical Practice* 27, no. 1 (2023): 25–34.

Aceituno, David, Norha Vera, A. Matthew Prina, and Paul McCrone. "Cost-Effectiveness of Early Intervention in Psychosis: Systematic Review." *British Journal of Psychiatry* 215, no. 1 (2019): 388–94.

Adams, Jared R., Robert E. Drake, and George L. Wolford. "Shared Decision-Making Preferences of People with Severe Mental Illness." *Psychiatric Services* 58, no. 9 (2007): 1219–21.

Adams, J. T. *The Epic of America*. New York: Blue Ribbon Books, 1931.

Addington, J., and D. Addington. "Patterns, Predictors, and Impact of Substance Use in Early Psychosis: A Longitudinal Study." *Acta Psychiatrica Scandinavica* 115, no. 4 (2007): 304–9.

Addington, Jean, Robert K. Heinssen, Delbert G. Robinson, Nina R. Schooler, Patricia Marcy, Mary F. Brunette, Cristoph U. Correll, Sue Estroff, Kim T. Mueser, David Penn, James A. Robinson, Robert A. Rosenheck, Susan T. Azrin, Amy B. Goldstein, Joanne Severe, and John M. Kane. "Duration of Untreated Psychosis in Community Treatment Settings in the United States." *Psychiatric Services* 66, no. 7 (2015): 753–56.

Addington, Jean, Sarah Van Mastrigt, J. Hutchinson, and Donald Addington. "Pathways to Care: Help Seeking Behaviour in First Episode Psychosis." *Acta Psychiatrica Scandinavica* 106, no. 5 (2002): 358–64.

Afiya. *Afiya Peer Respite: Annual Report FY '17.* 2018. WHO QualityRights. Accessed April 1, 2024. https://qualityrights.org/wp-content/uploads/Afiya-annual-report-fy-17-alt.pdf.

Alang, Sirry M., and Donna D. McAlpine. "Pathways to Mental Health Services and Perceptions about the Effectiveness of Treatment." *Society and Mental Health* 9, no. 3 (2019): 388–407.

Allen, Leslie. "Short-Term Emergency Commitment Laws Require Police to Assess Symptoms of Mental Illness." *Bill of Health* (blog), November 25, 2014. Petrie-Flom Center, Harvard Law School. https://blog.petrieflom.law.harvard.edu/2014/11/25/short-term-emergency-commitment-laws-require-police-to-assess-symptoms-of-mental-illness/#.VEkPpiLF98F.

Alvidrez, J., L. R. Snowden, and D. M. Kaiser. "The Experience of Stigma among Black Mental Health Consumers." *Journal of Health Care for the Poor and Underserved* 19, no. 3 (2008): 874–93.

Amar, Mohamed Ben. "Cannabinoids in Medicine: A Review of Their Therapeutic Potential." *Journal of Ethnopharmacology* 105, nos. 1–2 (2006): 1–25.

Amaro, Hortensia, Mariana Sanchez, Tara Bautista, and Robynn Cox. "Social Vulnerabilities for Substance Use: Stressors, Socially Toxic Environments, and Discrimination and Racism." *Neuropharmacology* 188 (2021).

American Psychiatric Association, "New Report Calls for Research on 988 Crisis Line Effectiveness, Caller Demographics, and More." January 6, 2023. https://www.psychiatry.org/news-room/apa-blogs/more-research-needed-on-988-crisis-line.

Ames, Donna, Zachary Erickson, Chelsea Geise, Suchi Tiwari, Sergii Sakhno, Alexander C. Sones, Chaplain Geoffrey Tyrrell, et al. "Treatment of Moral Injury in US Veterans with PTSD Using a Structured Chaplain Intervention." *Journal of Religion and Health* 60, no. 5 (2021): 3052–60.

Anderson, K. K., N. Flora, S. Archie, C. Morgan, and K. McKenzie. "A Meta-analysis of Ethnic Differences in Pathways to Care at the First Episode of Psychosis." *Acta Psychiatrica Scandinavica* 130, no. 4 (2014): 257–68.

Anderson-Fye, Eileen P. and Jerry Floersch. "'I'm Not Your Typical Homework Stresses Me out Kind of Girl': Psychological Anthropology in Research on the Usage of Psychiatric Medications and Mental Health Services." *Ethos* 29, no. 4 (2011): 501–521.

Anglin, Deidre M., Bruce G. Link, and Jo C. Phelan. "Racial Differences in Stigmatizing Attitudes toward People with Mental Illness." *Psychiatric Services* 57 (2006): 857–62.

Anglin, Deidre M., Sabrina Ereshefsky, Mallory J. Klaunig, Miranda A. Bridgwater, Tara A. Niendam, Lauren M. Ellman, Jordan DeVylder, Griffin Thayer, Khalima Bolden, Christie W. Musket, Rebecca E. Grattan, Sarah Hope Lincoln, Jason Schiffman, Emily Lipner, Peter Bachman, Cheryl M. Corcoran, Natália B. Mota, and Els van der Ven. "From

Womb to Neighborhood: A Racial Analysis of Social Determinants of Psychosis in the United States." *American Journal of Psychiatry* 178, no. 7 (2021): 599–610.

Aoki, Ai, Yuta Aoki, Robert Goulden, Kiyoto Kasai, Graham Thornicroft, and Claire Henderson. "Change in Newspaper Coverage of Schizophrenia in Japan over 20-Year Period." *Schizophrenia Research* 175, nos. 1–3 (2016): 193–97.

Archie, Suzanne, Brian R. Rush, Noori Akhtar-Danesh, Ross Norman, Ashok Malla, Paul Roy, and Robert B. Zipursky. "Substance Use and Abuse in First-Episode Psychosis: Prevalence before and after Early Intervention." *Schizophrenia Bulletin* 33, no. 6 (2007): 1354–63.

Arnett, Jeffrey Jensen. *Emerging Adulthood: The Winding Road from the Late Teens through the Twenties*. Oxford: Oxford University Press, 2014.

Azrin, Susan T., Amy B. Goldstein, and Robert K. Heinssen. "Early Intervention for Psychosis: The Recovery after an Initial Schizophrenia Episode Project." *Psychiatric Annals* 45, no. 11 (2015): 548–53.

Balfour, Margaret E., Arlene Hahn Stephenson, Ayesha Delany-Brumsey, Jason Winsky, and Matthew L. Goldman. "Cops, Clinicians, or Both? Collaborative Approaches to Responding to Behavioral Health Emergencies." *Psychiatric Services* 73, no. 6 (2021): 658–69.

Bao, Yuhua, Michelle A. Papp, Rufina Lee, David Shern, and Lisa B. Dixon. "Financing Early Psychosis Intervention Programs: Provider Organization Perspectives." *Psychiatric Services* 72, no. 10 (2021): 1134–38.

Barnes, Arnold. "Race, Schizophrenia, and Admission to State Psychiatric Hospitals." *Administration and Policy in Mental Health and Mental Health Services Research* 31, no. 3 (2004): 241–52.

Barrett, Robert J. *The Psychiatric Team and the Social Definition of Schizophrenia: An Anthropological Study of Person and Illness*. Cambridge: Cambridge University Press, 1996.

Bazargan, Mohsen, Sharon Cobb, and Shervin Assari. "Discrimination and Medical Mistrust in a Racially and Ethnically Diverse Sample of California Adults." *Annals of Family Medicine* 19, no. 1 (2021): 4–15.

Beavan, Vanessa, John Read, and Claire Cartwright. "The Prevalence of Voice-Hearers in the General Population: A Literature Review." *Journal of Mental Health* 20, no. 3 (2011): 281–92.

Bebbington, P., and L. Kuipers. "The Clinical Utility of Expressed Emotion in Schizophrenia." *Acta Psychiatrica Scandinavica* 89 (1994): 46–53.

Béhague, Dominique Pareja. "Psychiatry, Bio-epistemes, and the Making of Adolescence in Southern Brazil." *História, Ciências, Saúde-Manguinhos* 23 (2016): 131–54.

Bellah, Robert N., Richard Madsen, William M. Sullivan, Ann Swidler, and Steven M. Tipton. *Habits of the Heart: Individualism and Commitment in American Life*. Berkeley: University of California Press, 2007.

Bellamy, Chyrell, Timothy Schmutte, and Larry Davidson. "An Update on the Growing Evidence Base for Peer Support." *Mental Health and Social Inclusion* 21, no. 3 (2017): 1–7.

Bennett, Daniel, and Robert Rosenheck. "Socioeconomic Status and the Effectiveness of Treatment for First-Episode Psychosis." *Health Services Research* 56, no. 3 (2021): 409–17.

Berglund, Nils, and Åke Edman. "Family Intervention in Schizophrenia." *Social Psychiatry and Psychiatric Epidemiology* 38, no. 3 (2003): 116–21.

Bergner, Erin, Amy S. Leiner, Tandrea Carter, Lauren Franz, Nancy J. Thompson, and Michael T. Compton. "The Period of Untreated Psychosis before Treatment Initiation: A Qualitative Study of Family Members' Perspectives." *Comprehensive Psychiatry* 49, no. 6 (2008): 530–36.

Bergström, Tomi, Birgitta Alakare, Jukka Aaltonen, Pirjo Mäki, Päivi Köngäs-Saviaro, Jyri J. Taskila, and Jaakko Seikkula. "The Long-Term Use of Psychiatric Services within the Open Dialogue Treatment System after First-Episode Psychosis." *Psychosis* 9, no. 4 (2017): 310–21.

Bergström, Tomi, Jaakko Seikkula, Birgitta Alakare, Pirjo Mäki, Päivi Köngäs-Saviaro, Jyri J. Taskila, Asko Tolvanen, and Jukka Aaltonen. "The Family-Oriented Open Dialogue Approach in the Treatment of First-Episode Psychosis: Nineteen–Year Outcomes." *Psychiatry Research* 270 (2018): 168–75.

Berkhout, Suze G., Juveria Zaheer, and Gary Remington. "Identity, Subjectivity, and Disorders of Self in Psychosis." *Culture, Medicine and Psychiatry* 43, no. 3 (2019): 442–67.

Berwick, Donald M., and Martha E. Gaines. "How HIPAA Harms Care, and How to Stop It." *Journal of the American Medical Association* 320, no. 3 (2018): 229–30.

"The Best Television Series of 2022." *The Economist*, December 2, 2022. https://www.econo mist.com/culture/2022/12/02/the-best-television-series-of-2022.

Bidois, Egan. "A Cultural and Personal Perspective of Psychosis." In *Experiencing Psychosis*, edited by Jim Geekie, Patte Randal, Debra Lampshire, and John Read, 55–63. Oxfordshire, UK: Routledge, 2011.

Biehl, João, Byron Good, and Arthur Kleinman, eds. *Subjectivity: Ethnographic Investigations*. Ethnographic Studies in Subjectivity 7. Berkeley: University of California Press, 2007.

Biehl, João, Stefan Ecks, Byron J. Good, Mary-Jo Del Vecchio–Good, Janis H. Jenkins, Tanya Luhrmann, Emily Martin, Jonathan M. Metzl, and A. Jamie Saris. *Pharmaceutical Self: The Global Shaping of Experience in an Age of Psychopharmacology*. Edited by Janis H. Jenkins. Santa Fe: School for Advanced Research Press, 2010.

Blacksher, Erika. "On Being Poor and Feeling Poor: Low Socioeconomic Status and the Moral Self." *Theoretical Medicine and Bioethics* 23 (2002): 455–70.

Bleuler, Eugen. *Dementia Praecox; or, The Group of Schizophrenias*. Translated by Joseph Zinkin and Nolan D. C. Lewis. New York: International Universities Press, 1950.

Bloom, Sandra L., and Brian Farragher. *Destroying Sanctuary: The Crisis in Human Service Delivery Systems*. Oxford: Oxford University Press, 2010.

Borgen, Linda, and Rubén G. Rumbaut. "Coming of Age in 'America's Finest City': Transitions to Adulthood among Children of Immigrants in San Diego." In *Coming of Age in America: The Transition to Adulthood in the Twenty-First Century*, edited by Mary C. Waters, 133–68. Berkeley: University of California Press, 2011.

Boscarato, Kara, Stuart Lee, Jon Kroschel, Yitzchak Hollander, Alice Brennan, and Narelle Warren. "Consumer Experience of Formal Crisis-Response Services and Preferred Methods of Crisis Intervention." *International Journal of Mental Health Nursing* 23, no. 4 (2014): 287–95.

Bouchery, Ellen E., Michael Barna, Elizabeth Babalola, Daniel Friend, Jonathan D. Brown, Crystal Blyler, and Henry T. Ireys. "The Effectiveness of a Peer-Staffed Crisis Respite Program as an Alternative to Hospitalization." *Psychiatric Services* 69, no. 10 (2018): 1069–74.

Bower, Karen, Adriana Furuzawa, and Dina Tyler. "Back to School: Toolkits to Support the Full Inclusion of Students with Early Psychosis in Higher Education." Campus Staff and Administrator Version. National Association of the State Mental Health Program Directors (NASMHPD) Publications, 2016.

Boyd, Rhea W. "Police Violence and the Built Harm of Structural Racism." The Lancet 392, no. 10,144 (2018): 258–59.

Bradbury, Joanne, Marie Hutchinson, John Hurley, and Helen Stasa. "Lived Experience of Involuntary Transport under Mental Health Legislation." International Journal of Mental Health Nursing 26, no. 6 (2017): 580–92.

Briggs, Ernestine C., Johanna K. P. Greeson, Christopher M. Layne, John A. Fairbank, Angel M. Knoverek, and Robert S. Pynoos. "Trauma Exposure, Psychosocial Functioning, and Treatment Needs of Youth in Residential Care: Preliminary Findings from the NCTSN Core Data Set." Journal of Child and Adolescent Trauma 5, no. 1 (2012): 1–15.

Brodwin, Paul. Everyday Ethics: Voices from the Front Line of Community Psychiatry. Berkeley: University of California Press, 2013.

Brown, Julia E. H. "The Stories We Tell or Omit: How Ethnographic (In)Attention can Obscure Structural Racism in the Anthropology of Mental Healthcare." Medicine Anthropology Theory 10, no. 1 (2023): 1–15.

Brown, Julia E. H., Michael D'Arcy, Neely L. Myers, and Tali Ziv. "Experimental Engagements with Ethnography, Moral Agency, and Care." Special section in Medicine Anthropology Theory 10, no. 1 (2023).

Bruner, Jerome. "The Narrative Construction of Reality." Critical Inquiry 18, no. 1 (1991): 1–21.

Bryson, Stephanie A., Emma Gauvin, Ally Jamieson, Melanie Rathgeber, Lorelei Faulkner Gibson, Sarah Bell, Jana Davidson, Jennifer Russel, and Sharlynne Burke. "What Are Effective Strategies for Implementing Trauma-Informed Care in Youth Inpatient Psychiatric and Residential Treatment Settings? A Realist Systematic Review." International Journal of Mental Health Systems 11, no. 1 (2017): 1–16.

Bury, Michael. "Chronic Illness as Biographical Disruption." Sociology of Health and Illness 4, no. 2 (1982): 167–82.

Butler, Lisa D., Filomena M. Critelli, and Elaine S. Rinfrette. "Trauma-Informed Care and Mental Health." Directions in Psychiatry 31, no. 3 (2011): 197–212.

Butzlaff, Ronald L., and Jill M. Hooley. "Expressed Emotion and Psychiatric Relapse: A Meta-analysis." Archives of General Psychiatry 55, no. 6 (1998): 547–52.

Cairns, Victoria A., Graeme S. Reid, and Craig Murray. "Family Members' Experience of Seeking Help for First-Episode Psychosis on Behalf of a Loved One: A Meta-synthesis of Qualitative Research." Early Intervention in Psychiatry 9, no. 3 (2015): 185–99.

Calvo, Ana, Miguel Moreno, Ana Ruiz-Sancho, Marta Rapado-Castro, Carmen Moreno, Teresa Sánchez-Gutiérrez, Celso Arango, and María Mayoral. "Psychoeducational Group Intervention for Adolescents with Psychosis and Their Families: A Two-Year Follow-Up." Journal of the American Academy of Child and Adolescent Psychiatry 54, no. 12 (2015): 984–90.

Carbon, Maren, John M. Kane, Stefan Leucht, and Christoph U. Correll. "Tardive Dyskinesia Risk with First- and Second-Generation Antipsychotics in Comparative Randomized Controlled Trials: A Meta-analysis." World Psychiatry 17, no. 3 (2018): 330–40.

Cardoso, Jodi Berger, Kalina Brabeck, Randy Capps, Tzuan Chen, Natalia Giraldo-Santiago, Anjely Huertas, and Nubia A. Mayorga. "Immigration Enforcement Fear and Anxiety in Latinx High School Students: The Indirect Effect of Perceived Discrimination." *Journal of Adolescent Health* 68, no. 5 (2021): 961–68.

Carter, C. Sue. "Oxytocin Pathways and the Evolution of Human Behavior." *Annual Review of Psychology* 65, no. 1 (2014): 17–39.

Cechnicki, Andrzej, Anna Bielańska, Igor Hanuszkiewicz, and Artur Daren. "The Predictive Validity of Expressed Emotions (EE) in Schizophrenia: A 20-Year Prospective Study." *Journal of Psychiatric Research* 47, no. 2 (2013): 208–14.

Centers for Disease Control and Prevention (CDC). "About Teen Pregnancy." CDC.gov. Last reviewed November 15, 2021. https://www.cdc.gov/teenpregnancy/about/index.htm.

Centers for Disease Control and Prevention. "New CDC Data Illuminate Youth Mental Health Threats during the COVID-19 Pandemic." CDC.gov, 2022. https://www.cdc.gov/media/releases/2022/p0331-youth-mental-health-covid-19.html.

Centers for Disease Control and Prevention. "Youth Risk Behavior Surveillance Data Summary and Trends Report: 2009–2019." CDC.gov, 2020. https://www.cdc.gov/nchhstp/dear_colleague/2020/dcl-102320-YRBS-2009-2019-report.html.

Cerdeña, Jessica P., Luisa M. Rivera, and Judy M. Spak. "Intergenerational Trauma in Latinxs: A Scoping Review." *Social Science and Medicine* 270 (2021): 113662.

Cès, Agathe, Bruno Falissard, Nine Glangeaud-Freudenthal, Anne-Laure Sutter-Dallay, and Florence Gressier. "Pregnancy in Women with Psychotic Disorders: Risk Factors Associated with Mother-Baby Separation." *Archives of Women's Mental Health* 21, no. 6 (2018): 699–706.

Chamary, J. V. "'Work Hard, Play Hard' Lifestyle Is Real, Says Science." *Forbes*, June 2016.

Chambers, Angelina N. "Impact of Forced Separation Policy on Incarcerated Postpartum Mothers." *Policy, Politics, and Nursing Practice* 10, no. 3 (2009): 204–11.

Chaumba, Josphine. "Health Status, Use of Health Care Resources, and Treatment Strategies of Ethiopian and Nigerian Immigrants in the United States." *Social Work in Health Care* 50, no. 6 (2011): 466–81.

Cheng, Alice W., Ora Nakash, Mario Cruz-Gonzalez, Mirko K. Fillbrunn, and Margarita Alegría. "The Association between Patient-Provider Racial/Ethnic Concordance, Working Alliance, and Length of Treatment in Behavioral Health Settings." *Psychological Services* 20, no. S1 (2023): 145.

Chien, Wai-Tong, and Ian Norman. "The Effectiveness and Active Ingredients of Mutual Support Groups for Family Caregivers of People with Psychotic Disorders: A Literature Review." *International Journal of Nursing Studies* 46, no. 12 (2009): 1604–23.

Chien, Wai-Tong, and Sally W. C. Chan. "The Effectiveness of Mutual Support Group Intervention for Chinese Families of People with Schizophrenia: A Randomised Controlled Trial with 24-Month Follow-Up." *International Journal of Nursing Studies* 50, no. 10 (2013): 1326–40.

Chinman, Matthew, Preethy George, Richard H. Dougherty, Allen S. Daniels, Sushmita Shoma Ghose, Anita Swift, and Miriam E. Delphin-Rittmon. "Peer Support Services for Individuals with Serious Mental Illnesses: Assessing the Evidence." *Psychiatric Services* 65, no. 4 (2014): 429–41.

Claxton, Melanie, Juliana Onwumere, and Miriam Fornells-Ambrojo. "Do Family Interventions Improve Outcomes in Early Psychosis? A Systematic Review and Meta-analysis." *Frontiers in Psychology* 8 (2017): 371.

CNN. "Anderson Cooper Tries a Schizophrenia Simulator." YouTube, June 9, 2014. Video, 5:03. https://www.youtube.com/watch?v=yL9UJVtgPZY.

Cocaine Cowboys: The Kings of Miami. Directed by Billy Corben. 2006.

Codjoe, Louisa, Sarah Barber, Shalini Ahuja, Graham Thornicroft, Claire Henderson, Heidi Lempp, and Joelyn N'Danga-Koroma. "Evidence for Interventions to Promote Mental Health and Reduce Stigma in Black Faith Communities: Systematic Review." *Social Psychiatry and Psychiatric Epidemiology* 56 (2021), 895–911.

Cohen, Laura J. "Psychiatric Hospitalization as an Experience of Trauma." *Archives of Psychiatric Nursing* 8, no. 2 (1994): 78–81.

Cohen, Mark A., and Alex R. Piquero. "An Outcome Evaluation of the YouthBuild USA Offender Project." *Youth Violence and Juvenile Justice* 8, no. 4 (2010): 373–85.

Colizzi, Marco, Elena Carra, Sara Fraietta, John Lally, Diego Quattrone, Stefania Bonaccorso, Valeria Mondelli, Olesya Ajnakina, Paola Dazzan, Antonella Trotta, Lucia Sideli, Anna Kolliakou, Fiona Gaughran, Mizanur Khondoker, Anthony S. David, Robin M. Murray, James H. MacCabe, and Marta Di Forti. "Substance Use, Medication Adherence, and Outcome One Year following a First Episode of Psychosis." *Schizophrenia Research* 170, nos. 2–3 (2016): 311–17.

Colizzi, Marco, Mirella Ruggeri, and Antonio Lasalvia. "Should We Be Concerned about Stigma and Discrimination in People at Risk for Psychosis? A Systematic Review." *Psychological Medicine* 50, no. 5 (2020): 705–26.

Compton, Michael T., and Beth Broussard. *The First Episode of Psychosis: A Guide for Patients and their Families*. Oxford: Oxford University Press, 2009.

Compton, Michael T., Andrew C. Furman, and Nadine J. Kaslow. "Preliminary Evidence of an Association between Childhood Abuse and Cannabis Dependence among African American First-Episode Schizophrenia-Spectrum Disorder Patients." *Drug and Alcohol Dependence* 76, no. 3 (2004): 311–16.

Compton, Michael T., Brooke Halpern, Beth Broussard, Simone Anderson, Kelly Smith, Samantha Ellis, Kara Griffin, Luca Pauselli, and Neely Myers. "A Potential New Form of Jail Diversion and Reconnection to Mental Health Services: I. Stakeholders' Views on Acceptability." *Behavioral Sciences and the Law* 35, no. 5–6 (2017): 480–91.

Compton, Michael T., Francisco Fantes, Claire Ramsay Wan, Stephanie Johnson, and Elaine F. Walker. "Abnormal Movements in First-Episode, Nonaffective Psychosis: Dyskinesias, Stereotypies, and Catatonic-Like Signs." *Psychiatry Research* 226, no. 1 (2015): 192–197.

Compton, Michael T., Mary E. Kelley, and Dawn F. Ionescu. "Subtyping First-Episode Nonaffective Psychosis Using Four Early-Course Features: Potentially Useful Prognostic Information at Initial Presentation." *Early Intervention in Psychiatry* 8, no. 1 (2014): 50–58.

Compton, Michael T., Neil E. Whicker, and Karen M. Hochman. "Alcohol and Cannabis Use in Urban, African American, First-Episode Schizophrenia-Spectrum Patients: Associations with Positive and Negative Symptoms." *Journal of Clinical Psychiatry* 68, no. 12 (2007): 1939–45.

Compton, Michael T., Roger Bakeman, Beth Broussard, Dana Hankerson-Dyson, Letheshia Husbands, Shaily Krishan, Tarianna Stewart-Hutto, Barbara M. D'Orio, Janet R. Oliva, Nancy J. Thompson, and Amy C. Watson. "The Police-Based Crisis Intervention Team (CIT) Model: II. Effects on Level of Force and Resolution, Referral, and Arrest." *Psychiatric Services* 65, no. 4 (2014): 523–29.

Compton, Michael T., Sandra M. Goulding, Tynessa L. Gordon, Paul S. Weiss, and Nadine J. Kaslow. "Family-Level Predictors and Correlates of the Duration of Untreated Psychosis in African American First-Episode Patients." *Schizophrenia Research* 115, no. 2–3 (2009): 338–45.

Cooke, Anne, ed. "Understanding Psychosis and Schizophrenia (Revised)." British Psychological Society, 2017. Accessed January 29, 2024. https://doi.org/10.53841/bpsrep.2017.rep03.

Corcoran, Cheryl, Elaine Walker, Rebecca Huot, Vijay Mittal, Kevin Tessner, Lisa Kestler, and Dolores Malaspina. "The Stress Cascade and Schizophrenia: Etiology and Onset." *Schizophrenia Bulletin* 29, no. 4 (2003): 671–92.

Corin, Ellen, and Gilles Lauzon. "Positive Withdrawal and the Quest for Meaning: The Reconstruction of Experience among Schizophrenics." *Psychiatry* 55, no. 3 (1992): 266–78.

Corin, Ellen, Rangaswami Thara, and Ramachandran Padmavati. "Living through a Staggering World: The Play of Signifiers in Early Psychosis in South India." In *Schizophrenia, Culture, and Subjectivity: The Edge of Experience*, edited by Janis H. Jenkins and Robert John Barrett, 110–45. Cambridge: Cambridge University Press, 2003.

Correll, Christoph, Brita Galling, Aditya Pawar, Anastasia Krivko, Chiara Bonetto, Mirella Ruggeri, Thomas J. Craig, Merete Nordentoft, Vinod H. Srihari, Sinan Guloksuz, Christy L. M. Hui, Eric Y. H. Chen, Marcelo Valencia, Francisco Juarez, Delbert G. Robinson, Nina R. Schooler, Mary F. Brunette, Kim T. Mueser, Robert A. Rosenheck, Patricia Marcy, Jean Addington, Sue E. Estroff, James Robinson, David Penn, Joanne B. Severe, and John M. Kane. "Comparison of Early Intervention Services vs Treatment as Usual for Early-Phase Psychosis: A Systematic Review, Meta-analysis, and Meta-regression." *JAMA Psychiatry* 75, no. 6 (2018): 555–65.

Corrigan, Patrick W. "How Stigma Interferes with Mental Health Care." *American Psychologist* 59, no. 7 (2004): 614–25.

Corrigan, Patrick W., and Amy C. Watson. "The Paradox of Self-Stigma and Mental Illness." *Clinical Psychology: Science and Practice* 9, no. 1 (2002): 35–53.

Cotes, Robert O., Justin M. Palanci, Beth Broussard, Stephanie Johnson, M. Alejandra Grullón, Grayson S. Norquist, C. Christina Mehta, Keith Wood, Lauren Cubellis, Maryam Gholami & Douglas Ziedonis. "Feasibility of an Open Dialogue–Inspired Approach for Young Adults with Psychosis in a Public Hospital System." *Community Mental Health Journal* 59 (2023): 1428–35.

Croft, Bevin, Anne Weaver, and Laysha Ostrow. "Self-Reliance and Belonging: Guest Experiences of a Peer Respite." *Psychiatric Rehabilitation Journal* 44, no. 2 (2021): 124–131.

Croft, Bevin, and Nilüfer İsvan. "Impact of the 2nd Story Peer Respite Program on Use of Inpatient and Emergency Services." *Psychiatric Services* 66, no. 6 (2015): 632–37.

Crouch, Julie L., Rochelle F. Hanson, Benjamin E. Saunders, Dean G. Kilpatrick, and Heidi S. Resnick. "Income, Race/Ethnicity, and Exposure to Violence in Youth: Results from the National Survey of Adolescents." *Journal of Community Psychology* 28, no. 6 (2000): 625–41.

Cusack, Karen J., B. Christopher Frueh, Thom Hiers, Samantha Suffoletta-Maierle, and Sandy Bennett. "Trauma within the Psychiatric Setting: A Preliminary Empirical report." *Administration and Policy in Mental Health and Mental Health Services Research* 30, no. 5 (2003): 453–60. <It seems inconsistent to me when you are adding page numbers and when you are deleting the number and adding it so maybe just check on that when you finalize?>

D'Arcy, Michael. "'Swallow Them All, and It's Just like Smack': Comorbidity, Polypharmacy, and Imagining Moral Agency alongside Methadone and Antipsychotics." *Medicine Anthropology Theory* 10, no. 1 (2023): 1–25.

Damour, Lisa. *Untangled: Guiding Teenage Girls through the Seven Transitions into Adulthood*. New York: Ballantine Books, 2016.

Darmi, E., T. Bellali, I. Papazoglou, I. Karamitri, and D. Papadatou. "Caring for an Intimate Stranger: Parenting a Child with Psychosis." *Journal of Psychiatric and Mental Health Nursing* 24, no. 4 (2017): 194–202.

Dart, Tom. "Three Cops, a 17-Year-Old and 'a Cry for Help': Why Did Kristiana Coignard Die?" *The Guardian* (US edition), January 28, 2015. https://www.theguardian.com/us-news/2015/jan/28/kristiana-coignard-longview-texas-police-killing.

Davis, Elizabeth A. *Bad Souls: Madness and Responsibility in Modern Greece*. Durham, NC: Duke University Press, 2012.

Deegan, Pat. 2023. Common Ground Program Outcomes: Hearing Distressing Voices Simulation. Accessed April 22, 2024. https://s3.amazonaws.com/kajabi-storefronts-production/sites/41305/themes/793117/downloads/9ufrnx23TlKoJxOMKhMB_voices_simulation_outcomes_2-6-2019.pdf.

Delva, Jorge, Pilar Horner, Ramiro Martinez, Laura Sanders, William D. Lopez, and John Doering-White. "Mental Health Problems of Children of Undocumented Parents in the United States: A Hidden Crisis." *Journal of Community Positive Practices* 3 (2013): 25–35.

De Mooij, Liselotte D., Martijn Kikkert, Jan Theunissen, Aartjan T. F. Beekman, Lieuwe De Haan, Pim W. R. A. Duurkoop, Henricus L. Van, and Jack J. M. Dekker. "Dying Too Soon: Excess Mortality in Severe Mental Illness." *Frontiers in Psychiatry* 10 (2019): 855.

DiAngelo, Robin. *White Fragility: Why It's So Hard for White People to Talk about Racism*. Boston: Beacon Press, 2018.

Digel Vandyk, Amanda, Lisa Young, Colleen MacPhee, and Katharine Gillis. "Exploring the Experiences of Persons Who Frequently Visit the Emergency Department for Mental Health–Related Reasons." *Qualitative Health Research* 28, no. 4 (2018): 587–99.

Dillinger, Rachel L., and Jonathan M. Kersun. "Caring for Caregivers: Understanding and Meeting Their Needs in Coping with First Episode Psychosis." *Early Intervention in Psychiatry* 14, no. 5 (2020): 528–34.

Dixon, Lisa. "What It Will Take to Make Coordinated Specialty Care Available to Anyone Experiencing Early Schizophrenia: Getting over the Hump." *Journal of the American Medical Association Psychiatry* 74, no. 1 (2017): 7–8.

Dixon, Lisa, and Scott Stroup. "Medications for First-Episode Psychosis: Making a Good Start." *American Journal of Psychiatry* 172, no. 3 (2015): 209–11.

Docherty, Nancy M., Annie St-Hilaire, Jennifer M. Aakre, James P. Seghers, Amanda McCleery, and Marielle Divilbiss. "Anxiety Interacts with Expressed Emotion Criticism in the Prediction of Psychotic Symptom Exacerbation." *Schizophrenia Bulletin* 37, no. 3 (2011): 611–18.

Dole, Christopher, and Thomas J. Csordas. "Trials of Navajo Youth: Identity, Healing, and the Struggle for Maturity." *Ethos* 31, no. 3 (2003): 357–84.

Douglass, Frederick. *Narrative of the Life of Frederick Douglass, an American Slave*. Oxford: Oxford University Press, 1999.

Downen, Robert. "Unlicensed Religious Chaplains May Counsel Students in Texas' Public Schools after Lawmakers OK Proposal." *Texas Tribune* (Austin), May 24, 2023. https://www.texastribune.org/2023/05/24/texas-legislature-chaplains-schools/.

Doyle, Roisin, Niall Turner, Felicity Fanning, Daria Brennan, Laoise Renwick, Elizabeth Lawlor, and Mary Clarke. "First-Episode Psychosis and Disengagement from Treatment: A Systematic Review." *Psychiatric Services* 65, no. 5 (2014): 603–11.

DuBrul, Sascha Altman. *Maps to the Other Side: Adventures of a Bipolar Cartographer*. Portland, OR: Microcosm, 2013.

DuBrul, Sascha Altman. "The Icarus Project: A Counter Narrative for Psychic Diversity." *Journal of Medical Humanities* 35, no. 3 (2014): 257–71.

Duhig, Michael, Sue Patterson, Melissa Connell, Sharon Foley, Carina Capra, Frances Dark, Anne Gordon, Saveena Singh, Leanne Hides, John J. McGrath, and James Scott. "The Prevalence and Correlates of Childhood Trauma in Patients with Early Psychosis." *Australian and New Zealand Journal of Psychiatry* 49, no. 7 (2015): 651–59.

Duncan, Whitney. *Transforming Therapy: Mental Health Practice and Cultural Change in Mexico*. Nashville: Vanderbilt University Press, 2018.

Edwards, Frank, Michael H. Esposito, and Hedwig Lee. "Risk of Police-Involved Death by Race/Ethnicity and Place, United States, 2012–2018." *American Journal of Public Health* 108, no. 9 (2018): 1241–48.

Elisseou, Sadie, Sravanthi Puranam, and Meghna Nandi. "A Novel, Trauma-Informed Physical Examination Curriculum for First-Year Medical Students." *MedEdPORTAL: The Journal of Teaching and Learning Resources* 15 (2019). doi: 10.15766/mep_2374-8265 .10799.

Erikson, Erik. *Identity: Youth and Crisis*. New York: W. W. Norton, 1968.

Esterberg, Michelle, and Michael Compton. "Family History of Psychosis Negatively Impacts Age at Onset, Negative Symptoms, and Duration of Untreated Illness and Psychosis in First-Episode Psychosis Patients." *Psychiatry Research* 197, no. 1–2 (2012): 23–28.

Estroff, Sue E. *Making It Crazy: An Ethnography of Psychiatric Clients in an American Community*. Berkeley: University of California Press, 1981.

Evans, Arthur C., and Clarence E. Anthony. "Gun Violence: A Public Health Problem." *The Hill*, April 6, 2018. https://thehill.com/blogs/congress-blog/healthcare/381874-gun -violence-a-public-health-problem/.

Ezeobele, I., A. Malecha, P. Landrum, and L. Symes. "Depression and Nigerian-Born Immigrant Women in the United States: A Phenomenological Study." *Journal of Psychiatric and Mental Health Nursing* 17, no. 3 (2010): 193–201.

Falkenburg, Jara, and Derek K. Tracy. "Sex and Schizophrenia: A Review of Gender Differences." *Psychosis* 6, no. 1 (2014): 61–69.

Faridi, Kia, Nicole Pawliuk, Suzanne King, Ridha Joober, and Ashok K. Malla. "Prevalence of Psychotic and Non-psychotic Disorders in Relatives of Patients with a First Episode Psychosis." *Schizophrenia Research* 114, nos. 1–3 (2009): 57–63.

Fein, Elizabeth. *Living on the Spectrum: Autism and Youth in Community*. New York: New York University Press, 2020.

Feldman, Justin M., Jarvis T. Chen, Pamela D. Waterman, and Nancy Krieger. "Temporal Trends and Racial/Ethnic Inequalities for Legal Intervention Injuries Treated in Emergency Departments: US Men and Women Age 15–34, 2001–2014." *Journal of Urban Health* 93, no. 5 (2016): 797–807.

Fleming, Charles B., Katarina Guttmannova, Christopher Cambron, Isaac C. Rhew, and Sabrina Oesterle. "Examination of the Divergence in Trends for Adolescent Marijuana Use and Marijuana-Specific Risk Factors in Washington State." *Journal of Adolescent Health* 59, no. 3 (2016): 269–75.

Fletcher, Erica Hua. "Uncivilizing 'Mental Illness': Contextualizing Diverse Mental States and Posthuman Emotional Ecologies within the Icarus Project." *Journal of Medical Humanities* 39, no. 1 (2018): 29–43.

Fletcher, Erica Hua, and Adriane Barroso. "'It's a Much More Relaxed Atmosphere': Atmospheres of Recovery at a Peer Respite." *Emotion, Space, and Society* 36 (2020): 100705.

Florence, Ana Carolina, Gerald Jordan, Silvio Yasui, Daniela Ravelli Cabrini, and Larry Davidson. "'It Makes Us Realize That We Have Been Heard': Experiences with Open Dialogue in Vermont." *Psychiatric Quarterly* 92, no. 4 (2021): 1771–83.

Flores, Elaine C., Daniela C. Fuhr, Angela M. Bayer, Andres G. Lescano, Nicki Thorogood, and Victoria Simms. "Mental Health Impact of Social Capital Interventions: A Systematic Review." *Social Psychiatry and Psychiatric Epidemiology* 53 (2018): 107–19.

Flournoy, Edward Brian. "The Rising of Systemic Racism and Redlining in the United States of America." *Journal of Sustainable Social Change* 13, no. 1 (2021): 6.

Fortuna, Lisa R., Michelle V. Porche, and Margarita Alegria. "Political Violence, Psychosocial Trauma, and the Context of Mental Health Services Use among Immigrant Latinos in the United States." *Ethnicity & Health* 13, no. 5 (2008): 435–463.

Francey, Shona M., Brian O'Donoghue, Barnaby Nelson, Jessica Graham, Lara Baldwin, Hok Pan Yuen, Melissa J. Kerr, Aswin Ratheesh, Kelly Allott, Mario Alvarez-Jimenez, Alex Fornito, Susy Harrigan, Andrew D. Thompson, Stephen Wood, Michael Berk, and Patrick D. McGorry. "Psychosocial Intervention with or without Antipsychotic Medication for First-Episode Psychosis: A Randomized Noninferiority Clinical Trial." *Schizophrenia Bulletin Open* 1, no. 1 (2020): sgaa015.

Frank, A. W. *The Wounded Storyteller: Body, Illness, and Ethics.* Chicago: University of Chicago Press, 1995.

Franz, Lauren, Tandrea Carter, Amy S. Leiner, Erin Bergner, Nancy J. Thompson, and Michael T. Compton. "Stigma and Treatment Delay in First-Episode Psychosis: A Grounded Theory Study." *Early Intervention in Psychiatry* 4, no. 1 (2010): 47–56.

Frueh, B. Christopher, Karen J. Cusack, Thomas G. Hiers, Susan Monogan, Victoria C. Cousins, and S. Diane Cavenaugh. "Improving Public Mental Health Services for Trauma Victims in South Carolina." *Psychiatric Services* 52, no. 6 (2001): 812–14.

Frueh, B. Christopher, Marc E. Dalton, Michael R. Johnson, Thomas G. Hiers, Paul B. Gold, Kathryn M. Magruder, and Alberto B. Santos. "Trauma within the Psychiatric Setting: Conceptual Framework, Research Directions, and Policy Implications." *Administration and Policy in Mental Health and Mental Health Services Research* 28, no. 2 (2000): 147–54.

Frueh, B. Christopher, Rebecca G. Knapp, Karen J. Cusack, Anouk L. Grubaugh, Julie A. Sauvageot, Victoria C. Cousins, Eunsil Yim, Cynthia S. Robins, Jeannine Monnier, and Thomas G. Hiers. "Special Section on Seclusion and Restraint: Patients' Reports of Traumatic or Harmful Experiences within the Psychiatric Setting." *Psychiatric Services* 56, no. 9 (2005): 1123–33.

Fuller, Doris A., H. Richard Lamb, Michael Biasotti, and John Snook. *Overlooked in the Undercounted: The Role of Mental Illness in Fatal Law Enforcement Encounters.* Arlington, VA: Treatment Advocacy Center, 2015. https://www.treatmentadvocacycenter.org/overlooked-in-the-undercounted.

Gangi, C. "On the Gravity of Mental Illness Stigma." *Philosophy, Psychiatry, and Psychology* 28, no. 4 (2021): 385–95.

Garcia, Angela. *The Pastoral Clinic: Addiction and Dispossession along the Rio Grande.* Berkeley: University of California Press, 2010.

Garcia, Myriam, Itziar Montalvo, Marta Creus, Ángel Cabezas, Montse Solé, Maria José Algora, Irene Moreno, Alfonso Gutiérrez-Zotes, and Javier Labad. "Sex Differences in the Effect of Childhood Trauma on the Clinical Expression of Early Psychosis." *Comprehensive Psychiatry* 68 (2016): 86–96.

Garro, Linda C. "Enacting Ethos, Enacting Health: Realizing Health in the Everyday Life of a California Family of Mexican Descent." *Ethos* 39, no. 3 (2011): 300–330.

Gatov, Evgenia, Nicole Koziel, Paul Kurdyak, Natasha R. Saunders, Maria Chiu, Michael Lebenbaum, Simon Chen, and Simone N. Vigod. "Epidemiology of Interpersonal Trauma among Women and Men Psychiatric Inpatients: A Population-Based Study." *Canadian Journal of Psychiatry* 65, no. 2 (2020): 124–35.

Gee, Dylan G., and Tyrone D. Cannon. "Prediction of Conversion to Psychosis: Review and Future Directions." *Brazilian Journal of Psychiatry* 33 (2011): S129–S142.

Gee, Gilbert C., and Chandra L. Ford. "Structural Racism and Health Inequities: Old Issues, New Directions." *Du Bois Review: Social Science Research on Race* 8, no. 1 (2011): 115–32.

George, Preethy, Nev Jones, Howard Goldman, and Abram Rosenblatt. "Cycles of Reform in the History of Psychosis Treatment in the United States." *SSM–Mental Health* 3 (2023): 100205.

Gibbs, Jada S., Sydney Kriegsman, and Hannah E. Brown. "Dismantling Racial Inequities in Early Psychosis Family Psychoeducation." *Psychiatric Services* 73, no. 9 (2022).

Gidugu, Vasudha, E. Sally Rogers, Christopher Gordon, A. Rani Elwy, and Mari-Lynn Drainoni. "Client, Family, and Clinician Experiences of Open Dialogue-Based Services." *Psychological Services* 18, no. 2 (2021): 154–63.

Gilligan, Carol. *In a Different Voice: Psychological Theory and Women's Development.* Cambridge, MA: Harvard University Press, 1993.

Gillon, Leah, Marcia Valenstein, Frederic C. Blow, John E. Zeber, John F. McCarthy, and C. Raymond Bingham. "Ethnicity and Diagnostic Patterns in Veterans with Psychoses." *Social Psychiatry and Psychiatric Epidemiology* 39 (October 2004): 841–51. https://doi.org/10.1007/s00127-004-0824-7.

Giordano, Cristiana. *Migrants in Translation: Caring and the Logics of Difference in Contemporary Italy.* Oakland: University of California Press, 2014.

Girl, Interrupted. Directed by James Mangold. Culver City, CA: Columbia Pictures, 1999.

Godress, Julia, Salih Ozgul, Cathy Owen, and Leanne Foley-Evans. "Grief Experiences of Parents Whose Children Suffer from Mental Illness." *Australian and New Zealand Journal of Psychiatry* 39, no. 1–2 (2005): 88–94.

Good, Byron J. *Medicine, Rationality, and Experience: An Anthropological Perspective.* Cambridge: Cambridge University Press, 1993.

Good, Byron J., Michael M. J. Fischer, Sarah S. Willen, and Mary-Jo DelVecchio Good, eds. *A Reader in Medical Anthropology: Theoretical Trajectories, Emergent Realities.* Malden, MA: Blackwell, 2010.

Good, Mary-Jo DelVecchio. "The Biotechnical Embrace." *Culture, Medicine, and Psychiatry* 25, no. 4 (2001): 395–410.

Good, Mary-Jo DelVecchio, ed. *Postcolonial Disorders.* Berkeley: University of California Press, 2008.

Gorczynski, Paul, and Wendy Sims-Schouten. "Evaluating Mental Health Literacy amongst US College Students: A Cross Sectional Study." *Journal of American College Health* (2022): 1–4.

Goulding, Sandra M., Victoria H. Chien, and Michael T. Compton. "Prevalence and Correlates of School Drop-Out Prior to Initial Treatment of Nonaffective Psychosis: Further Evidence Suggesting a Need for Supported Education." *Schizophrenia Research* 116, nos. 2–3 (2010): 228–33.

Greenfield, Thomas K., Beth C. Stoneking, Keith Humphreys, Evan Sundby, and Jason Bond. "A Randomized Trial of a Mental Health Consumer-Managed Alternative to Civil Commitment for Acute Psychiatric Crisis." *American Journal of Community Psychology* 42, no. 1 (2008): 135–44.

Greenwald, Ricky, Lynn Siradas, Thomas A. Schmitt, Summar Reslan, Julia Fierle, and Brad Sande. "Implementing Trauma-Informed Treatment for Youth in a Residential Facility: First-Year Outcomes." *Residential Treatment for Children and Youth* 29, no. 2 (2012): 141–53.

Griffen, Adrienne, Teresa Twomey, and Kristina Dulaney. "Survivors of Pregnancy and Postpartum Psychosis Speak Out." Maternal Mental Health Leadership Alliance, February 14, 2024. https://www.mmhla.org/articles/survivors-of-pregnancy-and-postpartum-psychosis-speak-out.

Griffith, James L., Neely Myers, and Michael T. Compton. "How Can Community Religious Groups Aid Recovery for Individuals with Psychotic Illnesses?." *Community Mental Health Journal* 52, no. 7 (2016): 775–780.

Grof, Stanislav. *Psychology of the Future: Lessons from Modern Consciousness Research.* Albany: State University of New York Press, 2019.

Grof, Stanislav, and Christina Grof, eds. *Spiritual Emergency: When Personal Transformation Becomes a Crisis.* New York: Jeremy P. Tarcher, 1989.

Guarnaccia, Peter J. "*Ataques de Nervios* in Puerto Rico: Culture-Bound Syndrome or Popular Illness?" *Medical Anthropology* 15, no. 2 (1993): 157–70.

Gutmann, Matthew C. *The Meanings of Macho: Being a Man in Mexico City.* Tenth anniversary edition. Men and Masculinity 3. Berkeley: University of California Press, 2006.

Guzmán, Eleonora M., Katherine M. Tezanos, Bernard P. Chang, and Christine B. Cha. "Examining the Impact of Emergency Care Settings on Suicidal Patients: A Call to Action." *General Hospital Psychiatry* 63 (2020): 9–13.

Haenfler, Ross. "The Entrepreneurial (Straight) Edge: How Participation in DIY Music Cultures Translates to Work and Careers." *Cultural Sociology* 12, no. 2 (2018): 174–92.

Hailes, Helen P., Rongqin Yu, Andrea Danese, and Seena Fazel. "Long-Term Outcomes of Childhood Sexual Abuse: An Umbrella Review." *The Lancet Psychiatry* 6, no. 10 (2019): 830–39.

Hall, Granville Stanley. *Adolescence: Its Psychology and Its Relations to Physiology, Anthropology, Sociology, Sex, Crime, Religion, and Education.* Vol. 2. New York: D. Appleton, 1905.

Halliburton, Murphy. *Mudpacks and Prozac: Experiencing Ayurvedic, Biomedical, and Religious Healing.* New York: Routledge, 2009.

Hamann, Johannes, Gabi Pitschel-Walz, and Werner Kissling. "Medication Adherence Studies in Schizophrenia." *American Journal of Psychiatry* 161, no. 3 (2004): 582.

Hammond, W. P. "Psychosocial Correlates of Medical Mistrust among African American Men." *American Journal of Community Psychology* 45 (2010): 87–106.

Hansen, Helena, and Jonathan Metzl, eds. *Structural Competency in Mental Health and Medicine: A Case-Based Approach to Treating the Social Determinants of Health*. Cham, Switzerland: Springer Nature, 2019.

Hansen, Helena, Philippe Bourgois, and Ernest Drucker. "Pathologizing Poverty: New Forms of Diagnosis, Disability, and Structural Stigma under Welfare Reform." *Social Science and Medicine* 103 (February 2014): 76–83. doi: 10.1016/j.socscimed.2013.06.033.

Harris, Barbara, Ross Beurmann, Samantha Fagien, and Mona M. Shattell. "Patients' Experiences of Psychiatric Care in Emergency Departments: A Secondary Analysis." *International Emergency Nursing* 26 (2016): 14–19.

Harris, Maxine, and R. Fallot. *Using Trauma Theory to Design Service Systems*. New Directions for Mental Health Services. San Francisco: Jossey-Bass, 2001.

Hart, Brian. "Terrell State Hospital." In *Handbook of Texas Online*. Updated July 1, 1995. https://www.tshaonline.org/handbook/entries/terrell-state-hospital.

Hartmann, Jessica, Barnaby Nelson, Aswin Ratheesh, Devi Treen, and Patrick D McGorry. "At-Risk Studies and Clinical Antecedents of Psychosis, Bipolar Disorder, and Depression: A Scoping Review in the Context of Clinical Staging." *Psychological Medicine* 49, no. 2 (2019): 177–89.

Hasan, Alkomiet, Rupert von Keller, Chris Maria Friemel, Wayne Hall, Miriam Schneider, Dagmar Koethe, F. Markus Leweke, Wolfgang Strube, and Eva Hoch. "Cannabis Use and Psychosis: A Review of Reviews." *European Archives of Psychiatry and Clinical Neuroscience* 270, no. 4 (2020): 403–12.

Haynes, T. F., A. M. Cheney, J. G. Sullivan, K. Bryant, G. M. Curran, M. Olson, N. Cottoms, and C. Reaves. "Addressing Mental Health Needs: Perspectives of African Americans Living in the Rural South." *Psychiatric Services*, 68, no. 6 (2017): 573–78.

Hedman, Leslie C., John Petrila, William H. Fisher, Jeffrey W. Swanson, Deirdre A. Dingman, and Scott Burris. "State Laws on Emergency Holds for Mental Health Stabilization." *Psychiatric Services* 67, no. 5 (2016): 529–35.

Heinssen, Robert K., Amy B. Goldstein, and Susan T. Azrin. "Evidence-Based Treatments for First Episode Psychosis: Components of Coordinated Specialty Care." National Institute of Mental Health, April 14, 2014. https://www.nimh.nih.gov/health/topics/schizophrenia/raise/evidence-based-treatments-for-first-episode-psychosis-components-of-coordinated-specialty-care.

Hejtmanek, Katie Rose. *Friendship, Love, and Hip Hop: An Ethnography of African American Men in Psychiatric Custody*. New York: Palgrave Macmillan, 2015.

Hendy, Corrine, and Mark Pearson. "Peer Supported Open Dialogue in a UK NHS Trust–A Qualitative Exploration of Clients' and Network Members' Experiences." *Journal of Mental Health Training, Education, and Practice* 15, no. 2 (2020): 95–103.

Herman, Judith Lewis. *Trauma and Recovery: The Aftermath of Violence—From Domestic Abuse to Political Terror*. New York: Basic Books, 1997.

Hirota, Tomoya, Diana Paksarian, Jian-Ping He, Sachiko Inoue, Emma K. Stapp, Anna Van Meter, and Kathleen R. Merikangas. "Associations of Social Capital with Mental Disorder Prevalence, Severity, and Comorbidity among US Adolescents." *Journal of Clinical Child and Adolescent Psychology* 51, no. 6 (2022): 970–81.

Hodgson, Dorothy L., *Once Intrepid Warriors: Gender, Ethnicity, and the Cultural Politics of Maasai Development*. Bloomington: Indiana University Press, 2001.

Holland, Dorothy. *Identity and Agency in Cultural Worlds*. Edited by William Lachicotte Jr., Debra Skinner, and Carole Cain. Cambridge, MA: Harvard University Press, 1998.

Hopper, Kim. "Interrogating the Meanings of Culture in the WHO International Studies of Schizophrenia." In *Schizophrenia, Culture, and Subjectivity: The Edge of Experience*, edited by Janis H. Jenkins and Robert John Barrett, 62–86. Cambridge: Cambridge University Press, 2003.

Hopper, Kim. *Reckoning with Homelessness*. Ithaca, NY: Cornell University Press, 2019.

Hopper, Kim. "Rethinking Social Recovery in Schizophrenia: What a Capabilities Approach Might Offer." *Social Science and Medicine* 65, no. 5 (2007): 868–79.

Hornstein, Gail A. "Bibliography of First-Person Narratives of Madness in English (5th edition)." ResearchGate. Updated December 2011. https://www.researchgate.net/publication/272477644_Bibliography_of_First-Person_Narratives_of_Madness_in_English_5th_edition.

"How Drug Trafficking Is (And Isn't) to Blame for Violence in Latin America." *The Economist*, February 8, 2022. https://www.economist.com/the-economist-explains/2022/02/08/how-drug-trafficking-is-and-isnt-to-blame-for-violence-in-latin-america.

Howes, Oliver D., Thomas Whitehurst, Ekaterina Shatalina, Leigh Townsend, Ellis Chika Onwordi, Tsz Lun Allenis Mak, Atheeshaan Arumuham et al. "The Clinical Significance of Duration of Untreated Psychosis: An Umbrella Review and Random-Effects Meta-analysis." *World Psychiatry* 20, no. 1 (2021): 75–95.

Huguelet, Philippe, Sylvia Mohr, Laurence Borras, Christiane Gillieron, and Pierre-Yves Brandt. "Spirituality and Religious Practices among Outpatients with Schizophrenia and Their Clinicians." *Psychiatric Services* 57, no. 3 (2006): 366–72.

Humensky, Jennifer L., Ilana Nossel, Iruma Bello, and Lisa B. Dixon. "Supported Education and Employment Services for Young People with Early Psychosis in OnTrackNY." *Journal of Mental Health Policy and Economics* 22, no. 3 (2019): 95–108.

Hummer, Victoria Latham, Norín Dollard, John Robst, and Mary I. Armstrong. "Innovations in Implementation of Trauma-Informed Care Practices in Youth Residential Treatment: A Curriculum for Organizational Change." *Child Welfare* 89, no. 2 (2010): 79–95.

The Icarus Project. *Friends Make the Best Medicine: A Guide to Creating Community Mental Health Support Networks*. The Icarus Project NYC. Accessed March 23, 2023. nycicarus.org/articles/friends-best-medicine/.

Imtiaz, Aysha. "The Way We View Free Time Is Making Us Less Happy." *BBC*, September 16, 2021. https://www.bbc.com/worklife/article/20210914-the-way-we-view-free-time-is-making-us-less-happy.

"Inner Compass Initiative." The Inner Compass. Accessed August 22, 2023. https://www.theinnercompass.org/.

Indigo Girls. *1200 Curfews*. Epic E2K 68229, 1995.

Jacobson, Nora. "Dignity and Health: A Review." *Social Science and Medicine* 64, no. 2 (2007): 292–302.

Jansen, Jens Einar, John Gleeson, and Sue Cotton. "Towards a Better Understanding of Caregiver Distress in Early Psychosis: A Systematic Review of the Psychological Factors Involved." *Clinical Psychology Review* 35 (2015): 56–66.

Jarvis, G. Eric, Laurence J. Kirmayer, George K. Jarvis, and Rob Whitley. "The Role of Afro-Canadian Status in Police or Ambulance Referral to Emergency Psychiatric Services." *Psychiatric Services* 56, no. 6 (2005): 705–10.

Jenkins, Janis H. "Ethnopsychiatric Interpretations of Schizophrenic Illness: The Problem of *Nervios* within Mexican-American Families." *Culture, Medicine, and Psychiatry* 12, no. 3 (1988): 301–29.

Jenkins, Janis H. *Extraordinary Conditions: Culture and Experience in Mental Illness.* Berkeley: University of California Press, 2015.

Jenkins, Janis H., ed. *Pharmaceutical Self: The Global Shaping of Experience in an Age of Psychopharmacology.* Santa Fe: School for Advanced Research Press, 2010.

Jenkins, Janis H. "Psychopharmaceutical Self and Imaginary in the Social Field of Psychiatric Treatment." In Jenkins, *Pharmaceutical Self,* 17–40.

Jenkins, Janis H., and Bridget M. Haas. "Trauma in the Lifeworlds of Adolescents." In *Culture and PTSD: Trauma in Global and Historical Perspective,* edited by Devon E. Hinton and Byron J. Good, 215–45. Philadelphia: University of Pennsylvania Press, 2015.

Jenkins, Janis H., and Elizabeth A. Carpenter-Song. "Awareness of Stigma among Persons with Schizophrenia: Marking the Contexts of Lived Experience." *Journal of Nervous and Mental Disease* 197, no. 7 (2009): 520–29.

Jenkins, Janis H., and Elizabeth Carpenter-Song. "The New Paradigm of Recovery from Schizophrenia: Cultural Conundrums of Improvement without Cure." *Culture, Medicine, and Psychiatry* 29, no. 4 (December 2005): 379–413.

Jenkins, Janis H., and Robert John Barrett, eds. *Schizophrenia, Culture, and Subjectivity: The Edge of Experience.* Cambridge: Cambridge University Press, 2003.

Jenkins, Janis H., and Thomas J. Csordas. *Troubled in the Land of Enchantment: Adolescent Experience of Psychiatric Treatment.* Oakland: University of California Press, 2020.

Jennings, Ann, and Ruth O. Ralph. "In Their Own Words: Trauma Survivors and Professionals They Trust Tell What Hurts, What Helps, and What Is Needed for Trauma Services." *Maine Trauma Advisory Groups Report,* 1997. https://www.theannainstitute.org/ITOW.pdf.

Jindal, Monique, Kamila B. Mistry, Maria Trent, Ashlyn McRae, and Rachel L. J. Thornton. "Police Exposures and the Health and Well-Being of Black Youth in the US: A Systematic Review." *JAMA Pediatrics* 176, no. 1 (2021): 78–88.

Johannessen, Lars E. F., Erik Børve Rasmussen, and Marit Haldar. "Educational Purity and Technological Danger: Understanding Scepticism towards the Use of TelepresenceRobots in School." *British Journal of Sociology of Education* 44, no. 4 (2023): 703–19.

Jones, Nev, Karen Bower, Adriana Furuzawa, and Dina Tyler. "Back to School: Toolkits to Support the Full Inclusion of Students with Early Psychosis in Higher Education." Student and Family Version. National Association of the State Mental Health Program Directors (NASMHPD) Publications, 2016.

Jones, Nev, Mona Shattell, Timothy Kelly, Robyn Brown, LaVome Robinson, Richard Renfro, Barbara Harris, and Tanya Marie Luhrmann. "'Did I Push Myself over the Edge?': Complications of Agency in Psychosis Onset and Development." *Psychosis* 8, no. 4 (2016): 324–35.

Jones, Nev, Shannon Pagdon, Ikenna Ebuenyi, Howard Goldman, and Lisa Dixon. "Recovering the Vocational Self? Service User Accounts of Barriers to Work and School and the Role of Early Psychosis Services in Supporting Career Development." *Community Mental Health Journal* 59 (2023): 1452–64. https://doi.org/10.1007/s10597-023-01149-3.

Jones, Nev, Timothy Kelly, and Mona Shattell. "God in the Brain: Experiencing Psychosis in the Postsecular United States." *Transcultural Psychiatry* 53, no. 4 (2016): 488–505.

Jones, Simon R., and Charles Fernyhough. "A New Look at the Neural Diathesis-Stress Model of Schizophrenia: The Primacy of Social-Evaluative and Uncontrollable Situations." *Schizophrenia Bulletin* 33, no. 5 (2007): 1171–77.

Judge, Abigail M., Sue E. Estroff, Diana O. Perkins, and David L. Penn. "Recognizing and Responding to Early Psychosis: A Qualitative Analysis of Individual Narratives." *Psychiatric Services* 59, no. 1 (2008): 96–99.

Kane, John M., Nina R. Schooler, Patricia Marcy, Christoph U. Correll, Mary F. Brunette, Kim T. Mueser, Robert A. Rosenheck et al. "The RAISE Early Treatment Program for First-Episode Psychosis: Background, Rationale, and Study Design." *Journal of Clinical Psychiatry* 76, no. 3 (2015): 16590.

Kavanaugh, Philip R., and Tammy L. Anderson. "Solidarity and Drug Use in the Electronic Dance Music Scene." *Sociological Quarterly* 49, no. 1 (2008): 181–208.

Keating, Frank. "Racialized Communities, Producing Madness and Dangerousness." *Intersectionalities: A Global Journal of Social Work Analysis, Research, Polity, and Practice* 5, no. 3 (2016): 173–85.

Keller, Allen, Amy Joscelyne, Megan Granski, and Barry Rosenfeld. "Pre-migration Trauma Exposure and Mental Health Functioning among Central American Migrants Arriving at the US Border." *PLoS One* 12, no. 1 (2017): e0168692.

Kendi, Ibram X. *Stamped from the Beginning: The Definitive History of Racist Ideas in America.* London: Hachette UK, 2016.

Kendig, Sarah M., Marybeth J. Mattingly, and Suzanne M. Bianchi. "Childhood Poverty and the Transition to Adulthood." *Family Relations* 63, no. 2 (2014): 271–86.

Kennedy, John F. "Address at the Free University of Berlin" (speech), June 26, 1963, John F. Kennedy Presidential Library and Museum, audio file. https://www.jfklibrary.org/asset-vie wer/archives/JFKWHA/1963/JFKWHA-201-001/JFKWHA-201-001.

Kernan, Luke James Leo. "Psychotic Bodies/Embodiment of Suicidal Bipolar Poets: Navigating through the Sensorium of Immersive Worlds and Psychoscapes." *Liminalities* 16, no. 1 (2020): 1–31.

Khalifa, Wiz. "Work Hard, Play Hard." Atlantic Records, 2012.

Khan, Arif, James Faucett, Shaneta Morrison, and Walter A. Brown. "Comparative Mortality Risk in Adult Patients with Schizophrenia, Depression, Bipolar Disorder, Anxiety Disorders, and Attention-Deficit/Hyperactivity Disorder Participating in Psychopharmacology Clinical Trials." *JAMA Psychiatry* 70, no. 10 (2013): 1091–99.

Kindy, Kimberly, Julie Tate, Jennifer Jenkins, and Ted Mellnik. "Fatal Police Shootings of Mentally Ill People Are 39 Percent More Likely to Take Place in Small and Midsized Areas." *Washington Post*, October 17, 2020. Sale

Kirkbride, James B., and Peter B. Jones. "The Prevention of Schizophrenia—What Can We Learn from Eco-epidemiology?" *Schizophrenia Bulletin* 37, no. 2 (2011): 262–71.

Kirmayer, Laurence J., and Ian Gold. "Re-socializing Psychiatry: Critical Neuroscience and the Limits of Reductionism." *Critical Neuroscience: A Handbook of the Social and Cultural Contexts of Neuroscience* (2011): 305–30.

Kitanaka, Junko. *Depression in Japan: Psychiatric Cures for a Society in Distress*. Princeton, NJ: Princeton University Press, 2012.

Kleinman, Arthur. "Experience and Its Moral Modes: Culture, Human Conditions, and Disorder." In *The Tanner Lectures on Human Values*, vol. 20, edited by Grethe B. Peterson. Salt Lake City: University of Utah Press, 1999.

Kleinman, Arthur, and Byron Good, eds. *Culture and Depression: Studies in the Anthropology and Cross-Cultural Psychiatry of Affect and Disorder*. Berkeley: University of California Press, 1985.

Kline, Nolan. *Pathogenic Policing: Immigration Enforcement and Health in the US South*. New Brunswick, NJ: Rutgers University Press, 2019.

Knight, Kelly R. *Addicted. Pregnant. Poor*. Durham, NC: Duke University Press, 2015.

Koike, Shinsuke, Sosei Yamaguchi, Yasutaka Ojio, Takafumi Shimada, Kei-ichiro Watanabe, and Shuntaro Ando. "Long-Term Effect of a Name Change for Schizophrenia on Reducing Stigma." *Social Psychiatry and Psychiatric Epidemiology* 50, no. 10 (2015): 1519–26.

Korbin, Jill E., and Eileen P. Anderson-Fye. "Adolescence Matters: Practice- and Policy-Relevant Research and Engagement in Psychological Anthropology." Introduction to "Psychological Anthropology and Adolescent Well-Being." Special issue, *Ethos* 39, no. 4 (2011): 415–25.

Kraan, Tamar, Eva Velthorst, Laura Koenders, Kimberley Zwaart, Helga K. Ising, David van den Berg, Lieuwe de Haan, and Mark van der Gaag. "Cannabis Use and Transition to Psychosis in Individuals at Ultra-high Risk: Review and Meta-analysis." *Psychological Medicine* 46, no. 4 (2016): 673–81.

Kranke, Derrick, Sarah Elizabeth Jackson, Jerry Floersch, Lisa Townsend, and Eileen Anderson-Fye. "'I feel like it improves everything': Empowering Experiences of College Students Utilizing Psychiatric Treatment." *American Journal of Psychiatric Rehabilitation* 16, no. 3 (2013): 213–31.

Kranke, Derrick, Sarah E. Jackson, Debbie A. Taylor, Eileen Anderson-Fye, and Jerry Floersch. "College Student Disclosure of Non-apparent Disabilities to Receive Classroom Accommodations." *Journal of Postsecondary Education and Disability* 26, no. 1 (2013): 35–51.

Krupala, Katie. "The Evolution of Uneven Development in Dallas, TX." *Human Geography* 12, no. 3 (2019): 17–30.

Ku, Benson S., Luca Pauselli, Marc Manseau, and Michael T. Compton. "Neighborhood-Level Predictors of Age at Onset and Duration of Untreated Psychosis in First-Episode Psychotic Disorders." *Schizophrenia Research* 218 (2020): 247–54.

Kuipers, Elizabeth, and Paul Bebbington. "Cognitive Behaviour Therapy for Psychosis." *Epidemiology and Psychiatric Sciences* 15, no. 4 (2006): 267–75.

Kusters, Wouter. *A Philosophy of Madness: The Experience of Psychotic Thinking*. Cambridge, MA: MIT Press, 2020.

Laing, Ronald David. *The Politics of Experience and the Bird of Paradise*. Westminster: Penguin UK, 1967.

Lakoff, Andrew. *Pharmaceutical Reason: Knowledge and Value in Global Psychiatry*. Cambridge: Cambridge University Press, 2006.

Lambek, Michael. "Introduction." In *Ordinary Ethics: Anthropology, Language, and Action*, edited by Michael Lambek, 1–38. New York: Fordham University Press, 2010.

Langlois, Stephanie, Adria Zern, Mary E. Kelley, and Michael T. Compton. "Adversity in Childhood/Adolescence and Premorbid Tobacco, Alcohol, and Cannabis Use among First-Episode Psychosis Patients." *Early Intervention in Psychiatry* 15, no. 5 (2021): 1335–42.

Large, Matthew M., and Olav Nielssen. "Violence in First-Episode Psychosis: A Systematic Review and Meta-analysis." *Schizophrenia Research* 125, nos. 2–3 (2011): 209–20.

Larsen, John Aggergaard. "Finding Meaning in First Episode Psychosis: Experience, Agency, and the Cultural Repertoire." *Medical Anthropology Quarterly* 18, no. 4 (2004): 447–71.

Lavis, Anna, Helen Lester, Linda Everard, Nicholas Freemantle, Tim Amos, David Fowler, Jo Hodgekins, Peter Jones, Max Marshall, Vimal Sharma, John Larsen, Paul McCrone, Swaran Singh, Jo Smith, and Max Birchwood. "Layers of Listening: Qualitative Analysis of the Impact of Early Intervention Services for First-Episode Psychosis on Carers' Experiences." *British Journal of Psychiatry* 207, no. 2 (2015): 135–42.

Lawson, William B., Nancy Hepler, Jack Holladay, and Brian Cuffel. "Race as a Factor in Inpatient and Outpatient Admissions and Diagnosis." *Psychiatric Services* 45, no. 1 (1994): 72–74.

LeClair, Amy, Brian C. Kelly, Mark Pawson, Brooke E. Wells, and Jeffrey T. Parsons. "Motivations for Prescription Drug Misuse among Young Adults: Considering Social and Developmental Contexts." *Drugs: Education, Prevention, and Policy* 22, no. 3 (2015): 208–16.

"Legal Medical Marijuana States and DC." Britannica ProCon. Updated June 22, 2021. https://medicalmarijuana.procon.org/legal-medical-marijuana-states-and-dc/.

Leggatt, Margaret, and Gina Woodhead. "Family Peer Support Work in an Early Intervention Youth Mental Health Service." *Early Intervention in Psychiatry* 10, no. 5 (2016): 446–51.

Lesley, Elena. "The Anthropologist as Audience: Engaged Listening among Khmer Rouge Survivors and Ukrainian War Refugees." *Medicine Anthropology Theory* 10, no. 1 (2023): 1–12.

Lester, Rebecca J. *Famished: Eating Disorders and Failed Care in America*. Berkeley: University of California Press, 2019.

LeVine, Robert A. "Traditions in Transition: Adolescents Remaking Culture." In "Psychological Anthropology and Adolescent Well-Being." Special issue, *Ethos* 39, no. 4 (2011): 426–31.

Lewis, Bradley. "Taking a Narrative Turn in Psychiatry." *The Lancet* 383, no. 9911 (2014): 22–23.

Lewis, Sara E. *Spacious Minds: Trauma and Resilience in Tibetan Buddhism*. Ithaca, NY: Cornell University Press, 2020.

Lewis, Sara E., and Rob Whitley. "A Critical Examination of 'Morality' in an Age of Evidence-Based Psychiatry." *Culture, Medicine, and Psychiatry* 36 (2012): 735–43.

Lewis, Sara E., Kim Hopper, and Ellen Healion. "Partners in Recovery: Social Support and Accountability in a Consumer-Run Mental Health Center." *Psychiatric Services* 63, no. 1 (2012): 61–65.

Lewis-Fernández, Roberto, and Laurence J. Kirmayer. "Cultural Concepts of Distress and Psychiatric Disorders: Understanding Symptom Experience and Expression in Context." *Transcultural Psychiatry* 56, no. 4 (2019): 786–803.

Lillie-Blanton, M., M. Brodie, D. Rowland, D. Altman, and M. McIntosh. "Race, Ethnicity, and the Healthcare System: Public Perceptions and Experiences." *Medical Care Research and Review* 57 (2000): 218–35.

Lipschitz, Deborah S., Robert K. Winegar, Elizabeth Hartnick, Brad Foote, and Steven M. Southwick. "Posttraumatic Stress Disorder in Hospitalized Adolescents: Psychiatric Comorbidity and Clinical Correlates." *Journal of the American Academy of Child and Adolescent Psychiatry* 38, no. 4 (1999): 385–92.

Lobban, Fiona, Adam Postlethwaite, David Glentworth, Vanessa Pinfold, Laura Wainwright, Graham Dunn, Anna Clancy, and Gillian Haddock. "A Systematic Review of Randomised Controlled Trials of Interventions Reporting Outcomes for Relatives of People with Psychosis." *Clinical Psychology Review* 33, no. 3 (2013): 372–82.

Longden, Eleanor. "The Voices in My Head." TED, February 2013. Video, 14:04. https://www.ted.com/talks/eleanor_longden_the_voices_in_my_head?language=en.

Lopez, William D., Daniel J. Kruger, Jorge Delva, Mikel Llanes, Charo Ledón, Adreanne Waller, Melanie Harner, Ramiro Martinez, Laura Sanders, Margaret Harner, and Barbara Israel. "Health Implications of an Immigration Raid: Findings from a Latino Community in the Midwestern United States." *Journal of Immigrant and Minority Health* 19, no. 3 (2017): 702–8.

Lopez-Garcia, Pilar, Stefania Ashby, Pooja Patel, Katherine M. Pierce, Monet Meyer, Adi Rosenthal, Madison Titone, Cameron Carter, and Tara Niendam. "Clinical and Neurodevelopmental Correlates of Aggression in Early Psychosis." *Schizophrenia Research* 212 (2019): 171–76.

"Lost Cause: 50 Years of the War on Drugs in Latin America." *Washington Post*, June 14, 2021. https://www.washingtonpost.com/opinions/2021/06/14/war-on-drugs-50-years-latin-america-violence-mexico-colombia/.

Lovell, Alice. "Some Questions of Identity: Late Miscarriage, Stillbirth, and Perinatal Loss." *Social Science and Medicine* 17, no. 11 (1983): 755–61.

Lucksted, Alicia, William McFarlane, Donna Downing, and Lisa Dixon. "Recent Developments in Family Psychoeducation as an Evidence-Based Practice." *Journal of Marital and Family Therapy* 38, no. 1 (2012): 101–21.

Luhrmann, Tanya M. "Diversity within the Psychotic Continuum." *Schizophrenia Bulletin* 43, no. 1 (2017): 27–31.

Luhrmann, Tanya M. *How God Becomes Real: Kindling the Presence of Invisible Others.* Princeton, NJ: Princeton University Press, 2020.

Luhrmann, Tanya M. *Of Two Minds: An Anthropologist Looks at American Psychiatry.* New York: Vintage, 2011.

Luhrmann, Tanya M. "'The Street Will Drive You Crazy': Why Homeless Psychotic Women in the Institutional Circuit in the United States Often Say No to Offers of Help." *American Journal of Psychiatry* 165, no. 1 (2008): 15–20.

Luhrmann, Tanya M. "Thinking about Thinking: The Mind's Porosity and the Presence of the Gods." *Journal of the Royal Anthropological Institute* 26, no. S1 (2020): 148–62.

Luhrmann, Tanya M., and Jocelyn Marrow, eds. *Our Most Troubling Madness: Case Studies in Schizophrenia across Cultures.* Oakland: University of California Press, 2016.

Luhrmann, Tanya M., R. Padmavati, H. Tharoor, and A. Osei. "Differences in Voice-Hearing Experiences of People with Psychosis in the USA, India, and Ghana: Interview-Based Study." *British Journal of Psychiatry* 206, no. 1 (2015): 41–44.

Malla, Ashok, and Patrick McGorry. "Early Intervention in Psychosis in Young People: A Population and Public Health Perspective." *American Journal of Public Health* 109 (2019): S181–S184.

Maniglio, R. "Severe Mental Illness and Criminal Victimization: A Systematic Review." *Acta Psychiatrica Scandinavica* 119, no. 3 (2009): 180–91.

Marconi, Arianna, Marta Di Forti, Cathryn M. Lewis, Robin M. Murray, and Evangelos Vassos. "Meta-analysis of the Association between the Level of Cannabis Use and Risk of Psychosis." *Schizophrenia Bulletin* 42, no. 5 (2016): 1262–69.

Martens, Laurie, and Jean Addington. "The Psychological Well-Being of Family Members of Individuals with Schizophrenia." *Social Psychiatry and Psychiatric Epidemiology* 36, no. 3 (2001): 128–33.

Martin, Brittney. "Texas' Crumbling State Mental Hospitals Need $1 Billion; Will They Get It?" *Dallas Morning News*, May 26, 2016. https://www.dallasnews.com/news/politics/2016/05/26/texas-crumbling-state-mental-hospitals-need-1-billion-will-they-get-it/.

Martin, Emily. *Bipolar Expeditions: Mania and Depression in American Culture.* Princeton, NJ: Princeton University Press, 2007.

Martins, Silvia S., Luis E. Segura, Natalie S. Levy, Pia M. Mauro, Christine M. Mauro, Morgan M. Philbin, and Deborah S. Hasin. "Racial and Ethnic Differences in Cannabis Use Following Legalization in US States with Medical Cannabis Laws." *JAMA Network Open* 4, no. 9 (2021).

Mattingly, Cheryl. *Moral Laboratories: Family Peril and the Struggle for a Good Life.* Berkeley: University of California Press, 2014.

Mattingly, Cheryl, and Linda C. Garro, eds. *Narrative and the Cultural Construction of Illness and Healing.* Berkeley: University of California Press, 2000.

Maura, Jessica, and Amy Weisman de Mamani. "Mental Health Disparities, Treatment Engagement, and Attrition among Racial/Ethnic Minorities with Severe Mental Illness: A Review." *Journal of Clinical Psychology in Medical Settings* 24, no. 3 (2017): 187–210.

May, Rufus. "Bringing an Inside Perspective to Mental Health Services." *Psychiatric Services* 73, no. 9 (2022).

Mazzoncini, Rodolfo, K. Donoghue, J. Hart, Craig Morgan, Gillian A. Doody, Paola Dazzan, Peter B. Jones, K. Morgan, Robin M. Murray, and Paul Fearon. "Illicit Substance Use and Its Correlates in First Episode Psychosis." *Acta Psychiatrica Scandinavica* 121, no. 5 (2010): 351–58.

McCormick, Katie A., Lalaine Sevillano, Vanessa V. Klodnick, Molly A. Lopez, and Deborah A. Cohen. "Virtual Technology's Critical Role in Sustaining Coordinated Specialty Care in Texas during the COVID-19 Pandemic." *Psychiatric Services* 73, no. 8 (2022), 962–29.

McGorry, Patrick. "Transition to Adulthood: The Critical Period for Pre-emptive, Disease-Modifying Care for Schizophrenia and Related Disorders." *Schizophrenia Bulletin* 37, no. 524 (2011).

McGough, Cecilia. "I Am Not a Monster: Schizophrenia." *YouTube*, March 27, 2017. Video, 14:40. https://www.youtube.com/watch?app=desktop&v=xbagFzcyNiM&bpctr=16736452.

McLean, Athena. "Contradictions in the Social Production of Clinical Knowledge: The Case of Schizophrenia." *Social Science and Medicine* 30, no. 9 (1990): 969–85.

McLeod, Melissa N., Daliah Heller, Meredith G. Manze, and Sandra E. Echeverria. "Police Interactions and the Mental Health of Black Americans: A Systematic Review." *Journal of Racial and Ethnic Health Disparities* 7, no. 1 (2020): 10–27.

McNamee, Stephen J., and Robert K. Miller. *The Meritocracy Myth.* Washington, DC: Rowman & Littlefield, 2009.

Mead, Margaret. *Coming of Age in Samoa*. New York: William Morrow and Co., 1928.

Meadows Mental Health Policy Institute. "Transforming Police Responses to Mental Health Emergencies: Rapid Integrated Group Healthcare Team (RIGHT Care)." May 2021. https://mmhpi.org/project/right-care/.

Meadows Mental Health Policy Institute, "Coordinated Specialty Care for Texans, June 2022." Emailed to author by Meadows Mental Health Policy Institute December 2023.

Merritt-Davis, Orlena B., and Matcheri S. Keshavan. "Pathways to Care for African Americans with Early Psychosis." *Psychiatric Services* 57, no. 7 (2006): 1043–44.

Mesic, Aldina, Lydia Franklin, Alev Cansever, Fiona Potter, Anika Sharma, Anita Knopov, and Michael Siegel. "The Relationship between Structural Racism and Black-White Disparities in Fatal Police Shootings at the State Level." *Journal of the National Medical Association* 110, no. 2 (2018): 106–16.

Metzl, Jonathan. *The Protest Psychosis: How Schizophrenia Became a Black Disease*. Boston: Beacon Press, 2010.

Meyers, Todd. *The Clinic and Elsewhere: Addiction, Adolescents, and the Afterlife of Therapy*. Seattle: University of Washington Press, 2013.

Mindlis, Irina, and Paolo Boffetta. "Mood Disorders in First- and Second-Generation Immigrants: Systematic Review and Meta-analysis." *British Journal of Psychiatry* 210, no. 3 (2017): 182–89.

Misra, Supriya, Valerie W. Jackson, Jeanette Chong, Karen Choe, Charisse Tay, Jazmine Wong, and Lawrence H. Yang. "Systematic Review of Cultural Aspects of Stigma and Mental Illness among Racial and Ethnic Minority Groups in the United States: Implications for Interventions." *American Journal of Community Psychology* 68, nos. 3–4 (2021): 486–512.

Mitchell, Sinéad, Ciaran Shannon, Ciaran Mulholland, and Donncha Hanna. "Reaching Consensus on the Principles of Trauma-Informed Care in Early Intervention Psychosis Services: A Delphi Study." *Early Intervention in Psychiatry* 15, no. 5 (2021): 1369–75.

Mohr, Sylvia, Pierre-Yves Brandt, Laurence Borras, Christiane Gilliéron, and Philippe Huguelet. "Toward an Integration of Spirituality and Religiousness into the Psychosocial Dimension of Schizophrenia." *American Journal of Psychiatry* 163, no. 11 (2006): 1952–59.

Molloy, Luke, Lorraine Fields, Baylie Trostian, and Grant Kinghorn. "Trauma-Informed Care for People Presenting to the Emergency Department with Mental Health Issues." *Emergency Nurse* 28, no. 2 (2020).

Moore, Sally F., and Barbara G. Myerhoff. "Introduction: Secular Ritual; Forms and Meanings." *Secular Ritual* (1977): 3–24.

Moran, Mark. "CMS Approves Payment for Coordinated Specialty Care of First-Episode Psychosis." *Psychiatric News*, September 28, 2023. https://psychnews.psychiatryonline.org/doi/10.1176/appi.pn.2023.11.11.18.

Morinis, Alan. "The Ritual Experience: Pain and the Transformation of Consciousness in Ordeals of Initiation." *Ethos* 13, no. 2 (1985): 150–74.

Mostaghim, Amir, and Andrew David Hathaway. "Identity Formation, Marijuana, and 'the Self': A Study of Cannabis Normalization among University Students." *Frontiers in Psychiatry* 4 (2013): 160.

Muench, John, and Ann M. Hamer. "Adverse Effects of Antipsychotic Medications." *American Family Physician* 81, no. 5 (2010): 617–22.

Murrie, Benjamin, Julia Lappin, Matthew Large, and Grant Sara. "Transition of Substance-Induced, Brief, and Atypical Psychoses to Schizophrenia: A Systematic Review and Meta-Analysis." *Schizophrenia Bulletin* 46, no. 3 (2020): 505–16.

Mustonen, Antti, Solja Niemelä, Tanja Nordström, Graham K. Murray, Pirjo Mäki, Erika Jääskeläinen, and Jouko Miettunen. "Adolescent Cannabis Use, Baseline Prodromal Symptoms, and the Risk of Psychosis." *British Journal of Psychiatry* 212, no. 4 (2018): 227–33.

Myers, Neely Anne Laurenzo. "Beyond the 'Crazy House': Mental/Moral Breakdowns and Moral Agency in First-Episode Psychosis." *Ethos* 47, no. 1 (2019): 13–34.

Myers, Neely Anne Laurenzo. *Recovery's Edge: An Ethnography of Mental Health Care and Moral Agency.* Nashville: Vanderbilt University Press, 2015.

Myers, Neely Anne Laurenzo. "Recovery Stories: An Anthropological Exploration of Moral Agency in Stories of Mental Health Recovery." *Transcultural Psychiatry* 53, no. 4 (2016): 427–44.

Myers, Neely Anne Laurenzo. "Update: Schizophrenia across Cultures." *Current Psychiatry Reports* 13 (2011): 305–11.

Myers, Neely Anne Laurenzo, and Tali Ziv. "'No One Ever Even Asked Me That Before': Autobiographical Power, Social Defeat, and Recovery among African Americans with Lived Experiences of Psychosis." *Medical Anthropology Quarterly* 30, no. 3 (2016): 395–413.

Myers, Neely Anne Laurenzo, Anubha Sood, Katherine E. Fox, Gillian Wright, and Michael T. Compton. "Decision Making about Pathways through Care for Racially and Ethnically Diverse Young Adults with Early Psychosis." *Psychiatric Services* 70, no. 3 (2019): 184–90.

Myers, Neely Anne Laurenzo, Justin Wilkey, Marne Chacon, Matthew Hutnyan, Claire Janssen, Halle Tarvin, Deborah Cohen, Imani Holmes, Vanessa Vorhies Klodnick, Mesganaw A. Mihiret, Samantha J. Rezik, Taylor Khouw Shimizu, Emily Stein, and Molly A. Lopez. "Perspectives of Young Adults Diagnosed with Early Psychosis Using Coordinated Specialty Care in Texas on Substance Use and Substance Use Interventions." *Early Intervention in Psychiatry*, Online First, November 29, 2023. doi:10.1111/eip.13488.

Myers, Neely Anne Laurenzo, Matthew Hutnyan, Tamara C. Daley, Iruma Bello, Marne Chacon, Ariel Currie, Beshaun J. Davis, Lisa B. Dixon, Preethy E. George, Anna Giannicchi, Anita N. Kwashie, Katie A. McCormick, Piper Meyer-Kalos, Arundati Nagendra, Swati Nayar, Deepak K. Sarpal, Tiana Y. Sepahpour, Daniel I. Shapiro, and Jessica Taylor-Zoghby. "Pathways through Early Psychosis Care for US Youths from Ethnically and Racially Minoritized Groups: A Systematic Review." *Psychiatric Services* 74, no. 8 (2023): 859–68.

Myers, Neely Anne Laurenzo, Robert Meeker, and Valerie Odeng. "Pastors as Partners in Care: African Immigrant Pastors' on Mental Health Care Referral Processes for Young Congregants Experiencing Symptoms of Psychosis in the US." *Community Mental Health Journal.* Online First.

Myers, Neely Anne Laurenzo, Yazeed Alolayan, Kelly Smith, Susan Alicia Pope, Beth Broussard, Nora Haynes, and Michael T. Compton. "A Potential Role for Family Members in Mental Health Care Delivery: The Family Community Navigation Specialist." *Psychiatric Services* 66, no. 6 (2015): 653–55.

Myles, Hannah, Nicholas Myles, and Matthew Large. "Cannabis Use in First Episode Psychosis: Meta-analysis of Prevalence, and the Time Course of Initiation and Continued Use." *Australian & New Zealand Journal of Psychiatry* 50, no. 3 (2016): 208–219.

Nabbali, Essya. "A 'Mad' Critique of the Social Model of Disability." *International Journal of Diversity in Organisations, Communities, and Nations* 9, no. 4 (2009).

Nadeem, Erum, Jane M. Lange, and Jeanne Miranda. "Mental Health Care Preferences among Low-Income and Minority Women." *Archives of Women's Mental Health* 11, no. 2 (2008): 93–102.

Nagendra, Arundati, Nina R. Schooler, John M. Kane, Delbert G. Robinson, Kim T. Mueser, Sue E. Estroff, Jean Addington, Patricia Marcy, and David L. Penn. "Demographic, Psychosocial, Clinical, and Neurocognitive Baseline Characteristics of Black Americans in the RAISE-ETP Study." *Schizophrenia Research* 193 (2018): 64–68.

Nakamura, Karen. *A Disability of the Soul: An Ethnography of Schizophrenia and Mental Illness in Contemporary Japan.* Ithaca, NY: Cornell University Press, 2013.

National Empowerment Center. "Directory of Peer Respites." Accessed April 1, 2024. https://power2u.org/directory-of-peer-respites/.

National Institute of Mental Health. "Understanding Psychosis." NIH Publication No. 20-MH-8110; 2019. https://www.nimh.nih.gov/health/publications/understanding-psychosis.

Newcomer, John W. "Antipsychotic Medications: Metabolic and Cardiovascular Risk." *Journal of Clinical Psychiatry* 64, no. 4 (2007): 8–13.

Newcomer, John W., and Charles H. Hennekens. "Severe Mental Illness and Risk of Cardiovascular Disease." *Journal of the American Medical Association* 298, no. 15 (2007): 1794–96.

New York Council of State Governments Justice Center. "Law Enforcement Mental Health Learning Sites." Accessed September 23, 2021. https://csgjusticecenter.org/projects/police-mental-health-collaboration-pmhc/law-enforcement-mental-health-learning-sites.

Nichols, Vanessa Cruz, Alana M. W. LeBrón, and Francisco I. Pedraza. "Policing Us Sick: The Health of Latinos in an Era of Heightened Deportations and Racialized Policing." *PS: Political Science and Politics* 51, no. 2 (2018): 293–97.

Nieuwsma, Jason A., Jeffrey E. Rhodes, George L. Jackson, William C. Cantrell, Marian E. Lane, Mark J. Bates, Mark B. Dekraai, et al. "Chaplaincy and Mental Health in the Department of Veterans Affairs and Department of Defense." *Journal of Health Care Chaplaincy* 19, no. 1 (2013): 3–21.

Nixon, Richard. "Remarks about an Intensified Program for Drug Abuse Prevention and Control," June 17, 1971. American Presidency Project. https://www.presidency.ucsb.edu/documents/remarks-about-intensified-program-for-drug-abuse-prevention-and-control.

Nogueira, Bruno Lima, Jair de Jesus Mari, and Denise Razzouk. "Culture-Bound Syndromes in Spanish Speaking Latin America: The Case of *Nervios, Susto,* and *Ataques de Nervios.*" *Archives of Clinical Psychiatry (São Paulo)* 42 (2015): 171–78.

Nussbaum, Martha Craven. *Frontiers of Justice: Disability, Nationality, Species Membership.* Cambridge, MA: Belknap Press of Harvard University Press, 2006.

Obama, Barack. "2013 State of the Union Address." Washington, DC, February 12, 2013. The White House, President Barack Obama. https://obamawhitehouse.archives.gov/the-press-office/2013/02/12/president-barack-obamas-state-union-address-prepared-delivery.

Ochoa, Susana, Judith Usall, Jesús Cobo, Xavier Labad, and Jayashri Kulkarni. "Gender Differences in Schizophrenia and First-Episode Psychosis: A Comprehensive Literature Review." *Schizophrenia Research and Treatment,* April 8, 2012. doi: 10.1155/2012/916198.

Ochs, Elinor, and Lisa Capps. *Living Narrative: Creating Lives in Everyday Storytelling.* Cambridge, MA: Harvard University Press, 2001.

O'Connor, Karen, Deirdre Muller Neff, and Steve Pitman. "Burnout in Mental Health Professionals: A Systematic Review and Meta-analysis of Prevalence and Determinants." *European Psychiatry* 53 (2018): 74–99.

O'Dougherty, Maureen. "Demoralizing Care: Moral and Ethical Dilemmas of Parenting a Young Adult Who Lives with a Borderline Diagnosis." *Ethos*, December 25, 2022. https://doi.org/10.1111/etho.12370.

Oedegaard, Christine H., Larry Davidson, Brynjulf Stige, Marius Veseth, Anne Blindheim, Linda Garvik, Jan-Magne Sørensen, Øystein Søraa, and Ingunn Marie Stadskleiv Engebretsen. "'It Means So Much for Me to Have a Choice': A Qualitative Study Providing First-Person Perspectives on Medication-Free Treatment in Mental Health Care." *BMC Psychiatry* 20, no. 1 (2020): 1–11.

Oh, Hans, Ravi Rajkumar, Rachel Banawa, Sasha Zhou, and Ai Koyanagi. "Illicit and Prescription Drug Use and Psychotic Experiences among University Students in the United States." *Journal of Substance Use* 28, no. 5 (2022): 797–802.

Ojagbemi, A. and Oye Gureje. "The Importance of Faith-Based Mental Healthcare in African Urbanized Sites." *Current Opinion in Psychiatry*, 33, no. 3 (2020): 271–77.

Oluwoye, Oladunni, Beshaun Davis, Franchesca S. Kuhney, and Deidre M. Anglin. "Systematic Review of Pathways to Care in the US for Black Individuals with Early Psychosis." *NPJ Schizophrenia* 7, no. 58 (2021).

Oluwoye, Oladunni, Dennis Dyck, Sterling M. McPherson, Roberto Lewis-Fernández, Michael T. Compton, Michael G. McDonell, and Leopoldo J. Cabassa. "Developing and Implementing a Culturally Informed Family Motivational Engagement Strategy (FAMES) to Increase Family Engagement in First Episode Psychosis Programs: Mixed Methods Pilot Study Protocol." *BMJ open* 10, no. 8 (2020): e036907.

O'Nell, Theresa DeLeane. *Disciplined Hearts: History, Identity, and Depression in an American Indian Community.* Berkeley: University of California Press, 1996.

Ostrow, Laysha, and Dan Fisher. *Peer-Run Crisis Respites: A Review of the Model and Opportunities for Future Developments in Research and Innovation.* 2011. Online at National Empowerment Center. Accessed April 1, 2024. https://power2u.org/wp-content/uploads/2017/01/Ostrow-Fisher-PRCR-12.20.2011.pdf.

Ouellet-Plamondon, C., A. Abdel-Baki, É. Salvat, and S. Potvin. "Specific Impact of Stimulant, Alcohol, and Cannabis Use Disorders on First-Episode Psychosis: 2-Year Functional and Symptomatic Outcomes." *Psychological Medicine* 47, no. 14 (2017): 2461–71.

Overhage, Lindsay, Ruth Hailu, Alisa B. Busch, Ateev Mehrotra, Kenneth A. Michelson, and Haiden A. Huskamp. "Trends in Acute Care Use for Mental Health Conditions during the Covid-19 Pandemic." *Journal of the American Medical Association Psychiatry* 80, no. 9 (2023): 924–32.

Ozawa–de Silva, Chikako. *The Anatomy of Loneliness: Suicide, Social Connection, and the Search for Relational Meaning in Contemporary Japan.* Berkeley: University of California Press, 2021.

Padgett, Deborah K. "There's No Place Like (a) Home: Ontological Security among Persons with Serious Mental Illness in the United States." *Social Science and Medicine* 64, no. 9 (2007): 1925–36.

Pandolfo, Stefania. *Knot of the Soul: Madness, Psychoanalysis, Islam.* Chicago: University of Chicago Press, 2018.

Pangle, Lorraine Smith. *The Political Philosophy of Benjamin Franklin.* Baltimore: Johns Hopkins University Press, 2007.

Parish, Steven M. "Between Persons: How Concepts of the Person Make Moral Experience Possible." *Ethos* 42, no. 1 (2014): 31–50.

Parker, Howard, and Lisa Williams. "Intoxicated Weekends: Young Adults' Work Hard–Play Hard Lifestyles, Public Health and Public Disorder." *Drugs: Education, Prevention and Policy* 10, no. 4 (2003): 345–67.

Pepper, Kevin Phillip. "You Are Hereby Called: An Ethnographic Study of Mormon Missionaries." PhD dissertation, Texas A&M University, 2014.

Pescosolido, Bernice A., Bianca Manago, and John Monahan. "Evolving Public Views on the Likelihood of Violence from People with Mental Illness: Stigma and Its Consequences." *Health Affairs* 38, no. 10 (2019): 1735–43.

Petersen, Anne C., Joshua Joseph, and Monica Feit, eds. *New Directions in Child Abuse and Neglect Research.* Washington, DC: National Academies Press, 2014.

Pharoah, Fiona, Jair J. Mari, John Rathbone, and Winson Wong. "Family Intervention for Schizophrenia." *Cochrane Database of Systematic Reviews* 12 (2010).

Phillips, Lisa J., Patrick D. McGorry, Belinda Garner, Katherine N. Thompson, Christos Pantelis, Stephen J. Wood, and Gregor Berger. "Stress, the Hippocampus, and the Hypothalamic-Pituitary-Adrenal Axis: Implications for the Development of Psychotic Disorders." *Australian and New Zealand Journal of Psychiatry* 40, no. 9 (2006): 725–41.

Pinto, Sarah. *Daughters of Parvati: Women and Madness in Contemporary India.* Philadelphia: University of Pennsylvania Press, 2014.

Powers, Albert R., III, Megan S. Kelley, and Philip R. Corlett. "Varieties of Voice-Hearing: Psychics and the Psychosis Continuum." *Schizophrenia Bulletin* 43, no. 1 (2017): 84–98.

Prine, John. "Angel from Montgomery." *John Prine,* recorded January 1, 1971.

Prinzhorn, Hans. *Artistry of the Mentally Ill: A Contribution to the Psychology an Psychopathology of Configuration.* Translated by James L. Foy. Eastford, CT: Martino Fine Books, 2019.

Putnam, Robert D. *Bowling Alone: The Collapse and Revival of American Community.* New York: Simon & Schuster, 2000.

Radua, Joaquim, Valentina Ramella-Cravaro, John P. A. Ioannidis, Abraham Reichenberg, Nacharin Phiphopthatsanee, Taha Amir, Hyi Yenn Thoo, et al. "What Causes Psychosis? An Umbrella Review of Risk and Protective Factors." *World Psychiatry* 17, no. 1 (2018): 49–66.

Raikhel, Eugene. *Governing Habits: Treating Alcoholism in the Post-Soviet Clinic.* Ithaca, NY: Cornell University Press, 2016.

Ramsay, Claire E., Peggy Flanagan, Stephanie Gantt, Beth Broussard, and Michael T. Compton. "Clinical Correlates of Maltreatment and Traumatic Experiences in Childhood and Adolescence among Predominantly African American, Socially Disadvantaged, Hospitalized, First-Episode Psychosis Patients." *Psychiatry Research* 188, no. 3 (2011): 343–49.

Ramsay, Claire E., Sandra M. Goulding, Beth Broussard, Sarah L. Cristofaro, Glen R. Abedi, and Michael T. Compton. "Prevalence and Psychosocial Correlates of Prior Incarcerations in an Urban, Predominantly African-American Sample of Hospitalized

Patients with First-Episode Psychosis." *Journal of the American Academy of Psychiatry and the Law* 39, no. 1 (2011): 57–64.

Raune, D., E. Kuipers, and P. E. Bebbington. "Expressed Emotion at First-Episode Psychosis: Investigating a Carer Appraisal Model." *British Journal of Psychiatry* 184, no. 4 (2004): 321–26.

Rawls, John. *A Theory of Justice*. Cambridge, MA: Harvard University Press. 1971.

Read, Halley, and Brandon A. Kohrt. "The History of Coordinated Specialty Care for Early Intervention in Psychosis in the United States: A Review of Effectiveness, Implementation, and Fidelity." *Community Mental Health Journal* 58 (2021): 835–46.

Read, Ursula M. "Rights as Relationships: Collaborating with Faith Healers in Community Mental Health in Ghana. *Culture, Medicine, and Psychiatry* 43, no. 4 (2019): 613–35.

"Religious Landscape Study: Racial and Ethnic Composition." Pew Research Center. 2014. https://www.pewresearch.org/religion/religious-landscape-study/racial-and-ethnic -composition/.

Reyes-Foster, Beatriz. *Psychiatric Encounters: Madness and Modernity in Yucatan, Mexico*. New Brunswick, NJ: Rutgers University Press, 2018.

Rhodes, Colin. *Outsider Art: Art Brut and Its Affinities*. London: Thames & Hudson, 2022.

Rhodes, Lorna A. *Emptying Beds: The Work of an Emergency Psychiatric Unit*. Berkeley: University of California Press, 1991.

Richardson, Meg, Vanessa Cobham, Judith Murray, and Brett McDermott. "Parents' Grief in the Context of Adult Child Mental Illness: A Qualitative Review." *Clinical Child and Family Psychology Review* 14, no. 1 (2011): 28–43.

Rikard, R. V., Jodi K. Hall, and Karen Bullock. "Health Literacy and Cultural Competence: A Model for Addressing Diversity and Unequal Access to Trauma-Related Health Care." *Traumatology* 21, no. 3 (2015): 227.

Roberts, Andrea L., Stephen E. Gilman, Joshua Breslau, Naomi Breslau, and Karestan C. Koenen. "Race/Ethnic Differences in Exposure to Traumatic Events, Development of Post-Traumatic Stress Disorder, and Treatment-Seeking for Post-Traumatic Stress Disorder in the United States." *Psychological Medicine* 41, no. 1 (2011): 71–83.

Robins, Cynthia S., Julie A. Sauvageot, Karen J. Cusack, Samantha Suffoletta-Maierle, and B. Christopher Frueh. "Special Section on Seclusion and Restraint: Consumers' Perceptions of Negative Experiences and 'Sanctuary Harm' in Psychiatric Settings." *Psychiatric Services* 56, no. 9 (2005): 1134–38.

Robinson, Cendrine, Elizabeth L. Seaman, LaTrice Montgomery, and Adia Winfrey. "A Review of Hip Hop–Based Interventions for Health Literacy, Health Behaviors, and Mental Health." *Journal of Racial and Ethnic Health Disparities* 5 (2018): 468–84.

Rohr, Richard. *On the Threshold of Transformation*. Chicago: Loyola Press, 2010.

Rose, Diana. *Mad Knowledges and User-Led Research*. Cham, Switzerland: Palgrave Macmillan, 2022.

Rose, Diana. "Service User/Survivor–Led Research in Mental Health: Epistemological Possibilities." *Disability and Society* 32, no. 6 (2017): 773–89.

Rose, Lacey. "Donald Trump on the American Dream." *Forbes*, March 22, 2007. https://www .forbes.com/2007/03/21/donald-trump-dream-oped-cx_lr_dream0307_0322trump .html?sh=5ce2dffe781b.

Rosenbaum, James, Caitlin Ahearn, Kelly Becker, and Janet Rosenbaum. "The New Forgotten Half and Research Directions to Support Them." William T. Grant Foundation. 2015. https://files.eric.ed.gov/fulltext/ED565750.pdf.

Rosenberg, Jaime. "Mental Health Issues on the Rise among Adolescents, Young Adults." *American Journal of Managed Care*, March 19, 2019. https://www.ajmc.com/view/mental-health-issues-on-the-rise-among-adolescents-young-adults.

Rosenheck, Robert, Douglas Leslie, Richard Keefe, Joseph McEvoy, Marvin Swartz, Diana Perkins, Scott Stroup, John K. Hsiao, Jeffrey Lieberman, and CATIE Study Investigators Group. "Barriers to Employment for People with Schizophrenia." *American Journal of Psychiatry* 163, no. 3 (2006): 411–17.

Rutherford, Alison, Anthony B. Zwi, Natalie J. Grove, and Alexander Butchart. "Violence: A Glossary." *Journal of Epidemiology and Community Health* 61, no. 8 (2007): 676–80.

Sah, Dharay, Prabhat Chand, Mrunal Bandawar, Vivek Benegal, and Pratima Murthy. "Cannabis Induced Psychosis and Subsequent Psychiatric Disorders." *Asian Journal of Psychiatry* 30 (2017): 180–84.

Saks, Elyn R. *The Center Cannot Hold: My Journey through Madness*. New York: Hyperion, 2008.

Saleh, Amam Z., Paul S. Appelbaum, Xiaoyu Liu, T. Scott Stroup, and Melanie Wall. "Deaths of People with Mental Illness during Interactions with Law Enforcement." *International Journal of Law and Psychiatry* 58 (2018): 110–16.

Sanchez, Helen F., Michael F. Orr, Ann Wang, Miguel Á. Cano, Ellen L. Vaughan, Laura M. Harvey, Saman Essa, et al. "Racial and Gender Inequities in the Implementation of a Cannabis Criminal Justice Diversion Program in a Large and Diverse Metropolitan County of the USA." *Drug and Alcohol Dependence* 216 (2020).

Sass, Louis A. "Delusion and Double Book-Keeping." *Karl Jaspers' Philosophy and Psychopathology* (2014): 125–47.

Sass, Louis A. "'Negative Symptoms,' Common Sense, and Cultural Disembedding in the Modern Age." In *Schizophrenia, Culture, and Subjectivity: The Edge of Experience*, edited by Janis H. Jenkins, and Robert John Barrett, 303–29. Cambridge: Cambridge University Press, 2003.

Sato, Mitsumoto. "Renaming Schizophrenia: A Japanese Perspective." *World Psychiatry* 5, no. 1 (2006): 53.

Saunders, Heather. "Taking a Look at 988 Suicide and Crisis Lifeline Implementation One Year after Launch." KFF, July 14, 2023. https://www.kff.org/mental-health/issue-brief/taking-a-look-at-988-suicide-crisis-lifeline-implementation-one-year-after-launch/.

Savage, Mark. "Lady Gaga Had a 'Psychotic Break' After Sexual Assault Left Her Pregnant." *BBC News*, May 21, 2021. https://www.bbc.com/news/entertainment-arts-57199018.

Saya, Anna, Chiara Brugnoli, Gioia Piazzi, Daniela Liberato, Gregorio Di Ciaccia, Cinzia Niolu, and Alberto Siracusano. "Criteria, Procedures, and Future Prospects of Involuntary Treatment in Psychiatry around the World: A Narrative Review." *Frontiers in Psychiatry* 10 (2019): 271.

Sayer, Andrew. *Why Things Matter to People: Social Science, Values, and Ethical Life*. Cambridge: Cambridge University Press, 2011.

Schechter, David, Jason Trahan, Chance Horner, and T. Nicole Waivers. "'They Underestimate What We Can Do': WFAA Finds Banks Exclude Blacks, Hispanics in Southern Dallas from Access to Loans." WFAA, Channel 8, ABC affiliate, November 22, 2020. https://bit.ly/3yiyRx3.

Schensul, Jean J., Cristina Huebner, Merrill Singer, Marvin Snow, Pablo Feliciano, and Lorie Broomhall. "The High, the Money, and the Fame: The Emergent Social Context of 'New Marijuana' Use among Urban Youth." *Medical Anthropology* 18, no. 4 (2000): 389–414.

"Schizophrenia Given New Japanese Name." *Japan Times*, January 21, 2002. https://www.japantimes.co.jp/news/2002/01/21/national/schizophrenia-given-new-japanese-name/.

Schoeler, Tabea, Anna Monk, Musa B. Sami, Ewa Klamerus, Enrico Foglia, Ruth Brown, Giulia Camuri, A. Carlo Altamura, Robin Murray, and Sagnik Bhattacharyya. "Continued versus Discontinued Cannabis Use in Patients with Psychosis: A Systematic Review and Meta-analysis." *Lancet Psychiatry* 3, no. 3 (2016): 215–25.

Schoeler, Tabea, Natalia Petros, Marta Di Forti, Ewa Klamerus, Enrico Foglia, Olesya Ajnakina, Charlotte Gayer-Anderson et al. "Effects of Continuation, Frequency, and Type of Cannabis Use on Relapse in the First 2 Years after Onset of Psychosis: An Observational Study." *The Lancet Psychiatry* 3, no. 10 (2016): 947–53.

Schoenbaum, Michael, Jason M. Sutherland, Andre Chappel, Susan Azrin, Amy B. Goldstein, Agnes Rupp, and Robert K. Heinssen. "Twelve-Month Health Care Use and Mortality in Commercially Insured Young People with Incident Psychosis in the United States." *Schizophrenia Bulletin* 43, no. 6 (2017): 1262–72.

Schulenberg, John E., and Jennifer L. Maggs. "A Developmental Perspective on Alcohol Use and Heavy Drinking during Adolescence and the Transition to Young Adulthood." Supplement, *Journal of Studies on Alcohol* 14 (2002): 54–70.

Schutze, Jim. *The Accommodation: The Politics of Race in an American City*. Secaucus, NJ: Citadel Press, 1986. Reprint, Dallas: Deep Vellum, 2021.

Seale, Clive, and Jonathan Charteris-Black. "The Interaction of Class and Gender in Illness Narratives." *Sociology* 42, no. 3 (2008): 453–69.

Seikkula, Jaakko, Birgitta Alakare, and Jukka Aaltonen. "The Comprehensive Open-Dialogue Approach in Western Lapland: II. Long-Term Stability of Acute Psychosis Outcomes in Advanced Community Care." *Psychosis* 3, no. 3 (2011): 192–204.

Seikkula, Jaakko, Jukka Aaltonen, Birgittu Alakare, Kauko Haarakangas, Jyrki Keränen, and Klaus Lehtinen. "Five-Year Experience of First-Episode Nonaffective Psychosis in Open-Dialogue Approach: Treatment Principles, Follow-Up Outcomes, and Two Case Studies." *Psychotherapy Research* 16, no. 2 (2006): 214–28.

Selten, Jean-Paul, Els Van Der Ven, and Fabian Termorshuizen. "Migration and Psychosis: A Meta-analysis of Incidence Studies." *Psychological Medicine* 50, no. 2 (2020): 303–13.

Selten, Jean-Paul, Jan Booij, Bauke Buwalda, and Andreas Meyer-Lindenberg. "Biological Mechanisms Whereby Social Exclusion May Contribute to the Etiology of Psychosis: A Narrative Review." *Schizophrenia Bulletin* 43, no. 2 (2017): 287–92.

Shakespeare, William. *As You Like It*. Edited by Horace Howard Furness. New York: Dover, 1963.

Shedd, Carla, and John Hagan. "Toward a Developmental and Comparative Conflict Theory of Race, Ethnicity, and Perceptions of Criminal Injustice." In *The Many Colors of Crime: Inequalities of Race, Ethnicity, and Crime in America*, edited by Ruth D. Peterson, Lauren J. Krivo, and John Hagan (NY, NY: NYU Press, 2006): 313–333.

Shim, Ruth S. "Dismantling Structural Racism in Psychiatry: A Path to Mental Health Equity." *American Journal of Psychiatry* 178, no. 7 (2021): 592–98.

Shinn, Ann K., Philip B. Cawkwell, Kirsten Bolton, Brian C. Healy, Rakesh Karmacharya, Agustin G. Yip, Dost Öngür, and Stephanie Pinder-Amaker. "Return to College after a First Episode of Psychosis." *Schizophrenia Bulletin Open* 1, no. 1 (2020): sgaa041.

Shonkoff, Jack P., and Deborah A. Phillips. *From Neurons to Neighborhoods*. Washington, DC: National Academy Press, 2000.

Siantz, Elizabeth, Benjamin Henwood, Nicole McGovern, Joelle Greene, and Todd Gilmer. "Peer Respites: A Qualitative Assessment of Consumer Experience." *Administration and Policy in Mental Health and Mental Health Services Research* 46, no. 1 (2019): 10–17.

Sidgwick, H. "A Census of Hallucinations." *New Review* 4, no. 20 (1981): 52–59.

Silton, N. R., K. J. Flannelly, G. Milstein, and M. L. Vaaler. "Stigma in America: Has Anything Changed?" *Journal of Nervous and Mental Disease* 199, no. 6 (2011): 361–66.

Smith, Jonathan D., Dinesh Mittal, Lakshminarayana Chekuri, Xiaotong Han, and Greer Sullivan. "A Comparison of Provider Attitudes toward Serious Mental Illness across Different Health Care Disciplines." *Stigma and Health* 2, no. 4 (2017): 327–37.

Smith, Thomas E., Margaret Kurk, Rishi Sawhney, Yuhua Bao, Ilana Nossel, Dana E. Cohen, and Lisa B. Dixon. "Estimated Staff Time Effort, Costs, and Medicaid Revenues for Coordinated Specialty Care Clinics Services Clients with First Episode Psychosis." *Psychiatric Services* 70 (2019): 425–27.

Snowden, Lonnie R., and Freda K. Cheung. "Use of Inpatient Mental Health Services by Members of Ethnic Minority Groups." *American Psychologist* 45, no. 3 (1990): 347–55.

Social Security Administration (SSA). "Disability Benefits." SSA.gov. Accessed March 30, 2024. https://www.ssa.gov/pubs/EN-05-10029.pdf.

Social Security Administration. "Disability Evaluation under Social Security." SSA.gov. https://www.ssa.gov/disability/professionals/bluebook/12.00-MentalDisorders-Adult.htm.

Social Security Administration. "SSR 18-3p: Titles II and XVI; Failure to Follow Prescribed Treatment." SSA.gov, October 29, 2018. https://www.ssa.gov/OP_Home/rulings/di/02/SSR2018-03-di-02.html#FN01.

Social Security Administration. "2023 Annual Report of SSI Program." Accessed January 25, 2024. https://www.ssa.gov/oact/ssir/SSI23/II_Highlights.html.

Sommer, Iris E. C., Kirstin Daalman, Thomas Rietkerk, Kelly M. Diederen, Steven Bakker, Jaap Wijkstra, and Marco P. M. Boks. "Healthy Individuals with Auditory Verbal Hallucinations—Who Are They? Psychiatric Assessments of a Selected Sample of 103 Subjects." *Schizophrenia Bulletin* 36, no. 3 (2010): 633–41.

Sondhi, Arun, Lisa Luger, Lina Toleikyte, and Emma Williams. "Patient Perspectives of Being Detained under Section 136 of the Mental Health Act: Findings from a Qualitative Study in London." *Medicine, Science, and the Law* 58, no. 3 (2018): 159–67.

Sotto-Santiago, Sylk. "Time to Reconsider the Word Minority in Academic Medicine." *Journal of Best Practices in Health Professions Diversity* 12, no. 1 (2019): 72–78.

Sousa, Amy June. "Diagnostic Neutrality in Psychiatric Treatment in North India." In *Our Most Troubling Madness: Case Studies in Schizophrenia across Cultures*, edited by Tanya M. Luhrmann and Jocelyn Marrow, 42–55. Berkeley: University of California Press, 2016.

Spear, Thomas, and Richard Waller, eds. *Being Maasai: Ethnicity and Identity in East Africa*. Athens: Ohio University Press, 1993.

Spidel, Alicia, Tania Lecomte, Caroline Greaves, Kimberly Sahlstrom, and John C. Yuille. "Early Psychosis and Aggression: Predictors and Prevalence of Violent Behaviour amongst Individuals with Early Onset Psychosis." *International Journal of Law and Psychiatry* 33, no. 3 (2010): 171–76.

Spiker, Douglas A., and Joseph H. Hammer. "Mental Health Literacy as Theory: Current Challenges and Future Directions." *Journal of Mental Health* 28, no. 3 (2019): 238–42.

Stacy, Christina, Karolina Ramos, Donovan Harvey, Sonia Torres Rodríguez, Jorge Morales-Burnett, and Sabina Morris. "Disrupting Structural Racism: Increasing Transportation Equity in South Dallas." Urban Institute, updated December 2022. https://www.urban.org/sites/default/files/2022-12/Disrupting%20Structural%20Racism.pdf.

Stein, Catherine H., Rosa Aguirre, and Marcia G. Hunt. "Social Networks and Personal Loss among Young Adults with Mental Illness and Their Parents: A Family Perspective." *Psychiatric Rehabilitation Journal* 36, no. 1 (2013): 15.

Stephensen, Helene, Annick Urfer-Parnas, and Josef Parnas. "Double Bookkeeping in Schizophrenia Spectrum Disorder: An Empirical-Phenomenological Study." *European Archives of Psychiatry and Clinical Neuroscience* (2023): 1–11.

Stewart, Francis. *Punk Rock Is My Religion: Straight Edge Punk and 'Religious' Identity.* Abingdon, UK: Routledge, 2017.

Strakowski, Stephen M., Richard C. Shelton, and Meridith L. Kolbrener. "The Effects of Race and Comorbidity on Clinical Diagnosis in Patients with Psychosis." *Journal of Clinical Psychiatry* (1993).

Suarez-Orozco, Carola, and Marcelo Suarez-Orozco. *Transformations: Immigration, Family Life, and Achievement Motivation among Latino Adolescents.* Palo Alto, CA: Stanford University Press, 1995.

Substance Abuse and Mental Health Services Administration (SAMHSA). *Coordinated Special Care for First Episode Psychosis: Costs and Financing Strategies.* HHS Publication No. PEP23-01-00-003 Rockville, MD: Substance Abuse and Mental Health Services Administration, 2023. https://store.samhsa.gov/sites/default/files/pep23-01-00-003.pdf.

Substance Abuse and Mental Health Services Administration. *First-Episode Psychosis and Co-occurring Substance Use Disorders.* Publication PEP19-PL-Guide-3. National Mental Health and Substance Use Policy Laboratory, 2019. https://store.samhsa.gov/product/First-Episode-Psychosis-and-Co-OccurringSubstance-Use-Disorders/PEP19-PL-Guide-3.

Substance Abuse and Mental Health Services Administration. *Key Substance Use and Mental Health Indicators in the United States: Results from the 2019 National Survey on Drug Use and Health.* 2020. Distributed by Center for Behavioral Health Statistics and Quality, SAMHSA. https://www.samhsa.gov/data/.

Substance Abuse and Mental Health Services Administration. *Supported Employment: Building Your Program.* 2009. https://store.samhsa.gov/sites/default/files/d7/priv/buildingyourprogram-se_0.pdf.

Tambling, R. R., C. D'Aniello, and B. S. Russell. "Mental Health Literacy: A Critical Target for Narrowing Racial Disparities in Behavioral Health." *International Journal of Mental Health and Addiction* 21, no. 3 (2023): 1867–81.

Taplin-Kaguru, Nora E. *Grasping for the American Dream: Racial Segregation, Social Mobility, and Homeownership.* Oxfordshire, UK: Routledge, 2021.

Texas Department of Health and Human Services. "State Hospitals." Accessed January 25, 2023. https://www.hhs.texas.gov/services/mental-health-substance-use/state-hospitals.

Texas Health and Safety Code. § 573 (2019).

Texas Young Lawyers Association. "Involuntary Commitment in Texas." *Court Basics* (blog). TexasLawHelp.org, April 20, 2018. https://texaslawhelp.org/article/involuntary-commitment-texas.

Thomas, Damafing Keita. "West African Immigrants' Attitudes toward Seeking Psychological Help." PhD diss., Georgia State University, 2008.

Tien, Allen Y. "Distribution of Hallucinations in the Population." *Social Psychiatry and Psychiatric Epidemiology* 26, no. 6 (1991): 287–92.

Tiihonen, Jari, Antti Tanskanen, and Heidi Taipale. "20-Year Nationwide Follow-Up Study on Discontinuation of Antipsychotic Treatment in First-Episode Schizophrenia." *American Journal of Psychiatry* 175, no. 8 (2018): 765–73.

Tocqueville, Alexis de. *Democracy in America*. Translated by Harvey C. Mansfield and Delba Winthrop. Chicago: University of Chicago Press, 2000.

Tranulis, Constantin, Lawrence Park, Laura Delano, and Byron Good. "Early Intervention in Psychosis: A Case Study on Normal and Pathological." *Culture, Medicine, and Psychiatry* 33 (2009): 608–22.

Tribe, Rachel H., Abigail M. Freeman, Steven Livingstone, Joshua C. H. Stott, and Stephen Pilling. "Open Dialogue in the UK: Qualitative Study." *British Journal of Psychology Open* 5, no. 4 (2019).

Trotta, A., R. M. Murray, and H. L. Fisher. "The Impact of Childhood Adversity on the Persistence of Psychotic Symptoms: A Systematic Review and Meta-analysis." *Psychological Medicine* 45, no. 12 (2015): 2481–98.

Turner, Victor. "Betwixt and Between: The Liminal Period in Rites de Passage." In *The Forest of Symbols: Aspects of Ndembu Ritual*, 93–111. Ithaca, NY: Cornell University Press, 1967.

Turner, Victor. *The Ritual Process: Structure and Anti-structure*. Ithaca, NY: Cornell University Press, 1977.

Twamley, Iseult, Maria Dempsey, and Nicola Keane. "An Open Dialogue–Informed Approach to Mental Health Service Delivery: Experiences of Service Users and Support Networks." *Journal of Mental Health* 30, no. 4 (2021): 494–99.

US Department of Health and Human Services (USDHHS), Office for Civil Rights. *HIPAA Privacy Rule and Sharing Information Related to Mental Health*. Accessed March 31, 2024. https://www.hhs.gov/sites/default/files/hipaa-privacy-rule-and-sharing-info-related-to-mental-health.pdf.

US Department of Health and Human Services. "2016 Poverty Guidelines." Office of the Assistant Secretary for Planning and Evaluation, January 25, 2016. https://aspe.hhs.gov/2016-poverty-guidelines.

US Department of Health and Human Services. *Protecting Youth Mental Health: The US Surgeon General's Advisory*. Washington, DC: GPO, 2021.

US Department of Health and Human Services. "Readmission Measures." CMS.gov:QualityNet. Accessed March 24, 2024. https://qualitynet.cms.gov/inpatient/measures/readmission.

US Department of Health and Human Services Office for Civil Rights. *Modifications to the HIPAA Privacy, Security, Enforcement, and Breach Notification Rules under the Health Information Technology for Economic and Clinical Health Act and the Genetic Information Nondiscrimination Act; Other Modifications to HIPAA Rules*. January 25, 2013. https://s3.amazonaws.com/public-inspection.federalregister.gov/2013-01073.pdf.

Usher, L., A. C. Watson, R. Bruno, S. Andiukaitis, D. Kamin, C. Speec, and S. Taylor. *Crisis Intervention Team (CIT) Programs: A Best Practice Guide for Transforming Community Responses to Mental Health Crises*. Memphis, TN: CIT International, 2019. https://www.citinternational.org/bestpracticeguide.

UvnäsMoberg, Kerstin, Anette Ekström-Bergström, Sarah Buckley, Claudia Massarotti, Zada Pajalic, Karolina Luegmair, Alicia Kotlowska, Luise Lengler, Ibone Olza, Susanne Grylka-Baeschlin, Patricia Leahy-Warren, Eleni Hadjigeorgiu, Stella Villarmea, and Anna Dencker. "Maternal Plasma Levels of Oxytocin during Breastfeeding: A Systematic Review." *PLoS One* 15, no. 8 (2020): 1–38.

Van der Kolk, Bessel A., Susan Roth, David Pelcovitz, Susanne Sunday, and Joseph Spinazzola. "Disorders of Extreme Stress: The Empirical Foundation of a Complex Adaptation to Trauma." *Journal of Traumatic Stress: Official Publication of the International Society for Traumatic Stress Studies* 18, no. 5 (2005): 389–99.

Van der Zeijst, Martine, Wim Veling, Elliot Mqansa Makhathini, Ezra Susser, Jonathan K. Burns, Hans W. Hoek, and Ida Susser. "Ancestral Calling, Traditional Health Practitioner Training, and Mental Illness: An Ethnographic Study from Rural KwaZulu-Natal, South Africa." *Transcultural Psychiatry* 58, no. 4 (2021): 471–85.

Van Gennep, Arnold. *The Rite of Passage.* Chicago: University of Chicago Press, 2019.

Van Os, Jim, Richard J. Linscott, Inez Myin-Germeys, Philippe Delespaul, and L. J. P. M. Krabbendam. "A Systematic Review and Meta-analysis of the Psychosis Continuum: Evidence for a Psychosis Proneness–Persistence–Impairment Model of Psychotic Disorder." *Psychological Medicine* 39, no. 2 (2009): 179–95.

Vermeulen, J., G. Van Rooijen, P. Doedens, E. Numminen, M. Van Tricht, and L. De Haan. "Antipsychotic Medication and Long-Term Mortality Risk in Patients with Schizophrenia: A Systematic Review and Meta-analysis." *Psychological Medicine* 47, no. 13 (2017): 2217–28.

Vernez, Georges, and Allan Abrahamse. *How Immigrants Fare in US Education.* Santa Monica, CA: Rand Corporation, 1996.

Vine, Phyllis. *Fighting for Recovery: An Activists' History of Mental Health Reform.* Boston: Beacon Press, 2022.

Volpe, Umberto, Mario Luciano, Claudia Palumbo, Gaia Sampogna, V. Del Vecchio, and A. Fiorillo. "Risk of Burnout among Early Career Mental Health Professionals." *Journal of Psychiatric and Mental Health Nursing* 21, no. 9 (2014): 774–81.

Wagner, Jacqueline Marie. "Deserving Asylum and Becoming 'Good' Refugees in Madrid." *Medicine Anthropology Theory* 10, no. 1 (2023): 1–10.

Walker, Elaine F., and Donald Diforio. "Schizophrenia: A Neural Diathesis-Stress Model." *Psychological Review* 104, no 4 (1997): 667.

Walker, Elaine F., Vijay Mittal, and Kevin Tessner. "Stress and the Hypothalamic Pituitary Adrenal Axis in the Developmental Course of Schizophrenia." *Annual Review of Clinical Psychology* 4 (2008): 189–216.

Walker, Margaret Urban. *Moral Repair: Reconstructing Moral Relations after Wrongdoing.* Cambridge: Cambridge University Press, 2006.

Walker, Margaret Urban. *Moral Understandings: A Feminist Study in Ethics.* Oxford: Oxford University Press, 2007.

Ware, Norma C., Kim Hopper, Toni Tugenberg, Barbara Dickey, and Daniel Fisher. "Connectedness and Citizenship: Redefining Social Integration." *Psychiatric Services* 58, no. 4 (2007): 469–74.

"The Wars Don't Work." *The Economist*, May 2, 2015. https://www.economist.com/leaders/2015/05/02/the-wars-dont-work.

Wasser, Tobias, Jessica Pollard, Deborah Fisk, and Vinod Srihari. "First-Episode Psychosis and the Criminal Justice System: Using a Sequential Intercept Framework to Highlight Risks and Opportunities." *Psychiatric Services* 68, no. 10 (2017): 994–96.

Waters, Mary C., ed. *Coming of Age in America: The Transition to Adulthood in the Twenty-First Century*. Berkeley: University of California Press, 2011.

Watters, Ethan. *Urban Tribes: A Generation Redefines Friendship, Family, and Commitment*. New York: Bloomsbury USA, 2003.

Weber, Max. *The Protestant Ethic and the Spirit of Capitalism*. New York: Routledge, 1930.

Weiner, Stacy. "A Growing Psychiatrist Shortage and an Enormous Demand for Mental Health Services." *Association of American Medical Colleges*, August 9, 2022. https://www.aamc.org/news/growing-psychiatrist-shortage-enormous-demand-mental-health-services.

Weingarten, Kaethe. "The 'Cruel Radiance of What Is': Helping Couples Live with Chronic Illness." *Family Process* 52, no. 1 (2013): 83–101.

Wentzell, Emily. "Aging Respectably by Rejecting Medicalization: Mexican Men's Reasons for Not Using Erectile Dysfunction Drugs." *Medical Anthropology Quarterly* 27, no. 1 (2013): 3–22.

WFAA Staff. "Former A&M Football Player Gets Life in Prison for Killing White Rock Runner with Machete." WFAA, Channel 8, ABC affiliate, April 30, 2019. https://www.wfaa.com/article/news/ex-am-player-who-attacked-white-rock-runner-found-guilty/287-bbcebb69-f3b3-4d7f-85f1-c85df8382902.

Whitaker, Robert. "Medication-free Ward in Tromsø, Norway, May Soon Close." *Mad in America*, November 2, 2023. https://www.madinamerica.com/2023/11/medication-free-ward-in-tromso-norway-may-soon-close/.

Whiting, Daniel, Gautam Gulati, John R. Geddes, and Seena Fazel. "Association of Schizophrenia Spectrum Disorders and Violence Perpetration in Adults and Adolescents from 15 Countries: A Systematic Review and Meta-analysis." *JAMA Psychiatry* 79, no. 2 (2022): 120–32.

Wiens, Sandra E., and Judith C. Daniluk. "Love, Loss, and Learning: The Experiences of Fathers Who Have Children Diagnosed with Schizophrenia." *Journal of Counseling and Development* 87, no. 3 (2009): 339–48.

Willen, Sarah S. *Fighting for Dignity: Migrant Lives at Israel's Margins*. Philadelphia: University of Pennsylvania Press, 2019.

Williams-Wengerd, Anne. "Grief in Parents of Adults Experiencing Early Psychosis." PhD diss., University of Minnesota, 2022.

Willis, Paul. *Learning to Labor: How Working-Class Kids Get Working-Class Jobs*. New York: Columbia University Press, 1977.

Wise-Harris, Deborah, Daniel Pauly, Deborah Kahan, Jason Tan de Bibiana, Stephen W. Hwang, and Vicky Stergiopoulos. "'Hospital Was the Only Option': Experiences of Frequent Emergency Department Users in Mental Health." *Administration and Policy in Mental Health and Mental Health Services Research* 44, no. 3 (2017): 405–12.

Wolf-Meyer, Matthew J. *Unraveling: Remaking Personhood in a Neurodiverse Age*. Minneapolis: University of Minnesota Press, 2020.

Worthman, Carol M. "Inside-Out and Outside-In? Global Development Theory, Policy, and Youth." In "Psychological Anthropology and Adolescent Well-Being." Special issue, *Ethos* 39, no. 4 (2011): 432–51.

Vargas, Sylvanna M., Richard S. John, Linda C. Garro, Alex Kopelowicz, and Steven R. López. "Measuring Congruence in Problem Definition of Latino Patients and Their

Psychotherapists: An Exploratory Study." *Hispanic Journal of Behavioral Sciences* 41, no. 3 (2019): 392–411.

Viddal, Grete. "Vodou and Voodoo as Alternative Religion." *Nova Religio: The Journal of Alternative and Emergent Religions* 26, no. 4 (2023): 1–7.

Xanthopoulou, Penny, Ciara Thomas, and Jemima Dooley. "Subjective Experiences of the First Response to Mental Health Crises in the Community: A Qualitative Systematic Review." *British Medical Journal Open* 12, no. 2 (2022).

Yahalom, Jonathan, Sheila Frankfurt, and Alison B. Hamilton. "Between Moral Injury and Moral Agency: Exploring Treatment for Men with Histories of Military Sexual Trauma." *Medicine Anthropology Theory* 10, no. 1 (2023): 1–21.

Yamaguchi, Sosei, Masashi Mizuno, Yasutaka Ojio, Utako Sawada, Asami Matsunaga, Shuntaro Ando, and Shinsuke Koike. "Associations between Renaming Schizophrenia and Stigma-Related Outcomes: A Systematic Review." *Psychiatry and Clinical Neurosciences* 71, no. 6 (2017): 347–62.

Yang, Ying, and Jeffrey A. Hayes. "Causes and Consequences of Burnout among Mental Health Professionals: A Practice-Oriented Review of Recent Empirical Literature." *Psychotherapy* 57, no. 3 (2020): 426.

Yarris, Kristin Elizabeth, and Carolyn Ponting. "Moral Matters: Schizophrenia and Masculinity in Mexico." *Ethos* 47, no. 1 (2019): 35–53.

Yates, Kathryn, Ulla Lång, Evyn M. Peters, Johanna T. W. Wigman, Fiona McNicholas, Mary Cannon, Jordan DeVylder, Hans Oh, and Ian Kelleher. "Sexual Assault and Psychosis in Two Large General Population Samples: Is Childhood and Adolescence a Developmental Window of Sensitivity?" *Schizophrenia Research* 241 (2022): 78–82.

Yeisen, Rafal A. H., Jone Bjørnestad, Inge Joa, Jan Olav Johannessen, and Stein Opjordsmoen. "Psychiatrists' Reflections on a Medication-Free Program for Patients with Psychosis." *Journal of Psychopharmacology* 33, no. 4 (2019): 459–65.

Zigon, Jarrett. *"HIV Is God's Blessing": Rehabilitating Morality in Neoliberal Russia.* Berkeley: University of California Press, 2011.

Zigon, Jarrett. "Moral Breakdown and the Ethical Demand: A Theoretical Framework for an Anthropology of Moralities." *Anthropological Theory* 7, no. 2 (2007): 131–50.

Zigon, Jarrett, and C. Jason Throop. "Moral Experience: Introduction." In "Moral Experience." Special issue, *Ethos* 42, no. 1 (2014): 1–15.

Ziv, Tali R. "'I'm Trapped Here': Ethnography, Structural Violence, and Moral Injury." *Medicine Anthropology Theory* 10, no. 1 (2023): 1–13.

ABOUT THE ARTISTS

LAUREN ANN VILLARREAL

laurenann703@gmail.com | Instagram: @laurensart42

Hispanic artist Lauren Ann Villarreal was born on May 22, 2001, and raised in McAllen, Texas. She is based in Dallas, Texas, and graduated in 2024 from Southern Methodist University with a major in Fashion Media and a minor in Arts Entrepreneurship. Lauren has been drawing since she was 4 years old and continued her art education in high school and college. Lauren's mediums include graphite, ink, and acrylic paint. Her art is influenced by depression, anxiety, sexual trauma, and mental illness. Identity is a common theme throughout her work.

"I never create with a picture in mind. I create because I have to. The thoughts were so severe they couldn't possibly come from my own mind. I had to get them out. I create to cope; if it moves people or makes them feel something, that's a bonus."

· · ·

JOSEPH STEVEN LAURENZO

josephlaurenzo03@gmail.com

Joseph Steven Laurenzo has been making art for more than thirty years. He says, "People with mental illness have the gift of seeing and imagining things differently. This is expressed in their art."

INDEX

Abilify (long-acting antipsychotic injection), 126, 128

abuse, 35, 41, 70, 101

Adams, James Truslow, 27–28

Adderall: Amy using, 113–14, 131, 132; prescribed for ADHD, 158; Sage using, 126, 127, 128, 129

addiction. *See* substance use

Addison, 40, 41

ADHD, 29, 41, 66, 104, 106, 113–14, 158

adolescent development, 24–25, 34

adulthood, transitions to: American context of, 14, 24, 148–49; crossroads in, 36–37; disrupted by hospital admissions, 92–93; lack of clarity in, 27, 28; lost opportunities in, 5; psychosis in navigating, 33; theory on, 25–26

adverse social experiences, 11–12, 33–34, 70. *See also* childhood traumatic events

Affordable Care Act, 176

Afiya House, 166, 168

African Americans, 9. *See also* Black Americans

aggressive behavior, 3, 73–74, 159. *See also* dangerous behavior; violent behavior

alcohol, 29. *See also* substance use

Alcoholics Anonymous, 99

alternatives to hospitalizations, 167–68. *See also* hospitalizations

American culture: alternative pathways to adulthood in, 194n53; challenges of work hard, play hard in, 38; investing in

trauma-informed care, 168; schizophrenia in, 116; on transitions to adulthood, 14, 24–25, 26, 27; wariness of mental confusion in, 62

American dream, 15–16, 27–28, 30

Amir, 21

amnesia, 87–88, 93

amphetamines, 158, 194n40

Amy: accepting medication, 169; engaging with police, 80; feelings after hospitalization, 131–32; on hospital admission, 82–83; on hospital release, 104; impact of psychosis on, 44; initial story of, 40–43, 57; insurance coverage of, 91; moral agency of, 113; on psychosis treatment, 74–75; social withdrawal of, 51; on transitions to adulthood, 148

Anderson, Lonnie, 29

Andre, 15, 16

Angela, 30, 31, 32, 87

Anglin, Deidre, 11

anthropology, 6, 12

anxiety, 47, 48

Ariana: on diagnostic process, 111–12; family support for, 136; on infantilization, 132; insurance coverage of, 92; introduction to, 88–91; pursuing peer support training, 150–51, 166; refusing medication, 121, 169; refusing treatment, 110; understanding of her problems, 113; working on moral agency, 150

Founded in 1893,
UNIVERSITY OF CALIFORNIA PRESS
publishes bold, progressive books and journals
on topics in the arts, humanities, social sciences,
and natural sciences—with a focus on social
justice issues—that inspire thought and action
among readers worldwide.

The UC PRESS FOUNDATION
raises funds to uphold the press's vital role
as an independent, nonprofit publisher, and
receives philanthropic support from a wide
range of individuals and institutions—and from
committed readers like you. To learn more, visit
ucpress.edu/supportus.